PARENTING LIKE A PRO

A COMPREHENSIVE PARENTING CLASS

Monique Couillard Nelson BS, RN, IgCN

Copyright © 2025 by Monique Couillard Nelson BS, RN, IgCN

All rights reserved.

No part of this book may be reproduced in any form or by any electronic or mechanical means, including information storage and retrieval systems, without written permission from the author, except for the use of brief quotations in a book review.

NO AI TRAINING: Without in any way limiting the author's exclusive rights under copyright, any use of this publication to train generative artificial intelligence (AI) technologies to generate text is expressly prohibited. The author reserves all rights to license uses of this work for generative AI training and development of machine learning language models.

In accordance with Article 4(3) of the Digital Single Market Directive 2019/790, the author expressly reserves this work from the text and data mining exception.

CONTENTS

About the Author: My "Why?" 1

Introduction 7

Chapter 1: Pregnancy 9

Chapter 2: Hospital Routine 20

Chapter 3: Cord Blood 42

Chapter 4: Newborn Necessities 52

Chapter 5: Newborn Care and Newborn Illness 66

Chapter 6: Breast and Bottle Feeding 84

Chapter 7: The Postpartum Period 111

Chapter 8: Postpartum Depression 129

Chapter 9: Sleep 133

Chapter 10: Growth and Development 165

Chapter 11: Safety 197

Chapter 12: Health Lecture 230

Chapter 13: Dental 263

Chapter 14: Social and Emotional Development 269

Chapter 15: Infant Nutrition 297

Chapter 16: Learning Play 315

Chapter 17: Infant Massage 334

Chapter 18: Choosing a Nanny / Sitter or Daycare Provider 339

Chapter 19: Summertime Lecture 353

Chapter 20: Swim lessons: Traditional vs. Survival Swimming 369

Chapter 21: Nature vs. Nurture 382

Chapter 22: Self-Esteem 401

Chapter 23: Discipline 412

Final words from the author 447

Special Thank You 448

Index 450

Bibliography 612

ABOUT THE AUTHOR

MY "WHY?"

I am so excited to take this journey with you! Thank you for sharing this special time in your life with me.

It is important for me to first state that this book is for educational purposes only and is not meant to replace medical advice from your trusted provider/s. If you have concerns about your little one, please seek medical advice.

I would like to tell you a little bit about myself so you will know what compelled me to write this book and share my knowledge and experience with all of you. I am a registered nurse and mother of two amazing kids. My parenting journey has not been smooth sailing. I have been through many swells and storms along the way, but those stormy seas have made me a better mom, nurse, and educator. Without the challenges I faced I would not be sitting here writing this book to share with all of you. I have also learned that I am not the one steering this ship, I am merely a co-captain on this journey of life. I truly believe, however, that this course was charted for me, and this voyage I have been on was meant to be.

Every year someone suggests I write a book to share my knowledge with others. Someone will say "my sister in another state would just love to take your parenting class", or "my friend would benefit from this information so much, but she works full time". It wasn't until I got one final push from some friends and coworkers, Brian and

Abbey. Brian is a pharmacist I work with, and his wife Abbey is a physician's assistant. When I found out they were expecting their first baby, along with another good friend and colleague of mine and his wife, I offered to teach them all a private parenting class in the evenings. This way they could get the benefit of a parenting class while working full-time. Both couples said, "Monique, you just have to write a book! You can't keep all this knowledge to yourself." After each class, Brian would ask me, "When are you going to write a book? I am going to keep bugging you until I convince you." So, thank you, Brian, for the push I needed. I realized there may be more new parents out there, who can't make it to a parenting class and who want this information too.

In this book, I will share some personal stories, as well as my own opinions, from my years of working as a nurse in pediatrics and being a mom of two. I will also offer expert advice from the American Academy of Pediatrics, as well as some tried and true advice from brilliant physicians across the country, like Dr. T. Berry Brazelton and Dr. Barton Schmidt. I will try to cite every source I can, but I have adapted so much into my lectures over the years that the sources have become meshed together to become my words and my lectures. I apologize if I have missed any citations. I have also adopted advice and wisdom from various other fabulous physicians I have had the privilege of knowing and working with over the years and tidbits from others I have only read about but whose opinions I value.

You may not always agree with me and that is ok. Raising kids is not a one-size-fits-all endeavor. I had to pivot from my original plan with my two kids on several occasions due to their individual temperaments and personalities. Hopefully, my stories will show you that you are not alone and, yes, even people teaching parenting classes year after year don't have all the answers and make mistakes. Kids are forgiving and resilient and realize Mom and Dad are human. None of us is perfect and, if you make a mistake, you say you are sorry and you will try to do better next time.

My higher education journey started at Arizona State University in 1988. I graduated with a bachelor of science degree in biology Pre-med. I was planning on becoming a pediatrician. That plan changed when I met my husband of almost 30 years in my senior year and I just couldn't move out of the state. I went back to school to obtain a nursing degree and started my long career in nursing, specializing in pediatrics. I started my career as a pediatric triage nurse, giving parents advice on all subjects from illness, to breastfeeding, to discipline. This is where I gained most of my knowledge about newborns and childcare. (The rest came from my own experiences with motherhood).

I also started teaching pregnancy, newborn, and toddler classes all over the state of Arizona 26 years ago. I am still teaching parenting classes and hope to continue for many more years to come. In addition to teaching, I work as a full-time nurse, advocating and educating patients in a national position. I have been blessed to work for a company that has allowed me to continue to pursue my passion for teaching new parents.

Now for my parenting journey in a condensed nutshell... Pregnancy was not easy for me. I had hyperemesis gravidarum during both pregnancies. This is why my kids are five years apart. ☺ I had a PICC line to feed me as I vomited day and night throughout both pregnancies. Because I was considered a high-risk pregnancy for both, the babies were monitored closely. Both stopped growing at

32 weeks. They call it inter-uterine growth restriction. Even though I was 36 weeks gestation with each, the babies were only measuring 32 weeks and didn't progress developmentally past 32 weeks. I was told I needed an immediate C-section with both.

My first, Taylor, weighed only 4 lbs. 11 oz when she was born. She was born without a suck reflex, and she needed supplemental oxygen at birth. She alternated between tachycardia (her heart was beating too fast) and bradycardia (her heart was beating too slow). She also had apnea (she would forget to breathe). She came home on an apnea/heart monitor one week later. Because she had no suck reflex, it took her an hour to feed, and she needed to eat every hour and a half due to her tiny little belly. I was one tired new mama. As she grew, most of her health concerns improved. She will have to see a cardiologist and neurologist for the rest of her life, and she struggled a bit academically due to her health issues, but overall she is doing great. She went on to college and graduated after being on the dean's list each semester.

My second and final child came along five years later. Unfortunately, I developed hyperemesis again during my second pregnancy. Although I was just as sick as the first time, being prepared for it made it a little better and my mom was an amazing help. Thanks, Mom!! My son, Dylan, was my bruiser weighing 5lbs 3 oz at birth. If you can believe it, he had his own set of medical conditions. He was born with thrombocytopenia (critically low platelets). He had to have an IV infusion of immunoglobulin (a plasma product) the day after he was born to replace his platelets. He, like his sister, did not have a suck reflex either, so breastfeeding was not an option, and he was too weak to nurse. He also had apnea and came home on a monitor like his sister did. Unlike his sister, Dylan did not outgrow his health challenges but seemed to add to them. He will need immunoglobulin infusions for the rest of his life. He also has a primary immune deficiency called Common Variable Immune Deficiency (CVID). CVID is a genetic condition where he can't produce enough antibodies on his own, making him susceptible to illness, especially pneumonia. As if that were not enough, he also has a rare form of muscular dystrophy.

Yes, parenthood has been challenging. My children have had multiple medical problems throughout their lives, and I think we have seen every specialist in the state and many other states. Kids, however, are resilient and my children are remarkable. Despite enormous obstacles, my daughter graduated from college and is now a third-grade teacher and my son is a sophomore in college and has been a competitive gymnast his entire life. Yes, even with muscular dystrophy. When the neurologist told me my son shouldn't be able to do gymnastics, when Dylan was doing great and winning state championships, I asked him if he was going to tell him that, because I wasn't! I asked, "Will it harm him?" He said it wouldn't harm him but he eventually wouldn't be able to do it. I said we would cross that bridge when we came to it then. That bridge has never come.

I have never told my kids they can't do something, so they don't feel they have limitations. I have learned to be an advocate for my children and, in turn, to be an advocate for other parents and my patients. I believe things happen for a reason and these challenges, as I mentioned before, have made me the strong mom and nurse advocate I am today. I also think that the challenges my kids faced and continue to face make them the compassionate, strong-willed, courageous, and independent young adults they are today. In case you were wondering, I did get their permission to use their names and stories about them in this book. They have become so used to me talking about them in my classes over the years that they thought it was a given that I would be including stories about them, when I told them I was writing a book.

I hope you enjoy this book and feel the love and passion I have for teaching and raising kids and sharing my knowledge with all the new parents out there. Parenting is not easy, but it is the most rewarding job you will ever do. "The days are long, but the years are short." (Gretchen Rubin). Try to celebrate the accomplishments and try not to sweat the small stuff. Remember, none of us are perfect! 😊

INTRODUCTION

This book is written to make you feel as if you, the parents, were taking my parenting class. It was crafted from my lectures from what I call Newborn A. This is a class that I teach with parents who typically start the class in the final months of pregnancy and continue biweekly for the next nine months. The course material in this book will cover the first year of your baby's life and a few months more.

I have been giving these lectures for the past 25 years and I modify them each year to fit the changes in pediatrics and the topics that parents are most interested in. At the beginning of each year, I hand out a questionnaire asking what topics are the most important to each parent and I create a syllabus around their needs.

What I have learned, however, is that, year after year, the topics don't really change. New parents want information about the same subjects. So, this book is broken down into those 23 subjects that parents are most interested in year after year. Each chapter is basically a lecture.

The purpose of this book is to give parents a resource where they can find multiple topics in one place, without having to buy several books to get this information.

As I mentioned previously, I am predominantly a pediatric nurse, so my specialty is pediatrics and not OB/GYN. This book is meant for new parents navigating the waters of parenthood, not pregnancy, so the information on pregnancy and postpartum will be minimal.

I will give advice by sharing stories and giving my opinion, which comes from years of experience and advice from multiple experts. As I also mentioned previously, this book is not meant to replace the advice of your own physician or healthcare professional. www.healthychildren.org is the American Academy of Pediatrics website and a great resource as well. Please consult your own doctor if you have any medical questions or concerns. Having said this, you need to trust the doctors you choose. You chose them for a reason and if you are questioning them or their advice, interview another. I have changed various providers for my kids over the years. You are your child's best advocate. Trust your parental gut! Your intuition is rarely wrong. I hope you enjoy this book / class.

CHAPTER I

PREGNANCY

"A baby is something you carry inside you for nine months, in your arms for three years, and in your heart until the day you die."

– Mary Mason

As I mentioned before, pregnancy was not easy for me, but as crazy as it may sound, it was one of the most magical times in my life. The hyperemesis part was not so magical but the feeling of the baby moving and the closeness I felt was indescribable. Pregnancy is truly a miracle and I feel blessed I was able to experience it twice.

I have listed several of the questions I am often asked in class.

So, what is the typical duration of pregnancy?

This has changed over time. The current definitions are listed below.

Dr. Frank Miller, professor, and chair of the Department of Obstetrics and Gynecology at the University of Kentucky, suggests parents should look at their estimated due date in terms of a due month, with the potential to deliver two weeks on either side of the "due date", since 80% of babies are born within this period of time.

According to the Journal of Obstetrics and Gynecology, the definitions of early term, full term, late term, and post term are as follows:

Early term: between 37 weeks and 38 weeks 6 days

Full-term: between 39 weeks and 40 weeks 6 days

Late-term between the 41st and 42nd week

Post-term: after 42 weeks

How much weight should you expect to gain during pregnancy?

According to the American College of Obstetrics and Gynecology, women can expect to gain up to 10 lbs. in the first 20 weeks of pregnancy and about 1 lb per week during the rest of their pregnancy.

Phoenix Perinatal Associates says you will gain approximately ½ lb. per week for a single and 1 lb. per week for twins before 24 weeks and, after 24 weeks, 1 lb. per week for a single and 2 lb. per week for twins.

The American College of Obstetricians and Gynecologists recommends gaining 25–35 lbs. for a woman beginning her pregnancy at her ideal weight.

Where do those pounds go?

Here is an approximate pound-by-pound breakdown of how that weight is distributed.

1.5 lbs.: the weight of the placenta

7 lbs.: maternal stores of fat, protein, and other nutrients

7.5 lbs.: the average size of a full-term baby (this can vary)

2 lbs.: breast tissue (I know it feels like so much more!)

4 lbs.: increased fluid volume

4 lbs.: increased blood volume

2 lbs.: the uterus

2 lbs.: amniotic fluid

Total = 30 pounds

What foods should Mom avoid?

Seafood with high amounts of mercury—because mercury is naturally present in the marine environment, there are certain species of marine life that may contain amounts of mercury that are harmful to pregnant and breastfeeding moms. The FSA and National Fisheries Institute recommend that pregnant and breastfeeding moms limit their consumption of swordfish, shark, tilefish, king mackerel, and fresh tuna. They suggest that canned chunk light tuna generally has less mercury than other tuna but should still be eaten in moderation. Fish caught in streams and lakes may also be risky for pregnant mamas to eat. Contact the local environmental protection agency in your area first before consuming fish you catch on your own, just to be safe. Certain sushi should also be avoided due to mercury and the risk of bacteria.

Smoked seafood (refrigerated smoked seafood labeled lox, nova style kippered, or jerky) should be avoided as it could contain listeria. Canned or shelf-safe smoked seafood is not included in this warning.

Seafood, however, is high in omega-3 fatty acids, so don't be afraid to eat salmon, cod, tilapia, and cooked shrimp.

Uncooked meats in general should be avoided—including seafood, beef, poultry, and pork. Unless thoroughly cooked, these foods should be avoided due to the risk of contamination with coliform bacteria, E. coli, toxoplasmosis, and salmonella.

Other things to avoid—unpasteurized juices, raw eggs, and sauces that might be made with raw eggs such as Hollandaise sauce or some Caesar dressings.

Listeria is also a concern when you are pregnant. Listeriosis can take up to three weeks to set in and can cross the placenta and infect the baby. Avoid cold cuts unless you can warm them in a microwave first.

As imported cheeses may contain listeria, avoid cheeses such as Brie, Camembert, Roquefort, feta, Gorgonzola, and Mexican-style cheeses that include queso blanco and queso franco, unless they clearly state they are made with pasteurized milk. All soft non-imported cheese made with pasteurized milk is safe to eat.

What should you know about caffeine intake?

Lisa,Signorello an epidemiologist in Maryland, found a twofold increased risk of miscarriage among Swedish women who ingested 500 mg or more of caffeine each day.

That is equivalent to 5 cups of American coffee. An 8 oz cup of caffeinated tea contains about 40 mg of caffeine and a 12 oz can of cola contains approximately 45 mg of caffeine.

The American College of Obstetrics and Gynecologists' position is that there is no proof that the small amounts of caffeine in 1–2 cups of coffee or tea will cause problems in a normal pregnancy. I do think it is important, however, to point out that caffeine is a diuretic (it can dehydrate you), as well as a stimulant, so many pregnant moms choose to play it safe and cut out caffeine, especially in the first trimester. If you do choose to drink caffeine, don't exceed 200 mg daily.

Did you know that many of the flavors of the foods you eat in the last trimester of pregnancy can pass through the placenta and into the breast milk of nursing moms?

Biologist Julie Mennella, Ph.D., of the Monell Chemical Senses Center in Philadelphia, says a fetus can taste and smell by the third trimester. She did a fascinating study where she gave a group of pregnant women carrot juice in their last trimester of pregnancy, another group carrot juice during breastfeeding, and another group only water throughout pregnancy and breastfeeding (no carrot juice at all for them). Later, when the babies were fed carrot juice mixed in their cereal, the babies who had been exposed to it by moms during pregnancy or while nursing ate the cereal without issue. Those babies whose moms only had water and were never exposed to carrot juice, either in utero or through breast milk, refused the cereal mixed with carrot juice. Dr. Mennella's advice is to enjoy eating a wide variety of flavors, especially fruits and vegetables, while pregnant and nursing. She also suggests you eat ethnic foods and family recipes. You will want your child to grow up eating traditional family recipes and, in this way, they become familiar with them even before they are able to eat solid foods.

Gerber Foods/ Gerber Products Company suggests the same thing.

In an article put out by Gerber, they also remind pregnant moms to eat a variety of foods. Many of the flavors in a mother's diet are transferred to her baby in the womb, during her pregnancy, and later in her breastmilk. This way, your own food preferences may already seem familiar to your baby when the time comes to introduce solid foods.

What foods should mom be eating?

There are a few superfoods you could add to your diet.

Apples are high in fiber to help prevent constipation. They are rich in vitamin C. Apples are high in iron and may help prevent childhood asthma.

Avocados are rich in B6, which might help with morning sickness. Avocados are also high in folate which helps to prevent neural tube defects.

Salmon and shrimp are both low in mercury, high in omega-3 fatty acids and high in DHA.

Eggs are a great source of protein and choline (choline also helps prevent neural tube defects).

Greek yogurt is high in calcium, vitamins D, E and K, and high in protein.

Asparagus is very high in folate.

Green leafy veggies, including spinach, kale, and broccoli are all rich in folate, which helps develop the neural tube. The neural tube will eventually become the brain and spinal cord. These leafy greens are also high in iron, vitamin C, vitamin K, magnesium, and fiber.

Meat and legumes are rich sources of iron. Pregnant women need approx. 27 mg per day.

Placental encapsulation / placentophagy

What is this?

Now, this may not be your cup of tea, but I do get asked about placental encapsulation from time to time in my classes, so I thought I would include a short excerpt on what it is, how it is done, and why someone would want to do it. That way, if you are interested you can navigate how to go about it.

Maternal human placentophagy, or ingesting your own placenta after delivery, is a century-old practice. It has been gaining in popularity over the past few decades here in the US. I want to point out, however, that there have been very few scientific studies to show the benefits or harm of the practice. I do not have any firsthand experience with this practice, so this information is solely based on my research.

"More than 4,000 species of mammals consume their placenta; only in humans and camelids (mammals having a 3-chambered stomach, including the camel, llama, guanaco, alpaca, and vicuña) has it been noted that the afterbirth is not routinely ingested." https://ncbi.nlm.nih.gov/pmc/articles/PMC6138470/ Geburtshilfe Frauenheilkd. 2018 Sep; 78(9): 846–852. Published online 2018 Sep 14. doi: 10.1055/a-0674-6275

So, how would one even go about eating their own placenta, you might ask?

Well, you might be surprised. I know I was. Some moms eat it raw, some cook with it, and some blend frozen pieces into a smoothie, but *most* people who consume their own placenta chose encapsulation as their method of choice. This is where the placenta is cleaned, dehydrated, and then ground into a fine powder and put into gelatin capsules.

The next question I am sure you are asking is why would someone want to do this?

One article published in the German Medical Journal, Geburtshilfe Frauenheilkd., explains several possible benefits seen in both the animal kingdom and benefits seen with human consumption. As I mentioned previously, I did not do this, so I have no personal feedback to give you, but this is probably the best article I found that offers clinical information.

Effects of placentophagy in humans

A historical study from 1918 describes the influence of ingesting desiccated placenta on lactation: Increased amounts of protein and lactose were measured in breast milk. Weight gain was also more rapid in the babies breastfed exclusively by the mothers in the placenta ingestion group.

Further benefits reported from the ingestion of placenta capsules are a stable mood postpartum, faster convalescence following parturition, increased milk production, and a subjective feeling of having "more energy" postpartum.

In the USA, almost a third of all mothers from community birth ingest the placenta either raw or dried: In more than 70% of cases, prevention of postpartum depression is given as the reason.

In my opinion, I feel that, if you are thinking about placental encapsulation, it is of *extreme* importance for you to do your homework when choosing a company to do the encapsulation. You want to make sure the company you chose is handling the placenta safely. Be sure to consult your healthcare provider to receive more information about proper procedures and a reputable company. It is also important to investigate state laws as well, to make sure it is legal to remove the placenta from the hospital where you are delivering.

Finding a pediatrician

The final thing I would like to talk about in this chapter is finding a pediatrician.

You do not want to wait until the last minute to find a pediatrician. You need to meet them and find one that you are comfortable with. This is a big decision. You are trusting the person you love the most with this individual. You need to feel comfortable with the advice you are getting. What may be a perfect fit for your friend may not always be the perfect fit for you. Set up interviews well in advance. Remember these doctors are busy seeing patients, so they have limited availability regarding when they can interview new parents and they may do this in a group setting. Have your list of questions ready to go so you can ask the same questions to each provider you interview.

Pediatrician interview questions

Here is a list of questions you might ask at your interview:

Do they have privileges at the hospital where you will be delivering the baby?

How soon will they see the baby at the hospital after they are born?

Will they see the baby themselves, or is there a chance their partner will?

Do they circumcise at the hospital or at the office?

How soon after the baby comes home will they want to see the baby?

When is the doctor available? What are their office hours?

Do they have sick hours every day?

What happens in the case of an emergency?

Is there a doctor on call 24/7?

Do they share on-call with another practice?

Do they have weekend hours?

Do they do basic labs in-house? For example, do they have rapid strep cultures? Rapid flu cultures? Covid tests? Can they take a quick look at urine to rule out an infection? Etc. I realize they will send tests out for confirmation, but you want answers as soon as possible when your little one is sick.

Do they have a sick and well side?

Do they have triage/advice nurses or how do they handle questions?

Does your pediatrician have their own kids?

Does your pediatrician listen to YOU?

How do they feel about your key values? Diet, antibiotics, alternative health, if that matters to you, vaccine schedule, etc.

Look around the office, is it clean?

Does it appear to run smoothly?

Does it appear kid-friendly and safe?

GO with your gut feeling.

If you find that the pediatrician you chose was not a good fit, you are not stuck! Find a new one. 😊

> *"There is no way to be a perfect mother, and a million ways to be a good one." Jill Churchill*

CHAPTER 2

HOSPITAL ROUTINE

"You will never know the amount of love you can give to somebody until you give birth to your first child."

— Unknown

What should you bring to the hospital?

What should you bring to the hospital for your delivery?

For you:

<u>Nursing pajamas</u>—otherwise you will just have a hospital gown.

<u>Slippers/socks with non-skid soles</u>—those hospital floors are cold. They can also be germy/dirty, and slick.

<u>A robe</u>—if you want to leave your room for any reason you will appreciate having a robe, especially for when visitors come. If you want to get up, or if you need to use the restroom and someone else is in the room, you will appreciate having a robe.

<u>A nursing bra and nursing pads</u>—nobody plans on being in the hospital long enough for your milk to come in, but you never know. Plan for the worst and hope for the best.

<u>Toiletries</u>—in my opinion, nothing helps you feel more normal than a shower with your own shampoo, body wash, and lotions after delivery.

<u>Hair tie</u>—if you have long hair, being able to pull it back and out of your face is a must.

<u>Contact lens case and glasses</u>—if needed.

<u>Maxi pads</u>—I like the thinnest pad possible and the ones with wings. So, if you are picky about your pads like me, pack your own just in case. Depending on the hospital where you deliver, you might end up with maxi pads that are more like a diaper than the thin store-bought pads you may be used to. Remember no tampons for quite some time.

<u>A pillow and blanket</u>—you might want to bring your own pillow from home as the ones in the hospital are not the soft, fluffy ones you may be used to. The pillows most hospitals have are flat and plastic-coated for easy cleaning.

I also brought a soft blanket from home when I delivered my kiddos. I have always done this with hospitalizations for myself and the kids to make it feel more home-like.

<u>Relaxing music and earbuds</u>—hospitals are noisy places, and it may be hard to relax or sleep without music or sound to drown out the hospital noise.

<u>Diffuser</u>—candles are not allowed in a hospital setting, so if you want a scent in your room, you can bring in an essential oil diffuser and baby-safe oils. Lavender is very calming and safe for babies.

Lip balm

Hard candies to suck on

A call list—for your partner to make calls once the baby arrives.

A recording device—typically your phone and/or camera.

Cord blood kit—if you are collecting or donating.

For your baby:

A couple of outfits—clothes are not necessary, but you may want some for photos.

Sleepers—otherwise your baby will just be in a diaper and receiving blanket, which may be fine with you, but you might want to pack a couple to give you options.

Onesies—similar to the above statement, having a couple of onesies to put the baby in if you want is a nice option.

Baby socks—nothing is provided except diapers, a blanket, and a hat. The hospital can be cold, and socks are nice to have.

Pacifier—the hospital will provide an Avent Soothie type pacifier, but if you want an orthodontic pacifier, you will need to bring one. The orthodontic pacifier is the dentist's preference. Once a baby becomes attached to one pacifier it is difficult to change. Some babies have a greater need to suck than others and may need a pacifier.

Receiving blanket—just one to go home with as they provide them while you are there.

Car seat—have the base fitted into your car weeks before your due date.

*Be careful to keep your baby's clothes separate from the hospital's laundry.

Keep your hospital bag packed and keep gas in your car at least two weeks before your due date.

What tests and/or procedures should I expect, if any?

Immediately after birth, there are several tests that will be performed on the baby. Some you may know about and some you may not know about unless you notice or ask.

The first test is called an Apgar score. This score lets the medical team know how the baby is doing clinically after birth and lets the hospital staff know if your newborn will need a little extra care.

This is a score given to the baby one minute after birth and five minutes after birth. The baby is assessed for five characteristics: color, heart rate, muscle tone, reflex responses, and breathing.

Each category receives a score and can range from 0–2 points per category for a maximum score of 10 points. Most babies receive a seven or higher. If they score lower than a seven, it does not necessarily mean there will be a long-term problem, it is just that the baby should be carefully watched for a while.

Below is a chart on how a baby is scored:

Score	0	1	2
Heart rate	Absent	<100/min	>100/min
Resp	Absent	slow, irregular Weak cry	Good strong Crying
Muscle tone	Limp	Some flexing Of arms and legs	Active motion
Reflex	Absent	Grimace	Grimace, cough and Sneeze
Color	Blue or pale	Body pink Hands/feet blue	Completely pink

Reflex: judged by placing a bulb syringe in the infant's nose and watching the response

The nurse will also borrow the baby for various other tests and measurements.

The baby will be weighed, their length measured and their head and possibly their chest will be measured and charted.

An antibiotic eye ointment will be applied shortly after birth to prevent eye infections. This is primarily done to prevent infections that can occur from passing through the birth canal. This is not optional and is required even for C-section babies, even though they did not pass through the birth canal. This is a standard hospital policy.

The baby will be given a vitamin K shot to prevent bleeding. Only one dose is given. This is done due to a recommendation by the AAP (American Academy of Pediatrics). Vitamin K is given to prevent serious bleeding or hemorrhage in infants. Vitamin K is naturally produced by bacteria in the colon as the baby gets older. Newborns have not yet acquired the ability to make the bacteria needed to create vitamin K and are born with inadequate stores of vitamin K from Mom. There is also relatively little vitamin K in breast milk. Vitamin K is essential for clotting blood. This leaves infants at risk of hemorrhage, particularly those occurring in the brain, which can cause serious damage or death.

Before you leave the hospital, you will be offered your first vaccination. You will be given the opportunity to give your newborn the first of three hepatitis B vaccines.

You will also notice a small clamp on the cord stump. This is called a cord clamp, and it remains in place for 24–48 hours after birth or until the cord is dry and no longer bleeds. This should be removed before you leave the hospital, as it requires a special tool to remove it.

Occasionally, if your baby is born very large, or very small, jittery, or lethargic, the hospital staff will need to check your newborn's blood sugar. If it is too low, they may want to offer supplemental formula. If you plan on breastfeeding, you may want to ask the hospital personnel to feed the baby with a syringe rather than a bottle. Breastfeeding is more work than taking a bottle so giving formula with a syringe gives you a better chance at breastfeeding later.

If the mom is RH negative, has type O blood or the blood type was not previously tested, the baby's umbilical cord blood will be checked for RH antibodies. If you are going to store cord blood or donate it, this will be done at the same time as the cord blood collection (more about cord blood collection to come in the next chapter).

Assessments and reflexes

When your pediatrician assesses the baby for the first time, he or she will be making sure the baby is in good health. One of the ways they evaluate this is by checking several reflexes present at birth. Some pediatricians also use neonatal assessment tools. I have listed a couple of assessments below. I have also listed some of the reflexes they may check.

Neonatal maturity assessment—this is an assessment that measures physical and neuromuscular characteristics. These characteristics are scored, and the values are totaled to determine the maturity of the infant.

The Brazelton Neonatal Behavioral assessment—this assessment is named after the world-renowned developmental pediatrician, T. Berry Brazelton. I will reference him on multiple occasions in this book. This assessment uses various stimuli, such as lights, sounds, etc., to test types of behavior, including motor ability and reaction to stress, in those babies with low birth weight or those that may have neurological problems. Some hospitals routinely test all babies.

<u>Rooting reflex</u>—this is the baby's natural tendency to search for the breast. This reflex is present at birth and disappears by four months. It can be assessed by rubbing the baby's cheek or chin and the baby turns in that direction and tries to suck.

<u>The grasping reflex is also called the palmar reflex</u>—your baby will grasp onto a finger when it is placed in the center of their palm. This reflex is present at birth and disappears around 5–6 months of age.

<u>Plantar grasp reflex</u>-your baby will curl his or her toes and arch their foot when a finger is placed in the center of the foot. This reflex is present at birth and disappears at about 9–12 months. Trying to put on shoes before this reflex disappears is tricky. ☺

<u>The Moro reflex</u>—also called the startle reflex—is present at birth and disappears by two months. With this reflex, the arms fly out if startled or if the head shifts positions abruptly.

<u>The walking/stepping reflex</u>—this is present at birth and disappears by two months. To assess this reflex, your provider will hold the baby under his or her arms while supporting the head and the baby will step one foot in front of the other as if stepping when the feet are placed on a flat surface.

<u>The tonic neck reflex</u>—this reflex is present at birth and disappears around 4–5 months of age. This is a subtle reflex seen when the baby's head is turned to one side. The arm on that side will straighten and the other arm will bend up.

Circumcision

You may or may not know the gender of your baby prior to delivery. However, if you have a boy, you will have to decide whether or not to have him circumcised.

The American Academy of Pediatrics (AAP) does not recommend that all males should be circumcised. They feel it should be a personal choice.

They believe that circumcision has potential medical advantages and risks, therefore they recommend that the decision is best made by the parents in consultation with their pediatrician.

Many parents chose to have their infant male circumcised for religious reasons, others because all other males in the family are circumcised and they don't want their son to feel different.

I will list some pros and cons to help you make a decision. If your mind has not been made up yet on whether or not to circumcise, this will hopefully help you decide.

Research suggests there may be some medical benefits to circumcision:

1. There is a lower risk of a urinary tract infection (UTI). A circumcised male has about a 1 in 1,000 chance, whereas an uncircumcised male has a 1 in 100 chance of a UTI.

2. A circumcised male has a lower risk of getting cancer of the penis although this is rare anyway.

3. A circumcised male has a slightly lower risk of getting a sexually transmitted disease or STD, including AIDS.

4. Circumcision prevents foreskin infections since there is no foreskin to get infected.

5. Circumcision also prevents phimosis, which is a condition that makes foreskin retraction impossible.

6. Circumcision makes genital hygiene easier.

A study done by Kaiser Permanente Medical Program in 2000 analyzed 15,000 male infants with urinary tract infections and found that circumcised boys have a health advantage. They are nine times less likely to get urinary tract infections, according to the results of their study.

The American Academy of Pediatrics says that cancer of the penis is a very rare condition that has long been known to occur almost exclusively in uncircumcised men and cervical cancer may be more common in females with uncircumcised partners.

Possible reasons parents may not want to have their son circumcised:

1. The presence of the foreskin protects the glans of the penis against urine and feces and other irritants.

2. Circumcision is a surgical procedure and there is always risk involved with surgery.

3. There is a risk of bleeding (although bleeding tends to be minimal unless there is a clotting issue).

4. There is risk of cutting the foreskin too short or not short enough.

5. There is a risk of improper healing.

6. The surgical site could become infected (although, with proper care, this is also very rare).

Circumcisions never became common practice in Asia, South America, Central America, or most of Europe.

Approximately 67% of the world's population is not circumcised.

Rates vary widely, from over 90% in Israel and many Muslim-majority countries to 86.3% in South Korea, 80% in the United States, 58% in Australia, 45% in South Africa, 20.7% in the United Kingdom, and under 1% in Japan and Honduras

https://worldpopulationreview.com/country-rankings/circumcision-by-country

The American Academy of Pediatrics recommends that a local anesthetic or topical anesthetic cream should be used for all circumcisions.

Your baby also needs to urinate within 6–8 hours after the circumcision. If there has been no urination, call the doctor. Also call your doctor if there is persistent bleeding, or redness increases after 3–5 days.

What is a newborn screening panel?

All babies born in the United States get a newborn screening. However, each state decides which conditions to screen babies born in their state for. This is called the state's newborn screening panel. In Arizona, the Arizona Newborn Screening Program screens for 33 rare and serious conditions. For more information about the Arizona Newborn Screening Program, visit: https://www.azdhs.gov/preparedness/state-laboratory/newborn-screening/index.php?#info-for-parents-disorder-info

The newborn screening panel looks for diseases that are not usually visibly recognizable after delivery. This test is often referred to as the PKU test, even though that is just one of the tests included in the screening panel. Some of these disorders are genetic, others are metabolic disorders, and some are hormone related. None of these disorders are contagious and none can be cured, but all can be treated. Treatment is typically a change in diet, so it is very important to find these disorders as early as possible. Most screenings cannot be performed until a baby has received at least 24 hours of breast milk or formula. Your baby may need follow-up testing if you are discharged before this time or if the baby is unable to be tested before discharge. Most babies will be tested again when they are up to birth weight or at the first pediatric visit, which usually occurs between days 5–7.

Categories that the screenings look at include immune system disorders, endocrine disorders, hemoglobinopathies, enzyme deficiencies, amino acid disorders, fatty acid oxidation disorders, lysosomal storage disorders, neuromuscular disorders, organic acid disorders and cystic fibrosis.

Typically, a heel prick is used to sample the baby's blood. Sometimes they will draw blood from the baby's hand. The blood drops are collected in a small vial or on a special piece of paper. The blood is then sent for testing. The baby's heel may have some redness and bruising at the pricked site, but this usually disappears in a few days.

In addition to the newborn screening panel, a drop of blood will be used to check for jaundice. This happens 36 hours after birth. The results of the test will help with discharge timing and follow up.

Check with your individual state to see exactly which tests your state screens for. To find out what conditions are on your state's newborn screening panel, go to: http://www.babysfirsttest.org/newborn-screening/states

Most states also screen for hearing loss and critical congenital heart disease.

Critical Congenital Heart Disease (CCHD)

CCHD is estimated to affect two out of every 1,000 babies born each year in the US. After a baby is at least 24 hours old, a small, painless sensor, called a pulse oximeter is placed on the baby's skin. The pulse oximeter measures how much oxygen is in the baby's blood. Babies who do not have enough oxygen in their blood could have a type of heart problem called Critical Congenital Heart Disease or Defect. This test helps identify babies before they leave the hospital.

What are the two newborn hearing screenings called and how are they performed?

Hearing screening: Nearly all states screen newborns for hearing loss. Hearing screening can be done any time after a baby is about 12 hours old. There are two different ways that the hearing screen can be done. Both methods measure how well the baby responds to sound, and both are quick and painless.

Otoacoustic emissions (OAEs):

OAEs measure responses coming from the inner ear organ (the cochlea). For this test, a small earbud, which contains a microphone and an earphone, is placed in the baby's ear. Sounds are played through the earbud and echo responses coming from the inner ear organ are measured. If a baby hears normally or near-normally, an echo is reflected into the inner ear which is measured by the microphone. If the baby has significant hearing loss, no echo or a reduced echo is measured.

Automated auditory brainstem response (AABR):

AABR testing measures responses coming from the inner ear organ (the cochlea) as well as the auditory brainstem, as sound travels up to the brain. This is the test most hospitals use. For this screening, sticker electrodes are placed on the baby's head and small earphones are placed in or around the baby's ear. Sounds are played through the earphones and the electrodes (that look like little stickers) measure whether there is a response coming from the baby's ear and auditory brainstem. They then send the response to a computer where data is stored and scored and a result of "pass" or "refer" is given. If a baby hears normally, a response will be detected, and the baby will pass. If the baby has significant hearing loss, no response will be detected, and the baby will get a score of "refer". If the baby does not pass the test the first time, the test is rerun and if the baby fails the test again, they are referred to a specialist.

Why screen newborns for hearing loss at birth?

Newborn hearing screenings are extremely important. From the moment a baby is born, they begin learning language by hearing language around them. If a baby is not hearing, this will hinder the baby's ability to learn to talk and pick up the spoken language. When newborns who have hearing loss are diagnosed early, effective intervention is available to help them achieve normal or near-normal speech, language, and hearing milestones.

Below are some statistics from the American Academy of Audiology:

Approximately 3-6 of every 1,000 newborns have significant hearing problems.

More than 95 percent of newborns who are born deaf have parents with normal hearing.

Hearing loss is invisible; it cannot be seen by examining your newborn's ears.

Most newborns with hearing loss have no signs or symptoms.

https://www.audiology.org/consumers-and-patients/children-and-hearing-loss/newborn-hearing-screening/American Academy of Audiology

What will your newborn look like?

Your baby will be the most beautiful human being you have ever laid eyes on. You will be so in love from the moment you see him or her that you may not see tiny anomalies that may occur from being trapped in a tight womb, or pressed up against a pubic bone, or pushed through a birth canal. Yet as the newness wears off and you start to inspect every inch of your tiny human, you might start to notice a few things that don't look quite right to you. I want to reassure you that these slight imperfections on your perfect human are most likely temporary and nothing to be alarmed about. Below, I will list a few things you might notice.

Newborn appearance is adapted from Your Child's Health by Dr. Barton Schmitt M.D.

Eyes and eyelids

Your baby's eyelids might look a bit swollen, puffy, or red. This could be due to the pressure from delivery, or it could be from the antibiotic eye drops that they are required to put in all newborns' eyes after delivery. This generally improves within three days of birth.

You might also notice what is called a subconjunctival hemorrhage. This looks like a little broken blood vessel in the white of the eye. This is not uncommon. It is harmless and due to birth trauma. The blood is reabsorbed by the eye in 2–3 weeks so the eye will be clear white again and this will not affect the baby's vision.

Barton Schmitt: "Your newborn's eye color or iris is usually blue, green, gray, brown, or a variation of those colors. Permanent color is often uncertain until your baby reaches six months of age." Caucasian babies are usually born with gray-blue eyes and African American babies are born with brown to gray eyes. Children who will have a dark iris often change by two months of age and those with light-colored eyes usually change by 5–6 months. If the iris is still light by six months of age, it will stay light for the remainder of their lives.

Ears

Your newborn's cartilage is very soft and malleable. The edge of the ear may be folded over, due to the baby's position in utero. The cartilage will harden and take on a regular shape in the next few weeks.

Nose

The nose, like the ears, is very soft and can be asymmetrical due to the position in the womb or during delivery. It will change gradually to its normal shape by the end of the first week.

Gums

Some babies are born with little cysts on their gums called epithelial pearls. These are blocked mucus glands and contain clear fluid. These little cysts may also look white. These typically disappear after 1-2 months. They are not painful and are harmless.

Female genitalia

Baby girls may be born with little flaps of extra skin called vaginal tags. They may also have swollen labia. This is due to extra estrogen from Mom that has crossed over the placenta.

The hymen may also be swollen and have smooth ½ inch projections of pink tissue. These occur in about 10% of newborn baby girls and they slowly shrink over 2-4 weeks as the estrogen from Mom decreases in the baby's blood.

A clear or white discharge may also be present from the baby's vagina any time between days 3 and 10. Occasionally, the discharge will become pink, or blood-tinged, and this should not last more than 2-3 days. Blood should not be seen in the urine.

Male genitalia

Baby boys might be born with clear fluid filling the scrotum. This is due to the scrotum being squeezed during the birth process. This fluid is reabsorbed over the next 6-12 months.

In 4% of newborn males, the testes have not descended into the scrotum. This may be a gradual process where the testicle or testicles gradually descend into a normal position within the next few months. If by one year, however, it has not descended, surgery will be required. The chance of this happening is only about 7%.

If your son is uncircumcised, the foreskin will be tight. The skin is so tight it does not allow you to see the head of the penis. This is normal and should *not* be retracted in babies.

If your son was circumcised, there may be a yellow scab at the incision line that will come off in 7–10 days. If a ring was used for the circumcision, it should fall off between 10 and 14 days.

Erections occur commonly in newborn boys. They are normally triggered by a full bladder and demonstrate that the nerves of the penis are normal. Get a diaper ready if you see this, as you are about to get sprayed.

Breasts

Swollen breast tissue may be present in both male and female babies for several months. This is due to the passage of estrogen across the placenta.

Some puffiness may persist if the infant is breastfed.

Call your pediatrician if you notice redness, streaking, or tenderness.

Head

Your newborn's head may be slightly misshapen at first. They might even appear to have a cone-shaped head, from sitting engaged in the birth canal or passing through the birth canal. Normal shape should return in a few days. Your newborn might also have a bit of swelling called "caput" on the top of the head or throughout the scalp. This is also due to squeezing through the birth canal and fluid being squeezed under the skin. This is not painful and will clear and reabsorb in a few days.

Sometimes, your little one will develop a bruising lump on the side of the head or an accumulation of blood in the form of a lump from friction against the pelvic bone. This is called a "cephalohematoma". It usually appears two days after delivery and may grow for up to five days. It may not completely go away for 2–3 months.

Soft spots or fontanels

Your baby will have two soft spots on his or her head. These soft spots allow for rapid brain growth. They also help the skull to be pliable during the delivery process.

The first one is on the top of the head. This soft spot is called the anterior fontanel. This one is diamond shaped. You can typically see a pulse with each beat of the heart. It is safe to touch. This soft spot typically closes between 12 and 18 months of age.

The second soft spot is on the back of the skull. This soft spot is called the posterior fontanel. The posterior fontanel is much smaller than the anterior fontanel and closes earlier around at 2–3 months of age.

Hair

Most newborns are born with dark hair. This newborn hair is not permanent and begins to fall out by one month of age. Some babies lose it gradually and you may not even notice it is falling out while his or her permanent hair is coming in. Others lose it rapidly and are temporarily bald.

The permanent hair will appear by six months of age, and it is not uncommon for it to be a different color from the newborn hair.

Body hair is called "lanugo". Lanugo is the soft, fine hair that may be present on babies' backs and shoulders. We see this more often in preemies. It rubs off with normal friction by about 2–4 weeks of age.

Legs

Your baby's lower legs usually curve in and your baby may look a bit bow-legged when you hold them up in a standing position. This is normal and caused by the cramped quarters of the uterus and the crossed-legged position the baby was in while in the womb. The legs will straighten out when your little one starts walking.

Feet

In addition to the legs turning in, the feet may also turn at awkward angles. This is also due to being cramped in the womb. As long as the feet are flexible and can be easily moved into a normal position without your baby fussing, they are normal. "Normal" direction will occur around 6–12 months.

Hips

When your pediatrician is doing your baby's assessment and giving him or her a once-over, they will also test your infant's hips for hip dislocation. They are checking that they are not too tight. The most common cause of a tight hip is dislocation. The good news is that, if a joint has been dislocated during delivery, putting the joint back into place involves a fairly simple procedure. Babies are very pliable.

Skin

Newborns can have rashes and bumps that look odd to us but are very normal and harmless in a newborn. One odd-looking skin condition is called "erythema toxicum".

More than 50% of babies get this rash on the 2–3rd day of life. This rash looks like red blotches about 0.5–1 inch in size. They look like they have a center to them, but they are not fluid filled. The blotches can be numerous and may keep occurring. If they are fluid filled, or pus filled, or if they are grouped in clusters, especially on the scalp, have your baby seen to rule out herpes simplex.

Erythema toxicum may be present anywhere except for the palms and soles of the feet. Although they may look scary, they are not harmful. The cause is unknown, and they usually resolve in two weeks.

"Milia" is another common rash seen in newborns. Milia are little white bumps that occur on the faces of approximately 40% of newborns, mainly on the nose and cheeks. Sometimes they are found on the chin and the forehead as well. They are abundant and occur equally on both sides of the face. They are teeny tiny, about the size of pinheads and are different from infant acne. They are the result of blocked-off skin pores, and they will disappear in 1–2 months, according to Dr. Barton Schmitt. The American Academy of Pediatrics says most milia will disappear in the first 2–3 weeks of life.

"A Mongolian spot is a normal bluish-green or bluish-gray flat birthmark found in over 90% of Native American, Oriental, Hispanic, and African American babies and 10% of Caucasians, especially in those of Mediterranean descent. This occurs mainly over the back and buttocks, although it can be on any part of the body. It may vary greatly in size. It is not related to disease. Most fade by 2–3 years of age, although traces may be present until adulthood." Dr. Barton Schmitt.

Flat pink birthmarks are often called "stork bites." These occur over the bridge of the nose, eyelids and the back of the neck, in more than 50% of newborns. All of those that occur on the bridge of the nose and eyelids clear completely. The ones occurring on the eyelids resolve by one year of age. Those on the nose may persist for a few more years. Those on the forehead that run from the bridge of the nose to the hairline usually persist into adulthood. Laser treatment during infancy should be considered for these types of birthmarks. Most birthmarks that are on the neck also clear up. However, 25% of those on the neck persist through adulthood. Dr. Barton Schmitt

The skin over bony prominences can be injured from the pressure of going through the birth canal. Fetal monitors can also cause scrapes. The bruises and scrapes are usually seen at the time of the baby's birth or the day after and disappear within 1–2 weeks. The injury to fatty tissue typically won't appear until days 5–10. For any breaks in the skin, apply an antibiotic ointment four times a day until the area is healed and monitor for signs and symptoms of infection.

Newborn behavior

Dr. Barton Schmitt feels most newborn behaviors are due to an immature nervous system and will disappear in 2–3 months. Some typical newborn behaviors include:

Hiccups—hiccups are very common in the first two months, and they bother us more than they do them. This is due to an immature digestive system.

"Newborns have irregular breathing patterns. Any irregular pattern is normal if the baby is peaceful, and the rate is less than 60 breaths per minute and the pause is less than six seconds. The baby should not have a color change such as blue or gray. Occasionally infants take rapid progressive deeper breaths to expand the lungs." Barton Schmitt MD

Passing gas—some babies are gassier than others. Mylicon drops prior to each feed may help with this if it seems to bother the baby. If you are bottle feeding, try Dr. Brown's bottles.

Quivers and shivers are normal, especially chin and lip quivers.

Sleep noises from breathing and moving are common. Babies are noisier than you think.

Sneezes—babies sneeze just like adults. It is how they clear their nose of irritants.

Spit-up (1 tbsp is a typical amount of spit-up).

Startle reflex or brief stiffening of the body, following noise or movement.

Straining with bowel movements. Stools should be soft. Some babies cry and turn red, grunt and strain. As long as the stool is soft, this is normal.

Throat clearing or gurgling sounds due to secretions in the throat.

"Trembling or jitteriness of arms and legs during crying is common but convulsions are rare. During convulsions, babies also jerk and blink their eyes rhythmically, make sucking movements with their mouths and don't cry. If your baby is trembling and not crying, give him or her a pacifier to suck on. If trembling doesn't stop during sucking, call your pediatrician immediately." (Barton Schmitt, MD)

During your hospital stay, take advantage of the help that is available to you. Ask for a lactation consultant right away if you know you want to try breastfeeding. Ask your nurses questions about newborn care. The staff are usually amazing. The more you ask when you are in the hospital, the more comfortable you will feel when you go home. I remember thinking, as I was leaving the hospital, how scary it was to be walking out with a little human that I was now 100% responsible for. It can feel overwhelming. So, use the resources that are available to you in the hospital and, in my opinion, don't be in too big of a hurry to rush home.

CHAPTER 3

CORD BLOOD

*"Making the decision to have a child is momentous.
It is to decide forever to have your heart go
walking around outside your body."*

– Elizabeth Stone

What is cord blood banking?

In the past 20 or so years, a new type of banking has been established for parents about to give birth, called cord blood banking.

Blood is removed from the umbilical cord and placenta right after birth. This does not hurt the baby in any way and, if not used for banking or donation, it becomes medical waste. Some parents bank their infant's cord blood as insurance. Some bank because of family history. Some donate cord blood for research or possibly to save another person's life.

Like bone marrow, cord blood is found to be rich in stem cells. Stem cells are the building blocks of the blood and immune system. A stem cell contains both red and white cells, as well as platelets and plasma.

Cord blood is currently used to treat about 80 conditions and life-threatening diseases, such as leukemia and other cancers, as well as certain blood and immune disorders. Stem cells from cord blood have proved to be a viable alternative to bone marrow transplants for many conditions.

The stem cells collected moments after birth haven't been exposed to other elements like disease or aging, that can impact them later in life. Research shows that transplants using stem cells from a sibling result in double the survival rate for certain diseases when compared to treatment using cord blood, or stem cells from an unrelated donor.

The first successful transplant was performed in 1988 on a six-year-old boy suffering from a blood disorder called "Fanconi anemia."

"Over 40,000 stem cell transplants worldwide used cord blood from both donor and private family banks." (Viacord.com)

"Stem cells were discovered in cord blood in 1978, and the first cord blood transplant followed ten years later. Since then, more than 40,000 cord blood transplants have been performed around the globe." (Cyrocell.com)

Cord blood does not require as close of a match as bone marrow, and it has fewer side effects.

"Cord blood has less of a chance of rejection because it is coming from a newborn and the stem cells have none of the immunity "programming" that is built into mature bone marrow stem cells." (Cryocell.com)

So many things factor into a bone marrow transplant, making the total actual cost of such a procedure—assuming the patient has no insurance—range from $80,000 up to $400,000. Complications, such as graft versus host disease, can make any procedure exponentially more expensive, not to mention life-threatening. https://www.

lymphomainfo.net/articles/treatment/how-much-does-a-bone-marrow-transplant-cost

- This year, more than 130,000 Americans will be diagnosed with a serious blood disease.

- Leukemia (a blood cancer) will strike 44,000 Americans this year, including 3,500 children. It will kill about half of the adults and about 700 of the children.

- Leukemia is the most common childhood cancer.

- Only 30 percent of patients who need a bone marrow transplant have a matching donor in their family.

- The remaining 70 percent must hope that a compatible stranger can be found using the national registry.

- At any given time, about 7,500 Americans are actively searching the national registry for an unrelated donor.

- Only two percent of the population is on the national registry.

- A significant number of those on the national bone marrow registry cannot be located or will not donate when asked to do so. The percentages of donors who are available and willing are: 65 for Caucasians; 47 percent for Hispanics; 44 percent for Asians; 34 percent for African Americans.

- African American patients find an unrelated donor 25 percent of the time.

- Asian patients find a donor about 40 percent of the time.

- Hispanic patients find a donor about 45 percent of the time.

- Caucasian patients find a donor about 75 percent of the time.

- Multi-racial people face the worst odds.

- At least 3,000 people die each year because they cannot find a matching donor.

https://ij.org/bonemarrowstatistics/ Institute of Justice Bone Marrow Statistics

Cord blood harvesting and storage can be very costly, so it is an individual decision, and you should do it thinking that you will most likely never need to use it. It is like an insurance policy, in my opinion. This is where I will share my own story. I had heard about cord blood banking when I was pregnant with my daughter, but we were a young family starting out. I had to stop working due to my hyperemesis, so money was tight, and we could not afford to bank her cord blood. I knew the potential value of stem cells, however, so I tried to donate. I called all over and I could not find anyone at that time who would take it for donation. It bothered me for five years that her cord blood went to waste. So, when Dylan was born, we were in better shape financially and we decided to bank Dylan's cord blood. Now, the weird thing is that I must have had a mother's intuition or something when I was pregnant with Taylor, because the likelihood of ever needing or using banked blood is very low. Yet when Dylan was diagnosed with a rare immune deficiency, a stem cell transplant came up. The crazy thing is that, since Dylan's condition is genetic, we can't use his own stem cells. If we had banked his sister's, we could have used hers. We still keep his stem cells stored, as his immunologist says we don't know what the future holds for science, so we don't want to destroy his banked cells. The amazing thing is the bank I chose said if I ever had another baby, they would bank the blood for free due to the possibility of a member of our family needing it. I thought that was pretty amazing of them.

Reputable cord blood banks

Below are a few reputable cord blood banks including the one we use:

Cord blood registry

1(888) 932-6568 or 1(888)-cord blood - University of Arizona

The website is www.cordblood.com

Cryo-Cell

www.cryo-cell.com Florida

1800786-7235/1800storcell

This is where I banked my son's cord blood. Cryo-Cell was the least expensive bank at the time, and I liked that it was publicly traded. I also knew they were opening a state-of-the-art facility that can withstand a level 5 hurricane. They store in a multi-compartment bag so some can be taken out if needed and the rest stored. They said this method has a better cell recovery. These were my personal reasons for choosing this company.

Via Cord

www.viacord.com Cambridge MA

1(800)998-4226 or 1(866)-393-9062

Celebration Stem Cell Center

www.celebrationstemcellcenter.com

For Banking or Donation Gilbert Az (480) 722-9963

Storage of cord blood is not for everyone. Most doctors don't recommend it for a family that is not high risk, meaning no family history of an immediate family member with leukemia, sickle cell anemia, certain types of cancers, etc.

The chances that a child will develop a disease such as leukemia are very small, approximately 1 in 10,000.

If you do have an immediate family member in remission or suffering from a disorder treatable with stem cells, many banks will offer services free of charge.

Because the technology is so new, they still don't know how long the cells can be stored and still remain viable. They know they are still viable after 20 years and, if cryopreserved, many experts feel they should remain viable for the life of the patient.

But if you are not going to store your child's cord blood, you may want to donate it.

I feel this is similar to donating blood or plasma or even organ donation. You could save someone's life.

One organization that will help you donate is called Give Life Twice at 1888 770-GIVE. These donations will be used for transplants.

Two organizations collect for both research and transplants:

Cryobanks International at www.cryo-intl.com 1800 869-8608

Lifebank USA at www.lifebankusa.com 1877543-3226 or 1877lifebankusa

The University of California will take samples for research.

The University of Arizona also takes samples for research, but their storage space for donor samples is limited.

Save the Cord Foundation is a 5-1c3 nonprofit whose mission is to bring fair, balanced, and factual information about the medical value of umbilical cord blood and options to parents and the public. www.savethecordfoundation.org

The American Academy of Pediatrics view on storage of cord blood:

American Academy of Pediatrics Encourages Use of Public Cord Blood Banks https://www.aap.org/en/news-room/news-releases/aap/2017/aap-encourages-use-of-public-cord-blood-banks/

Stem cell transplants from cord blood have risen over the past decade to save children with fatal diseases, most often through the use of public cord blood banks.

Cord blood is increasingly being used to treat fatal or debilitating diseases, prompting the American Academy of Pediatrics to release a policy statement that calls for renewed emphasis and education about the advantages and need for public cord blood banking.

The policy statement, "**Cord Blood Banking for Future Transplantation**," published in the November 2017 issue of Pediatrics, serves as an update to the Academy's 2007 policy and references the latest research on clinical outcomes from cord blood transplants. The statement, to be published online on October 30, observes that a growing number of states are requiring universal newborn screening for diseases that could be treated with stem cell transplantation.

"Most parents will never need cord blood for their own family's use, but they can donate this precious life-saving gift to benefit others," said William T. Shearer, MD, Ph.D., FAAP, lead author of the policy statement. "We expect the need for these therapies that rely on stem cell transplantation to grow and would like families to understand the choices they have."

Cord blood, taken from the placenta of healthy newborn infants, was routinely discarded until it was discovered to be an excellent source of stem cells for hematopoietic stem cell transplantation for some diseases. According to research, more than 30,000 stem cell transplants had been performed using cord blood worldwide by 2013.

Cord blood is used most often in transplantation in infants and children with fatal diseases, such as malignancies, blood disorders, immune deficiencies, and metabolic disorders.

Donating cord blood is safe for the baby and it doesn't interfere with labor and delivery. Because families must register ahead of time—so a collection kit can be sent and used after the baby's delivery—the AAP recommends that physicians talk with families during an early prenatal visit.

Also recommended is that physicians discuss the value of cord blood and the difference between public cord blood banks versus private, for-profit cord blood banks.

The AAP policy statement lists these differences between public and private cord blood banking:

- Public cord blood banks serve patients worldwide by matching individuals in need. Private banks store the cord blood for the donor family's potential self-use, although there is little evidence supporting this use, unless a family shares a known genetic defect.

- Donation to a public cord blood bank is free. Private cord blood banks charge a placement fee of $1,350 to $2,300 and an annual maintenance fee of $100-$175.

- Public cord blood banks are highly regulated by oversight accrediting institutions. Private cord blood banks may not meet stringent requirements, which can cause cord blood to be of lesser quality.

- The rate that cord blood stem cells are utilized from a public bank is 30 times higher compared with private cord blood banks. Yet more cord blood donations from ethnic/minority populations are needed to meet increasing needs.

"The research is evolving in this area, which is exciting news for patients whose lives may someday depend on a donation of cord blood," Dr. Shearer said. "The hope is that more doctors will discuss the options with expectant parents well in advance of their baby's birth, so they understand the tremendous potential to help others in medical need." Parents can find information about cord blood banking and many other topics from the American Academy of Pediatrics at www.healthychildren.org.

I hope this chapter encourages some of you, if not all of you, to donate your child's cord blood, if you are not banking it yourself. Every day we make new strides in medicine and medical advances. We can't possibly know what we will be able to do with cord blood transplants in the next decade. Yes, it can be an extra step or hassle to set up and you will probably never know if your efforts were able to help someone or not, but what an amazing gift you might be able to give to someone. I know how I felt when those precious stem cells of Taylor's were sent to medical waste.

"We are not put on this earth for ourselves but are placed here for each other. If you are always there for others, then in time of need, someone will be there for you." **(Jeff Warner)**

CHAPTER 4

NEWBORN NECESSITIES

"The most precious jewels you'll ever have around your neck are the arms of your children."

— Altaf Ul Qadri

Bottle types:

No one particular bottle is best. You have to find the one that is best for your baby. What worked best for your best friend's baby may not be best for your baby.

If your baby does not spit up much, does not have colic, gas, or feeding problems, the type of bottle you use will probably not make much difference.

Now, if you do have a baby that is prone to spit-up or very gassy, I do have a favorite bottle:

My favorite bottle on the market to reduce spit-up and help with reflux is Dr. Browns Although I have to say, I have not personally tried the new Avent bottle that competes with Dr. Browns, so I can't make a comparison between the two.

The only problems with Dr. Brown's bottles are that they may be slightly more expensive than other bottles. They are more work to clean them due to multiple parts, and they may be more difficult to find.

Dr Brown's claim their bottle prevents nipple collapse and decreases colic symptoms, gas, and spit-up, due to an internal vent that prevents air bubbles from forming in the formula or milk. It does not create a vacuum, so it helps prevent fluid in the inner ear. The bottle connects to most breast pumps and is dishwasher safe. This bottle also comes in an 8 oz wide-mouth bottle. The 4 oz and 8 oz sizes are available in their regular bottle.

I have suggested this bottle to many people when nothing else seemed to be working. I have had amazing results over the years with this bottle, making it my favorite.

When my niece was born, she had severe reflux. She was always spitting up and was in so much pain. She was extremely gassy and fussy. My brother and sister-in-law changed the formula and put her on medication, but nothing made much difference until we found these bottles, which were brand-new on the market. The difference they made for her was like night and day. I also got two other moms with similar stories to try the bottles and, just like my sister-in-law, they were sold. After spending time with my niece and seeing the change in her, I started telling all my parents about these bottles. I used nothing else with my son, who also had severe reflux like my daughter. Yet, unlike my daughter, I did not have to put my son on medication, and I credit these bottles for that. I wish these had been available when my daughter was a baby. I personally think they are worth the money.

There are also bottles that are literally shaped like the breast, like Mimijumi and Nanobebe, that might be helpful for babies who are refusing bottles and only want the breast. I also like Tommee Tippee and Nancom. So, if you have a baby who does not want to take a bottle and only breastfeed you might try one of these bottles.

- A couple of little tips to help a baby who will not take a bottle. You can warm the nipple and get an item of clothing that smells like Mom to put up against the person feeding the baby. It is also best if someone other than Mom tries to offer the bottle.

Pacifiers:

A Dartmouth Medical School review of several SIDS studies showed that routine use of pacifiers may lower the risk of SIDS by as much as 50%. Scientists are not sure how and why pacifiers protect against SIDS and are therefore not ready to recommend their use for all newborns. They suspect that sucking on a pacifier may help keep the airway open and discourage some babies from turning on their faces during sleep. It may also trigger the ability to rouse themselves from sleep easier.

If your baby will not take a particular pacifier, don't give up. Try a few different brands.

Pacifiers must be strong enough not to separate into small pieces. Never leave them in the heat. Discard them as the manufacturer recommends. Never use a pacifier with a tie around the neck or with a long string that could wrap around the neck. Make sure the pacifier shield has ventilation holes and the pacifier should be large enough for infants not to be able to get the entire thing in their mouth. Get an older size as the baby grows.

How much sucking babies do between feeds varies from baby to baby. Some babies almost constantly suck on their thumb or fingers. You may want to use an orthodontic pacifier instead to prevent sucking on fingers to help prevent future dental problems, if you have a little one with a strong need to suck. Pacifiers exert less pressure on the teeth than fingers and thumbs and help to avoid a severe overbite. It can also be taken away, unlike the thumb. The peak age for sucking is 2–4 months and it normally decreases in the months following. Limit pacifier use to encourage speech and normal babbling, especially during the day. After six months of age, it can become a comfort object. This may be the time to get rid of it, if you do not want to keep it long term.

Cribs:

Each year, thousands of infants are injured seriously enough to require treatment in hospital emergency rooms from accidents involving cribs. Over a million cribs are produced each year and these cribs are manufactured to meet crib regulations. However, there are still some things to keep in mind.

The main concerns involve old or used cribs. If you are using a hand-me-down crib, make sure the crib meets today's safety regulations. Slats should not be more than 2 ⅛ inches apart. Cribs built after 1999 should meet current standards. Make sure your mattress fits snugly. If you can fit more than two fingers between the edge of the mattress and the crib side, the mattress is too small.

An infant can suffocate if its head or body becomes wedged between the mattress and crib sides. When I spoke with Babies-R-Us, they told me the cribs and mattresses are all standard size, yet they can vary a fraction of an inch, so if you figure ¼ of an inch on both sides, that could be a big gap.

If you paint or refinish a crib, make sure you use only high-quality household enamel paint and let it dry thoroughly, so there are no residual fumes.

Try not to place the crib near the window. If you do, make sure there is no drapery or window blind cords within reach, as these can pose a strangulation hazard. Put a window lock on the window.

Some crib accessories can become dangerous for active and older babies, e.g., crib mobiles should be removed by five months of age. No bumpers or bedding in the crib except for a tight-fitting crib sheet.

When fully lowered, the top of the rail should be at least 4 inches above the mattress, even when the mattress is at the highest position.

If the crib has corner posts, they should not be higher than $1/16^{th}$ of an inch, to prevent the baby's clothes from getting caught and possibly strangling them.

You may want to look into the new mesh style mattresses that are breathable.

New mattresses can release many volatile organic compounds and toxins. Since your baby is lying on the mattress, this makes the concentration of chemicals twice as high for them. You may want to purchase an organic crib mattress, as they have fewer toxic chemicals. Or get a regular mattress several months before you put your baby into the nursery. Let it air out in the garage, without the plastic to allow the chemicals to dissipate. Or, let your mattress air out in an empty room, without the plastic, for at least a month, if possible, before putting your baby on it.

Your crib has three positions. High, middle, and low. The crib mattress should be lowered to the middle position when your baby starts to show signs of sitting up. This is typically after rolling in both directions. It needs to be in the lowest position when a baby can get to a sitting position on their own. They will soon be able to pull themselves up to a standing position. It is always best to be safe, so lower it sooner rather than later.

Baby walkers:

Baby walkers delay walking and are not safe. Research has found that babies who use walkers walk later than those who do not. Babies learn best to walk by crawling and pulling themselves up repeatedly. They develop coordination, balance, and the muscle groups needed for walking. If you picture the way a baby walks in a walker, they are not using the proper body mechanics and large motor skills. They are leaning forward and walking on their toes, as opposed to walking flat footed and balancing on their own. The main reason to avoid them, however, is that they are dangerous. Thousands of children are seen in ER every year due to an accident involving a walker.

An Exersaucer:

An Exersaucer (Evenflo Exersaucer is just one type of many), on the other hand, is a wonderful baby item and I would recommend one for every baby. It allows for the baby to stand with appropriate body mechanics and has various activities to hold the baby's interest. It is stationary, so although the baby can turn in circles, he or she cannot get into danger like a walker. It is a great place to keep your baby safe, so you can take a shower. Since it is lightweight and portable, you can bring it right into the bathroom with you. ☺ I call this one of my baby stations to keep your baby entertained.

Baby gates:

Baby gates can be wonderful safety devices to block off a doorway opening, if used correctly. Baby gates keep your little one out of a room that may not be fully child proofed. It can also keep babies away from the tops and bottoms of stairs. Yet some baby gates themselves are dangerous. If using a gate, choose one with a straight top edge and rigid mesh screen. Be sure the baby gate is securely anchored in the doorway or stairway. Children have pushed gates over and fallen downstairs. Gates that are held in place with an expanding pressure bar should be installed so the bar is on the side away from the child, as this can be used as a step for your child to get up and over. Pressure bar gates should not be the ones used on stairs. Stair gates should be securely mounted to the wall and banister.

Bath rings and bath seats:

Many bath seats have been recalled over the years, as there have been known drownings in infants, primarily in the age range of 6–9 months. These devices typically have suction cups that attach to the bottom of tubs. Drownings are caused by the seat tipping over when the suction cups release, allowing the device and baby to tip over in the water. Entrapment, such as babies slipping between the legs of the bath ring and becoming trapped underwater, has also occurred. Never rely on these products to keep your baby safe. Only fill water high enough to cover your baby's legs, although drownings can occur in as little as an inch of water. Securely attach the bath seat to a smooth surface as the suction cups will not stick to textured surfaces or non-slip tubs. These bath seats can be great and save your back, if used properly. They are a nice transition from a baby bathtub to a big tub, but the baby must be watched at all times. If you never take your eyes off the baby, and the seat is used properly, there should be no issue with using a bath seat.

Play pens:

Many playpen injuries occur when the drop side of mesh playpens and portable cribs are left in the down position. Because the mesh hangs loosely, infants can become trapped and suffocate. The newer playpens, such as the Pack and Play, have small mesh weave, smaller than the smallest baby button. Avoid items like blankets and stuffed animals, just as you would in a crib, and do not put a playpen up against window cords, which could be a strangulation hazard. I loved my Pack and Play. It can serve multiple purposes, from a travel bed to a temporary timeout spot (more on this in the discipline lecture).

Baby swings:

A swing can be a great way to keep your little one entertained. Keep your baby in view. Always fasten the seat belts as well as the tray or brace if there is one. Each swing is different. Stop using the swing when your baby can grab the leg or side of the swing or pump their legs. Follow the manufacturers' recommendations on size restrictions: generally it is under 25 pounds or nine months of age. You will probably want an adjustable seat, which reclines for a newborn, a quiet, battery-operated one, with washable fabric, non-slip legs, and both a seat belt and a brace between the legs for greater stability.

Swings are wonderful, just don't let your baby routinely fall asleep in one. You don't want to create a bad sleep habit that you later will need to break. You can use your swing as one of your "stations" to keep your baby occupied.

Highchairs:

Each year, thousands of children are treated in hospital emergency rooms for injuries associated with highchairs. The majority of these injuries result from falls, although deaths can occur when children wiggle beneath the tray and are strangled.

Falls from highchairs and injuries occur when restraining straps are not used and when children are not closely supervised. When children are eating and sitting in a highchair they should never be left alone. Children should never be left alone period when eating.

To help prevent falls, highchairs should have a waist strap and a strap or bar that runs between the legs.

While in the highchair, children should always be restrained by these straps and the tray should not be used as a restraining device in place of the straps.

Without these two straps, children can stand in the seat and topple from the highchair or wiggle beneath the tray and be strangled when their head becomes stuck between the tray and the seat.

Other accidents occur when the chair collapses or falls over.

Highchairs fall if an active child pushes off with the hands or feet from the table, stands up in highchair or rocks back and forth. Choose one with a wide base for stability.

You may want a small portable or folding chair that attaches to a kitchen chair (I used my little fold-up portable highchair more than my big one, as my little one could sit at the table with us, and it was great for travel too).

Back carriers / front carriers:

The key to infant carriers is making sure you follow the manufacturer's guidelines and choose one that fits your infant's age and size.

A framed back carrier should not be used before a baby is 4–5 months old. By then, the baby's neck is able to withstand jolts and not sustain injury.

Look for a back carrier with padded covering over the metal frame near your baby's face.

Restraining straps are essential.

Always bend from your knees while your infant is in the carrier.

Leg openings should not be too wide or too tight. I had a little preemie and he loved to be in his "Snuggly" style front carrier. One day, I looked down and noticed his little legs were bright red, almost purple in color. I freaked out. Even though he weighed all of about 10 pounds, his little legs were too chubby, and he had outgrown that carrier.

So, make sure you are constantly monitoring your carrier for the proper fit. An alternative would be an ergonomic wrap or sling instead of a carrier, that is adjustable.

Bassinets and cradles:

Look for one with a sturdy bottom and a strong base.

Check screws and bolts periodically as they can loosen.

The mattress and padding should fit snuggly and be firm and smooth. Never use a pillow, blanket or bumper pads. Sheets should also be tight fitting.

Hook-on chairs / chairs that hook onto countertops and tables:

Never place the chair where your child's feet can reach table supports, benches or the back of the kitchen bar area, where they could push off and dislodge the chair from the table or counter.

If your little one is a bouncer, keep a close eye so that they don't wiggle or bounce themselves right off the edge. (I am personally not a fan of these. I have seen too many accidents with them).

Strollers:

Choose a stroller where the leg opening can be closed when used in the carriage position, if this is an option with your stroller. The base needs to be wide enough to prevent tipping even if the baby leans out.

If the seat can be adjusted into a reclining position, make sure the stroller does not tip backward when the baby lies down.

If a stroller has a shopping basket for carrying packages, it should be low on the back of the stroller and in front of or directly over the rear wheels.

Don't hang anything over the back handles, as this can cause tipping.

Choose one with strong belts that are easy to fasten and unfasten and always use them. These are not optional. If you always clip your kids in, they will realize it is not a choice.

Make sure your stroller has working brakes.

Car seats:

There is not one car seat that is better than others. It is what fits best in your car and what fits your baby the best.

Look at your car manual to see where they recommend placing the infant seat in your vehicle. Every car is different.

Install your seat facing the rear for at least two years, if possible. More to come on this in the safety chapter.

Look at the manufacturer's height and weight restrictions. Most infants outgrow their infant car seat due to height before weight.

Here is a list of some of my other favorite things:

As previously mentioned, Dr Brown's bottles—do not get too many 4 oz bottles as they will most likely be over 4 oz after one month.

Diapers—do not buy too many of the "newborn" size. Stock up on size one and above. Some babies don't even fit into the newborn size.

NoseFrida—this is easier than the bulb syringe, but a bulb syringe works too.

Thermometer (digital with cover)—do not use the ear thermometer type; they are inaccurate in infants. A Thermoscan thermometer is nice to have but you also need a digital thermometer to take rectal temperatures.

Humidifier (cool mist) with a removable filter and basin, so you can change the filter with each new illness, and an easy-to-clean removable basin.

A diaper bag.

A bottle bag with a couple of gel ice packs that can also be used to keep the car seat cool in summer

Nail clippers (round top) and a nail file.

Lightweight receiving blankets.

Burp cloths or cloth diapers.

A bouncy seat that vibrates.

Velcro bibs (rather than ones that tie).

Waterproof pads or one large one that you can cut into pieces. You can put this on the changing table instead of having to wash the cover. I used these in the car seat, etc.

Baby Safe Feeder / Fresh Food Feeder.

A front carrier or wrap.

A Pack and Play is not necessary unless you travel frequently, however I think it is great to have one.

Safety gadgets of all types especially magnetic cabinet locks(more about these in the safety chapter).

Mylicon / simethicone gas drops.

Diaper rash cream.

Vanicream products.

Grocery cart cover.

Graco Bumper Jumper —hangs in the door frame and will be a station.

Video baby monitor—they are now so clear you can see the baby breathe.

Activity playmats / small activity gym—the kind the baby lies under and bats at and that can be used for tummy time as well. These will also be activity stations.

If you have a boy and circumcise, you want a tube of Vaseline or Aquaphor or Vanicream ointment and gauze pads.

Milk collector cups—Haacaa is great brand, but they all work the same.

NumNum self-feeding utensils.

A baby bathtub / foam bathmat—these are also not necessary but nice to have. The kitchen sink works well, too.

In all honesty, newborns don't need much. The items mentioned above are nice to have but not necessary. Babies need milk, warmth, love, and diapers (lots of diapers.) The rest you can gather and figure out over time.

CHAPTER 5

NEWBORN CARE AND NEWBORN ILLNESS

"The littlest feet make the biggest footprints in our hearts."

— Unknown

Newborn care

Cord care

The umbilical cord normally falls off at approximately 2–3 weeks of age. However, some newborns hang on to theirs until about four weeks (if has not fallen off by four weeks, call your doctor). Keep the diaper folded down, so it does not snag the umbilical cord stump, and allows for the most air exposure possible. Umbilical cord infections are serious! Early signs of infection include a foul odor, yellow or green discharge, and redness. One or all may be present and, if you notice any of these symptoms, you need to book an office visit with your pediatrician. A small amount of bleeding is normal when the cord falls off or if it snags on the diaper or clothing and is pulled a bit. Avoid submerging the area in water until the cord has fallen off and for approximately three days afterwards.

Bathing

Bathe approximately 2–3 times a week. Babies do not really get dirty until they start eating solid foods. Their skin is extremely sensitive, so bathing can dry the skin unnecessarily. Soap is not necessary. If you would like to use it, however, use a baby bath or soap for sensitive skin, without fragrance and dye, such as a Vanicream product. Make sure the cord remains dry by giving a sponge bath and clean it with an alcohol wipe afterwards for added protection. Once you do start bathing them in the tub, after the cord has fallen off, many babies feel very exposed and exhibit the startle reflex. I found that getting a hand towel wet with warm water and lying it over the baby for warmth really helps with this.

Urine

It is normal to see what appears to be little beads of gelatin in the diaper when using disposable diapers, due to a reaction between the urine and chemicals in some brands of disposable diapers. You may also occasionally see a spot of reddish orange (not pink or bright red) discoloration on the diaper. This is typically not blood but urate crystals. This is most common in breastfed babies in the first few days of life when the mom's milk is not yet in, and the baby is not yet up to birth weight. These crystals sit on top of the urine and smell like urine, not metallic like blood. If you are unsure if these are urate crystals or blood it never hurts to have the baby checked. Bring the diaper in question with you to the pediatrician's office. Your newborn boy should have a strong urine stream. If you notice that the urine stream is not strong, bring this up with your pediatrician as well.

Stools

Stools can range from seedy, yellow, watery, cottage cheese, which is typically found in breastfed babies, to green, bluish green, tan/light brown. All are normal color variations. Call if you see blood in the stool or black tarry stools after the meconium has passed. Meconium is the only time you should see those tarry black-colored stools. Once they pass, you will never see stools like that again. Many babies grunt, grimace, turn red, and even cry when having a bowel movement but do not worry as long as it remains soft. If your baby has hard, pellet-like stools, call the doctor. At one month of age, like magic, you may see a sudden decrease in stools. Your baby may go from seven stools a day to stooling as infrequently as one every seven days. As long as that stool is soft, don't worry about it. This just means the baby's digestive tract is maturing and there is very little waste with breast milk. Celebrate your savings on diapers. 😊

Hiccups

Hiccups are very common in the first two months. This is just an immature digestive system.

Rashes

During the first two weeks, your baby may have a splotchy red rash with what appears to be a clear to whitish or even yellowish center to the bumps. The rash almost looks like bug bites, but they are not. The rash comes and goes and then disappears. This is called erythema toxicum, as we discussed earlier. These spots don't occur on the bottom of the hands or feet. They typically go away after the first few weeks. Remember, the center should not be fluid-filled and the baby should not have a fever with this rash.

Dry and peeling skin

It is also normal for the skin to be dry and peeling in the first couple of weeks, especially around the wrists and ankles. This is most common with a full-term baby. Baby lotion is not necessary, but it can be used if you want to. If your baby has sensitive skin, you might want to avoid scented baby lotions and use a non-scented lotion with no dyes or perfumes, such as Vanicream ointment, cream or lotion.

Acne

At around one month of age, approximately 30% of newborns get small bumps that actually look like little pimples. They can appear on the face, scalp, and neck. This is called "neonatal acne." This rash is caused by excessive oils on the skin and maternal hormones.

Wash the area with a mild soap and water twice a day and avoid lotions or anything that will further clog the pores or add more oil. Acne will typically disappear by 6–8 weeks. Call the doctor if the rash is severe or the rash seems to be increasing rather than decreasing with warm water rinses.

Diaper rash

Almost all babies will get diaper rash. It is a rite of passage. If you have a little one with sensitive skin, you might see diaper rash more often than others. If you notice that your little one does have more rashes than you feel are normal, think about changing diaper brands, wipes, or moving to cloth diapers. If you are already using cloth diapers, try a new detergent such as All Free. A barrier diaper rash cream can be applied to the rash with each diaper change. This is usually enough to cure a typical diaper rash within several days.

Avoid diaper wipes. Just use warm water (maybe use your peri bottle to rinse) and a soft wet paper towel and pat the area. Expose the skin to air. If the rash is severe or there is a fever associated with the rash, or sores on the bottom call your doctor.

There is a prescription diaper rash cream that must be made at a compounding pharmacy that I used on my own sensitive kiddos when they would get a really bad diaper rash. It is called Questran 5% in Aquaphor. This got rid of a bleeding diaper rash in 24 hours on multiple occasions.

Occasionally babies can develop yeast diaper rashes. If a rash is not improving with diaper rash treatment, and it has been present for more than three days, it may be yeast. Yeast is usually bright red with what we call "satellite" spots, which is a rash spreading from the main area of the rash. For example, if the origin of the rash started on the anal area but now you are seeing the rash on the buttocks as well, these are satellite spots. Your doctor may prescribe an antifungal medication such as Nystatin cream or you can buy over-the-counter Lotromin antifungal cream at your local drug store. Put this cream on the rash four times a day about an inch past the border of the rash and continue for five days after the rash has cleared, so typically treatment takes a total of 7–10 days.

Call your doctor if you notice peeling skin, open sores, a fever, or purple color associated with the rash.

Another soothing remedy for a diaper rash is called a sitz bath. Put two tablespoons of baking soda in a baby bathtub of water or sink and let the baby's bottom soak.

Drooling rash

Many babies develop a rash on their chin and cheeks that comes and goes. This can be caused by acid in spit-up, or once they start solid foods. It can be related to sensitive skin. Rinse their face with water after feeding. You can use Aquaphor or Vanicream ointment as a barrier prior to feeding, especially with solids that might irritate sensitive skin.

Eczema

Eczema is a common skin condition that affects about 10% of infants. It is characterized by excessive dryness, and it can be itchy. You might notice your baby rubbing his or her cheeks on the sheet or blanket, or against your shoulder. With flare ups, you often see scaly red bumps or rough dry patches. Sometimes you don't even see the spots, but you feel them. Most eczema patches are usually found on the face and sometimes scalp of newborns and older kids and adults, on elbow bends and behind the knees, as well as the back, and ankles and wrists.

It is also common to see eczema in children who have allergies and asthma.

When I see a very young baby with severe eczema, the first thing I ask Mom is if she is breastfeeding. If she is, the next thing I ask her is if she has tried cutting out milk. If she has not, I have her try removing it from her diet for a couple of weeks and, if the baby is on a milk-based formula, I usually have her try a non-dairy formula to see if it helps. If there is no change in the skin, she can put dairy back in her diet. If there is a change, they should eliminate dairy and they may want to see a pediatric allergist.

About 80% of kids with eczema have other family members with allergies or eczema. Most babies will outgrow the condition. Try products such as Eucerin, Lubriderm, Vanicream, or Cetaphil.

My pediatric dermatologist told me it is best if applied minutes after a bath, as it will seal in moisture. He also said, with children with dry skin, you do not need to use soap with every bath. He gave me two choices when it came to bath time. He said you can either bathe less frequently, like twice a week, or every day for about 10 minutes, then apply moisturizer when the skin is still moist. Since Dylan loved his bath, and it was part of our bedtime routine (he was about a year and a half at this time), I chose the daily bath with Vanicream immediately after. It worked well for us.

If you do use soap, use baby soap or an unscented soap such as Vanicream or Cetaphil. Also, keep their nails short!

With small areas of flare-up, you can use hydrocortisone cream 0.5% on the face and 1% on the rest of the body twice a day, for no more than 1–2 weeks as it can cause skin thinning and discoloration. If you need this often or longer, see a doctor so they can give you a non-steroidal option. He or she may suggest a diet change or possibly a visit to a pediatric dermatologist or allergist.

Heat rash / prickly heat

Here in Arizona this is common in the summer months. Heat rash looks like tiny pink bumps mainly in the folds of the neck and legs, and the upper back. Heat rash is caused by blocked sweat glands. Many children get heat rash during hot or humid weather when sweat glands are overworked. Infants can also get in the winter if they are overdressed or have or had fevers. With treatment, heat rash usually clears in 2–3 days. It involves cooling-off techniques: cool baths every 2–3 hours without soap or rinse the skin with cool washcloths. Leave the affected area open to air exposure if possible. Baby cornstarch powder applied directly to the skin can prevent the rash as well, as it absorbs moisture and keeps the area dry (don't sprinkle the powder over the baby, as you do not want the baby to inhale the powder). Avoid lotions and oils.

Cradle cap

This is dry, flaky and often crusty skin on top of the scalp. It often looks yellow. Do not pick at it as it can get infected. Even though you will be tempted, DON'T.

You can massage 1–2 teaspoons of coconut oil onto the baby's scalp before bathing, three to four times per week (with a soft baby hairbrush). Wash out promptly with baby shampoo and pat dry.

If this does not work or the cradle cap is severe, you can use an anti-dandruff shampoo once every 10 days. Be very careful not to get the shampoo into your baby's eyes. This typically takes two people over the kitchen sink.

Clothing / how to dress your newborn

Every year new parents ask me, "How should I dress my baby?" They want to know if they need hats and socks. Although it is true that newborns cannot regulate their body temperature like adults, we really don't dress them differently than how we would dress. New parents have a tendency to dress their newborns too warmly. If you would be hot in pajamas and socks and a hat and wrapped in a swaddle, then so will they. A good rule of thumb is to dress your baby how you would dress. If you are comfortable in short sleeves, do the same with your baby. If your baby prefers to be swaddled and it is warm in your home, you may just use a light receiving blanket and leave the baby in just a diaper and light T-shirt or onesie and possibly use a ceiling fan or lower the temperature in the house to accommodate your baby who likes to be swaddled. At night or when sleeping, use a thin cotton receiving blanket and be sure that the baby is not in direct line with cooling or heating vents. A ceiling fan, however, has been shown to decrease the incidence of SIDS, so if you need to dress the baby slightly warmer to have that fan on, do it. There is a greater risk of SIDS, however, with the baby being too warm as opposed to too cool.

Genital care

Boys

If your son was circumcised, you will want to gently sponge the area with a wet washcloth or rinse with your peri bottle and warm water into the diaper and pat the area dry. Apply a gauze pad with Vaseline or Vanicream ointment with every diaper change for 4–5 days.

It is very normal for the site to look sore and red for 1–2 days, but it should not be painful for them.

It will then change to yellow and sticky for 1–2 days. Then a dry yellow scab forms.

Bleeding should be minimal. If there is more than spotting on the diaper, call the pediatrician.

Healing will be complete by the end of the first week.

Most doctors re-check the site in 5–7 days. This is typically when most pediatricians want to see the baby after birth anyway, so it is perfect timing if this was done in the hospital at birth.

If your son is uncircumcised there are no special instructions, except that you should not try to retract the foreskin to clean. This does not occur until four to five years of age, when boys should be taught to retract the foreskin with bathing.

Foreskin retraction happens on its own. It may take a few days, months, or even years. Forcing retraction can be painful and cause tearing and bleeding.

Girls

Part the labia with each diaper change and sponge off debris using a baby wipe or wet cloth. Again, you can use your peri bottle from the hospital if you have a particularly messy diaper to rinse without having to wipe too much on delicate skin.

Newborn girls may have a white discharge for several days and sometimes a small amount of blood for a day or two during the first week. This is coming from the vaginal area and not in the urine. The discharge is from maternal hormones.

There is also a thick, protective "Vaseline-like" coating around the labia. This will dissipate with time. Do not try to remove this protective coating, as this will irritate the skin and it is there for a reason.

Clogged tear duct

If your baby's eye continually waters, the tear duct may be clogged. I know this sounds a bit backwards. You would think if the duct was clogged nothing would come out, but a clogged tear duct leaks pretty consistently.

Some babies have only one side that is clogged but, in approximately 30% of babies, both eyes have clogged ducts.

The good news is that more than 90% of clogged tear ducts open by 12 months.

There is debate between pediatricians and pediatric ophthalmologists on what to do with a clogged duct. Some physicians recommend tear duct massage three to four times a day with a soft baby wash cloth or soft cotton pad and warm water: one or two gentle wipes down the side of the tear duct on the side of the nose, while also wiping away the discharge. Some recommend doing nothing at all. Both of my kids had clogged ducts, and I massaged them.

If the discharge turns thick yellow or green and is persistent throughout the day with lashes matting together, a fever develops, or swelling of the eye orbit itself, contact your pediatrician's office.

Flat heads / back sleeping

The bones of a baby's skull are soft and not connected during the first year of life to make room for the rapidly growing brain. This is the reason babies have soft spots. Constantly lying on their backs puts pressure on these soft, pliable bones causing a flat spot in some babies. It is a small price to pay to prevent SIDS, however.

For most babies, this goes away as they begin to sit up. There are several things you can do to help prevent this or decrease the severity of it. One easy thing you can do is change the position of your baby in the crib. One week you put the baby's head at the top of the crib and the next week the baby's head is at the bottom of the crib or bassinet. Babies want to look out, so this way they are not always putting pressure on one side or the other.

The other thing you can do is increase tummy time during the day. Burp on both sides. Move your baby's equipment or stations around the house so the baby is using different muscles to look around.

Many sounds and faces of babies from North Scottsdale Pediatric Associates

"Babies make a lot more noise than you would think! Besides crying, they also sneeze, cough, grunt, snort, squeak, and have endless series of facial grimaces to match. In your many hours of baby-gazing, you will get to know your baby's sounds and faces. Your baby will follow your face with his or her eyes and be alert to the sound of your voice within the first week or two. He or she may "startle" with a noise or jolt and may move his or her arms with jittery movements."

Signs of illness in your newborn—when to seek medical attention. Adapted from Dr. Barton Schmitt and his pediatric triage protocol.

Call the doctor immediately if your newborn has a fever, severe lethargy, a bulging soft spot, a sunken soft spot (not normal pulsing), purple rash, cries inconsolably or cries when you touch them, no urine for more than 8 hours, convulsions, difficulty breathing, joint swelling, refuses to take fluids, is too weak to suck, or his or her appearance just makes you feel uncomfortable.

Fever

What constitutes a fever? If your baby feels warm to the touch, use a digital thermometer and take the temperature under the arm or use a forehead scanning type of thermometer. If the baby's temperature is over 99 degrees, retake the temperature rectally, as it is more accurate. If you were to call your pediatrician's office and say you want to bring your baby in for a fever, they will ask you how you took the temperature. If it was any other method besides a rectal temperature, they will most likely have you retake it rectally, as any other method in infants is just not as accurate.

Ear thermometers are not accurate in infants and are discouraged.

A fever in an infant under two months can be a sign of a serious illness so contact your doctor immediately.

To take a rectal temperature, lubricate the tip with KY or Vaseline and carefully insert the tip about ½–1 inch. Leave in place until it beeps if it is digital, which is typically after about 30 seconds.

The definition of a fever:

Rectal temp >100.4

Oral temp/pacifier temp >99.5

Axillary temp >98.6

If you suspect your newborn has a fever, do not give fever-reducing medication. Speak with your doctor's office immediately if your baby is under two months of age or take them to an urgent care provider or ER if after hours.

Lethargy / excessive sleepiness

Sleeping through two consecutive feedings (>6 hours) could be a sign of a serious illness, so call your physician.

Jaundice

Bilirubin is a yellow pigment produced naturally in the body as red blood cells break down. As red blood cells live only a short time, when they die the body converts the waste into yellow bilirubin.

Normally bilirubin is removed from circulation by the liver and excreted in the stool. Jaundice occurs when bilirubin is inadequately cleared from the circulation by an immature liver.

Babies with a high bilirubin level in the blood are termed jaundiced. Yellow will first appear on the face, then move to the chest and stomach, and finally to the legs.

Look at the baby in daylight or fluorescent light. Press with your fingertip to the skin: if the skin looks white and not yellow, then the baby is probably not jaundiced. If the yellowish color continues, call your doctor for an appointment.

About 1/3 of infants develop mild jaundice on the 3rd – 5th day of life involving the eyes and face which is not typically a cause for concern.

As the bilirubin level rises, the yellow color deepens and moves downward to involve the trunk and legs.

If your baby's face looks yellow but the color does not extend to the body, place your baby near a window, but not in direct sunlight.

Forty years ago, in England, they discovered that babies near windows were less likely to be jaundiced because daylight aids the body in ridding itself of extra bilirubin.

If the yellow color is striking, and particularly if it extends onto the abdomen and legs, be sure to call your pediatrician immediately. Your doctor will usually do a blood test to measure the level of bilirubin.

In babies with high levels of bilirubin, treatment may include phototherapy (special lights) which can usually be done at home. Sometimes brief interruptions of nursing for up to 72 hours may be necessary (if you want to continue to nurse, you must continue to pump). Some doctors, however, may just have you increase nursing or formula feeding to increase stools, as the more the baby stools, the faster the bilirubin will be removed.

They will perform a blood test to see how high the bilirubin level is and treatments vary:

If levels are mild to moderate, they may recommend indirect sunlight or nothing at all.

If the level is high, the baby may be treated with special phototherapy lights called bili lights or a bili blanket will be used. These help babies get rid of bilirubin by altering it and making it easier for the body to get rid of it. This can usually be done at home. If the bilirubin is too high, your baby will be admitted to the hospital for careful monitoring. At elevated levels, over 25, bilirubin may cause damage to the brain.

There are several reasons a baby may develop jaundice. Dr. Barton Schmitt describes the four types in his book, Your Child's Health.

Types of jaundice: (adapted from Dr. Barton Schmitt)

Normal physiological jaundice

Occurs in more than 50% of babies. This type first appears on days 2–4 and disappears by 1–2 weeks. This type is due to immaturity of the liver which leads to slower processing of bilirubin.

Breast milk jaundice

Occurs in 1–2% of breastfed babies. It is caused by a special substance that some mothers produce in their milk. The substance, an enzyme, increases the reabsorption of bilirubin in the baby's intestines, so it is reabsorbed rather than excreted in stools. This type starts at days 4–7 and may last 3–10 weeks.

Breastfeeding jaundice

Occurs in 5 to 10% of newborns. It is caused by an inadequate intake of calories. It follows the same pattern as normal physiological jaundice.

Blood group incompatibility

If the baby and mother have different blood types (Rh factor) sometimes the mother produces antibodies that destroy the newborn's red blood cells. This causes a sudden build-up of bilirubin in the baby's blood. This type usually begins within 24 hours of birth.

Spit-up / reflux

Normal spit-up is 1–2 mouthfuls or wet burps. Spit-up occurs in 50% of infants.

If your infant is spitting up, make sure you are not overfeeding. Try 1 oz less next feed or nurse for a shorter time. Try to wait two and a half hours before the next feed as it takes this long for the stomach to empty itself.

Avoid tight-fitting clothing around the baby's stomach or a diaper being too tight.

After meals, try to keep your baby upright. Lying flat causes reflux to increase. Keep baby upright as long as possible after feeds. You may try propping up the mattress with a crib wedge under the mattress of the crib or bassinet during naps and at bedtime. Keep the changing table elevated, etc.

Many babies improve by seven months of age as this condition is due to an immature digestive system that they outgrow.

Be sure to burp well.

You might try gas drops. Use simethicone infant drops *prior* to each feeding to see if you can prevent gas from forming and causing spit-up. Simethicone is safe for newborns to take with each feeding.

If the spit-up is severe, or if the spit-up is projectile or coming out of the nose, contact your doctor. If the baby is having painful spit-up or does not appear to be gaining weight, speak to your physician as it may be a more serious condition called reflux. With babies who have reflux, there are things that can be done. If you are using a bottle, try the Dr. Brown's brand if you are not using them already.

Shaken baby syndrome

I frequently get questions about shaken baby syndrome from everyday things like swings, or a little extra jostling in a stroller or grocery cart. Child magazine had a wonderful article that talked about just this thing:

"Many parents fear shaken baby syndrome and worry if a bumpy road or stroller ride or playing horsey could cause this. Dr. Karen Kay Imagawa, Clinical Director of Child Abuse Prevention at Children's Hospital in LA, says that comparing the jostling that occurs during these activities with the shaking that produces injury is like night and day. With shaken baby syndrome, the shaking is so violent and intense that it is difficult for people to visualize. Most episodes of shaking last about 20 seconds or less but there can be 40–50 shakes during that brief period, causing internal bleeding of the brain, often behind the eyes and generally without any external injury." So, the regular jostling of childhood is safe for babies. Don't be afraid to put your baby in the swing or push them in the stroller over a bumpy sidewalk. Babies are tougher than you think.

I hope this chapter has made you feel more prepared for caring for your newborn. So many new parents tell me it is great to have these notes to refer to, so they don't feel like they are bothering the pediatrician for simple questions. Hopefully the summaries in this chapter will give you the confidence to know what is "normal" for your newborn and when you need to bring your baby in.

CHAPTER 6

BREAST AND BOTTLE FEEDING

"No woman should ever feel guilty about the choices she makes regarding childbirth, breastfeeding, or the manner in which she cares for her baby."

— Amy Tuteur

I always start my in-person classes by sharing my story on breastfeeding. So, I will start this chapter the same way. As a pediatric nurse I knew the benefits of breastfeeding and was determined to do it. However, having premature babies with no suck reflex put a bit of a kink in my plan. I had serious trouble. I could not let down with the pump. I was engorged and miserable and just could not get the milk out and then the milk started to dry up.

I went to see an endocrinologist who specialized in breastfeeding and who suggested things like mother's milk tea with fenugreek supplements and even a prescription that he wrote that could only be obtained in Canada or Mexico. I tried all the natural remedies meant to help with no luck, so I resorted to the medications.

Being in Arizona, Mexico was within driving distance. My brother offered to go with my husband. Now my brother is 6 feet tall and works out every day and was and still is quite an imposing figure. My husband is no small fry himself at 5'11½". So, these two strapping men go into Mexico to buy breastfeeding medication. Everything went smoothly at first. They found a pharmacy that had the medication. They purchased it and were on their way back across the border when the trouble occurred. The border patrol stopped them and asked them what they were doing in Mexico. They told them the reason, but the border patrol was not buying it. Due to their size, they thought they were transporting illegal steroids across the border. This story makes me giggle now, but my husband and brother were not laughing then. They put them in separate glass rooms facing each other and stripped them down to their underwear looking for contraband. My husband and brother can almost laugh about it now, saying they saw way too much of each other that day.

When they realized all they really had truly was breastfeeding medication with a valid prescription, they let them go. Now I wish I could tell you that the ordeal my brother and husband went through was worth it, but I would be lying if I did. The medication did not work. So, I kept pumping, getting literally half an ounce of breastmilk at a time and mixing it with formula. I was trying to pump longer to get my milk supply up. Feeding and pumping constantly was like feeding twins. I was beyond exhausted when my husband said to me, "Honey, I know how much you want to breastfeed, trust me I know, but what is more important for our daughter, breast milk or a mom who is not exhausted and is enjoying her baby?" It was like I had finally been hit upside the head with a dose of reality. I needed to hear what he was saying. He was right. I had been missing out on what was most important, enjoying my time with my daughter without extra stress. I share this story with all of you, because if breastfeeding does not work out for you, please do not beat yourself up over it.

Statistics show that approximately 15% of mothers will not be successful at nursing, so try not to take it personally if it does not work for you. Remember my story and just enjoy that baby. I continued to pump for a total of eight weeks with Taylor, mixing the breast milk with formula but after that conversation with my husband, the stress was gone, and I did not feel guilty about stopping after eight weeks. When Dylan was born without a suck reflex either and the same thing happened, I was not stressed at all. I pumped for six weeks, added it to the formula, and there was no trip to Mexico 😊

Having said this, I do need to point out that The American Academy of Pediatrics does advocate for breastfeeding when possible. So, my suggestion is to give it a try. There are many advantages, making it worth giving it a go.

Advantages of breastfeeding

Below I have listed some of the information from the American Academy of Pediatrics to support breastfeeding.

Because of its nutritional composition, human milk is the ideal food for human infants.

Human milk and infant formula are different. Breast milk is made up of sugar (lactose) and easily digestible proteins, whey and casein, and digestible fatty acids (fat), all properly balanced with various vitamins and minerals, as well as antibodies and enzymes that aid in digestion and absorption. It also helps protect your baby against certain illnesses / infections and diseases. Also, breastfed babies may be less likely to be obese in childhood.

Because of the protective substances in human milk, breastfed children are also less likely to have the following:

Ear infections (otitis media)

Allergies

Vomiting

Diarrhea

Pneumonia, wheezing, and bronchiolitis

Meningitis

Urinary tract infections

Colds / flu

They are less likely to develop insulin-dependent diabetes, some lymphomas, ulcerative colitis, Chron's disease, and breast and ovarian cancers later in life.

Medical researchers from the University of Arizona reviewed records of over 1,200 infants from birth through one year.

They found that infants who were exclusively breastfed for at least four months were half as likely to develop ear infections as were formula-fed infants.

Breastfed babies who did develop ear infections suffered fewer repeat episodes.

Those that received breast milk plus other sources were still less likely than strictly formula-fed infants to develop ear infections.

Some additional advantages include:

Breast milk is instantly available and always at the right temperature.

There is direct skin-to-skin contact, which aids in bonding and producing hormones that stimulate milk production. Breastfeeding promotes feelings that enhance motherhood.

You do not have the expense of as many bottles or formula.

Breastfeeding burns more calories and helps you get back to your pre-pregnancy weight more quickly. Breastfeeding helps your body get back in shape by using 500 calories per day and helping the uterus tighten and return to normal size quicker.

Mothers who breastfeed are at reduced risk of ovarian cancer and, in pre-menopausal women, breast cancer.

Breastfeeding builds bone strength to protect against bone fractures in older age especially hip fractures. It also reduces the risk of osteoporosis.

Breastfeeding delays the return of your menstrual period for most women. Although breastfeeding may postpone menstruation for many, it does not prevent pregnancy, so be sure to use another form of birth control.

The longer you breastfeed, the greater the benefits will be for your baby and you, and the longer these benefits will last. The World Health Organization (WHO) and many other experts encourage women to breastfeed for as long as possible, one year or even longer, because human milk provides the best nutrition and protection against infections.

The AAP recommends breastfeeding for the first year of life if you can do it.

Disadvantages of breastfeeding

It is Mom's responsibility, whether it is nursing or pumping.

You must watch your diet.

It may not be convenient if you have to go back to work and it may not work for you or your baby.

It is important not to feel guilty if you decide to bottle feed for whatever reason.

Infant formula is an acceptable and nutritious alternative to human milk.

Breastfeeding is not for everyone (breastfeeding is a learned skill for both mother and baby).

If you are unsure, you might want to think about at least giving it a try.

If it does not work for you, you can always give it up. However, once your milk has dried up you may not be able to go back.

Again, 15% of mothers will not be successful at nursing, so try not to take it personally if it does not work for you. Remember, I was one of these!

Should you choose to breastfeed? How do you do it?
How often to nurse

I believe in nursing on demand, within reason. Usually, every 2–3 hours and not more than every 1.5 hours, and not less than every

4–5 hours, until they are sleeping through the night. Until the baby is sleeping through the night, wake baby during the day if they are going longer than three hours without eating. We will cover this more during the sleep section, but this step sets you up for a good sleeper. A baby needs a set number of calories in 24 hours. If they don't get enough during the day, they will be up at night wanting to eat.

If your baby is wanting to nurse constantly, make sure you have enough milk and they are not using you as a pacifier and nursing for comfort rather than nutrition. You can evaluate this by offering a couple of ounces in a bottle after nursing. If your baby guzzles it down, you do not have enough milk. If your baby ignores the extra ounces offered, then offer a pacifier instead.

Some babies may empty the breast in 5 minutes, and some may take 20 minutes (yet by the fourth day, work up to 20 minutes).

On average, nursing takes between 10 and 20 minutes per breast. 15–20 minutes is considered an adequate amount of time to spend feeding but some babies take longer.

How long to nurse

Dr. Barton Schmitt suggests new mothers nurse for 10 minutes on the first breast and then as long as they want on the second breast, with a goal of 30 minutes for each feeding. Once your milk supply is established, 10 minutes per breast may be sufficient, since the baby is likely to get 90% of the milk in this time.

During that time there is:

The initial letdown, which accounts for approximately 60% of the milk volume, is called "skim" milk.

Then there is "whole" milk, which accounts for approximately 35% of the milk volume.

Then the rich "cream" or hind milk, which accounts for approximately 5% of the milk volume, is usually released 10–20 minutes into the feeding. This is rich and full of calories.

Alternate sides, starting on the opposite breast each time. *Especially if it is easier on one breast.* Use an app to keep track of which side you left off on and how long you nursed on each side, or you can use a notebook the old-fashioned way, but keep track somehow or you will forget.

If feeding multiples, it is very important, if one baby has a stronger suck, to deliberately alternate side to side to assure good emptying of both breasts throughout the day,

Count the time between feedings from the beginning of the last feeding.

Example: if you start feeding at 12:00 and it takes you 20 minutes per breast and 10 minutes to burp and 10 minutes to change, that is one hour and, if your baby eats every two hours, you will need to start all over again at 2:00.

This will gradually get better as you both get more comfortable and efficient. Nursing is a learned skill for both mom and Baby. If you are having trouble, get help from a lactation consultant or even a friend who has successfully nursed.

Most newborns nurse 8–12 times in a 24-hour period.

Typically, by the time an infant is two weeks old, most mothers will produce between 24 and 30 ounces of milk per 24 hours.

Milk supply fluctuates with demand.

Growth spurts

**Growth spurts occur at about 10 days, 6 weeks, 3 months and 4–6 months.

During these times, infants may fuss and nurse twice as often for about two days. It typically takes about two days to increase your milk supply this way.

With multiples, it may take 3–4 days to increase the milk supply during these growth spurts.

Newborn babies may not recognize hunger for several days and will nurse to meet a sucking need and eventually associate sucking with getting milk and feeling good. This is why you need to wake a newborn regularly for feedings.

Some general guidelines of waking babies at night in the first few weeks

Wake babies every four hours in the first two-three weeks. By then most babies are up to birth weight and have established a nice pattern of gaining weight. By six weeks if a baby is sleeping let them sleep. Many pediatricians feel that once normal weight gain is established, you can trust the baby to know when to wake and feed, this happens around the sixth week mark some later but sometimes earlier. Follow the above as guidelines rather than firm rules except for the first two-three weeks when we need to ensure that a baby sleeping longer is not due to dehydration or undernutrition.

Tips to help your baby latch on to the breast

Aim the nipple up toward the middle of the palate, then pull your baby close to you (move them not your body or you will have a very sore back). To help elicit the rooting reflex, brush the middle of the baby's lower lip with your nipple. This will encourage them to open their mouth wider, so you can put your nipple and areola in the mouth. Baby's chin should be pressed snuggly against the breast.

The key is to get as much of the nipple and areola into the mouth as possible.

Place the nipple on the center top of the tongue. If only the nipple is in the mouth, break the seal by placing your pinky finger in the corner of the mouth and try again or you will have sore, possibly bleeding nipples.

Wet diapers in the first few days

Until your milk comes in on day 3-4, you will not necessarily feel your breasts softening and filling like you will later on, and the baby may not have six wet diapers.

In the first few days when the baby is only getting colostrum this is what you can expect, if you are not offering any supplemental formula:

On day 1 of life: 1 wet diaper

On day 2 of life: 2 wet diapers

On day 3 of life: 3 wet diapers

On day 4 of life: 4 wet diapers

Day 5: a minimum of 6 wet diapers. Typically, it is more like 8–12 wet diapers per day.

Stools in the first few days

Here is the breakdown for stools in the first few days of life, for solely breastfed babies as well:

Stools for BF babies: 1 stool/day for the first few days

By days 4–5 and through 1 month of age: at least 3 stools per day yet typically 6–10 / day.

Between 4 and 8 weeks of age, stools change to an infrequent bowel movement pattern: babies may have 1 soft bowel movement every 4–12 days! Crazy, I know.

Meconium stools are dark greenish black, thick, sticky stools. These normally pass during the first three days of life. Once these pass, as I mentioned before, you should never see a stool like this again. If you do, call your pediatrician.

Transitional stools are a mix of greenish brown, loose stools passed on days 4–5 of life.

Milk stools are those after that.

Breastfed stools tend to be frequent and loose yellow or yellow-green at first and then may become as infrequent as one per week by the end of the first month.

Breastfed stools are about the consistency of watery cottage cheese and usually the color of mustard.

That is after the tarry black meconium passes through.

Infrequent bowel movements are not normal in the first month of life.

As they get older, however, some babies have stools every feeding, while others have one huge blowout a week / seven days.

Don't get alarmed unless it has been more than 10 days, the stools are hard little pellets, your baby is straining for more than 10 minutes with no results or there is blood in the stool (streaks, spots, or black and tarry.) If you suspect blood in the stool, save the diaper and bring it into the pediatrician so they can test it for blood.

Many researchers feel colostrum is a natural laxative that helps meconium pass through. Breastfed babies may have fewer stools after two months as breast milk is easily digested and leaves hardly any solid waste.

How do you know your baby is getting enough?

Most doctors do not recommend routine formula supplements unless the baby is feeding poorly or acts unsatisfied after nursing. If the baby is not satisfied call the pediatrician. You may need to offer a supplement after nursing. You also may want to have the baby's weight checked.

If the baby has an increased need to suck, offer a pacifier.

You may want to offer a bottle at about 2–3 weeks of age, 2–3 times per week, once breastfeeding is going well. This way, your baby can take a bottle in the future and Dad and other family members can feed too.

Most babies lose weight in the first few days.

AAP: When a baby is born, birth weight includes excess body fluid which is lost during the first few days. Most babies, especially breastfed babies, lose about 10% of their birth weight during the first five days and regain it over the next five days, so that by day 10, they are back up to birth weight.

On average, typical weight gain after that is ½ to 1 oz per day until birth weight doubles.

Your baby will approximately triple his or her birth weight during the first year.

Some indications breastfeeding is going well

Plenty of wet and stooled diapers once your milk is in.

The baby is sucking well and is happy and satisfied between feeds.

Your baby's cheeks are rounded and his or her jaw glides with each suck.

You feel tugging on your breast but not pain.

Your baby's shoulders and arms are relaxed.

Your breasts soften during feedings.

Your baby's mouth is wet at the end of each feeding.

You will see the pink inner part of your infant's lips not just the outer skin.

There is no gap at the corners of the mouth.

The baby does not make a clicking noise with sucking.

There is no dimple in the middle of the cheek, which would indicate a loss of suction caused by a poor seal.

During active sucking and swallowing, the muscles in front of a baby's ears move, making it look like the ears wiggle.

During the first few days, your infant may suck 5–10 times before a swallow. When the milk comes in you will hear a swallow after every 1–2 sucks.

Mom's diet while nursing

You need to continue with prenatal vitamins and a healthy, balanced diet, as well as 2–3 quarts of liquid a day (I suggest every time you sit down to nurse, you do so with an 8 oz glass of fluid).

You do not need to drink milk to make milk, so if the baby is extremely gassy or fussy you may cut out dairy for one week to see if it improves. A good rule of thumb is if you cut out a particular food from your diet for one week without change, it is probably not the food. You can put it back into your diet. There is no need to deprive yourself. Most nursing moms find that there are very few foods, if any, that they need to avoid.

Think about ethnic foods and different cultures. Babies from other countries are no gassier than babies from the United States even though their mothers might eat far spicier foods.

Having said this, however, it is important to know food affects milk 4–24 hours after it is eaten. Yet doctors recommend eliminating suspected food for a week to be safe.

Examples of foods labeled as gassy foods include cabbage, onions, garlic, broccoli, and turnips. Symptoms from foods, if any, last fewer than 24 hours.

As I mentioned previously in the pregnancy chapter, you may want to eliminate or limit caffeine. Infants don't eliminate caffeine from their bodies efficiently and it tends to build up in their systems.

Alcohol does pass through into breast milk. In large doses it can cause sedation, irritability, and a weak sucking motion. It may also give milk an odor which may make your baby disinterested in nursing.

Julie Menella, PhD, biopsychologist and expert on alcohol's effect on breastfeeding, believes nursing women should avoid all alcohol. She says, however, that 3–4 hours after having a drink, the alcohol should be gone from your breast milk. If you still feel the effects of the alcohol, however, it is still in the breast milk. You may want to pump and dump or get milk test strips to test the milk prior to feeding it to your baby.

Many of the flavors in a mother's diet are transferred to her baby in the womb, during pregnancy and later in breastmilk. That means your own food preferences may already seem familiar to your baby when the time comes to introduce solid foods.

Engorgement

When your milk comes in, you will experience what is called engorgement. This occurs the day your milk comes in, typically on about day 3–4. When your milk comes in, your breasts may swell and become painful. They may be hot and hard, shiny, and red from stretching. This not-so-fun occurrence is called engorgement and usually lasts 12–24 hours. It can be mild to severe.

You will notice the change in your milk from the thick yellowish colostrum to the thinner whiter milk.

The best way to relieve this pain and pressure is to empty the breast by nursing or pumping.

Sometimes the breasts are so stretched that the baby has a difficult time latching on. You can help this by placing a warm, moist cloth across the breast prior to nursing to aid letdown or you can pump slightly to soften the breast a bit so the baby can latch on.

After nursing, however, apply ice packs to relieve the pain and you can also take acetaminophen.

Cold cabbage leaves (after breaking the veins) may decrease swelling and act as a natural analgesic. However, only do this if you are not going to nurse, as it may decrease your milk supply.

Clogged milk duct

Sometimes ducts can get clogged, and it is difficult to get the milk out. You may feel a small pea-sized to marble-sized lump in the breast. This can be aided again with moist heat and gentle massage.

Massaging your breast while in the shower or while your breast is in a bowl of warm water works well. If you are massaging in a bowl of water and the duct opens, you will see the milk shoot out into the bowl of water.

Gravity also helps, so lean forward while massaging and feeding.

It is not uncommon for one breast to leak while nursing from the other. Use milk shells to collect that precious liquid gold. (Haakkaa's are one brand, as mentioned above.)

Shortly after delivery, bleeding will also most likely be heavier when nursing as this is causing uterine contractions. Think of this as a positive thing, as your body is getting your uterus back to its original shape.

Sore nipples

I wish I could sugarcoat this for you but that would not be fair. I say it like it is in this book. Your nipples are going to be sore at first.

If this becomes a problem for you, first make sure the baby is getting not only the nipple but also the areola in the mouth.

Other helpful tips are to leave the nipples open to air. Apply Lanolin cream. This is very soothing and helps heal cracked and irritated nipples.

If the nipples are cracked and bleeding, it may help to apply crushed ice just before nursing to numb and cause them to stand more erect, so they are easier for the baby to grab onto.

After nursing, dry off the nipples to remove your baby's saliva and express a few drops of your own breast milk onto the nipple. This acts as a natural lubricant. Then allow the nipple to air dry. I suggest you do this from the get-go to help prevent sore nipples.

You can also get nipple shields to wear that help pull the nipple out more, allowing the baby to grab hold of it easier.

Some women have also found that warm, steeped teabags blotted on nipples after feedings may help. The tannic acid in the tea promotes healing (tea must be regular, not herbal or decaf).

If you are breastfeeding and your nipples are bleeding, you may see slight blood in your baby's spit-up. Do not be alarmed and, yes, you can continue nursing.

Thrush

Thrush is a yeast infection that babies can get in their mouth.

Yeast infections may be found in your baby's mouth, on your nipples, in the form of a diaper rash or as a vaginal infection for Mom.

Your baby may be in pain with nursing and pull away or not want to latch on.

The baby will have a white tongue that will not wipe off, along with white patches on the gums or cheeks. If it is just a white tongue it is more likely just a milk tongue, so make sure to look at the baby's gums and cheeks as well.

If you suspect thrush, call your pediatrician for a prescription of Nystatin oral suspension. A helpful hint for applying the Nystatin is to dip a clean Q-tip into the solution and then, when you drip the solution into your baby's mouth, you can spread it with the Q-tip and the Q-tip will not soak up the needed medication.

If you develop yeast on your nipples, you can apply Lotromin cream after feeding (rinse first) four times a day, past the borders. If your baby gets thrush, you will need to boil all bottle nipples and pacifiers.

Mastitis

Mastitis is a serious breast infection that may or may not be accompanied by a plugged duct. It is not to be ignored and should be taken very seriously. Symptoms may include a red, swollen, tender area of the breast that does not respond to treatment for a plugged duct, generalized flu-like symptoms which usually come on suddenly, such as aching joints, HA, nausea, exhaustion, and/or fever.

You often have a severe headache that does not respond to the usual treatment.

You may also have red streaks on the breast.

You do not need to stop nursing, in fact, this could make it worse if you also have a clogged duct.

However, you do need a 10-day course of antibiotics and aggressive treatment to unclog that duct.

You need to be on complete bed rest for 48 hours. This is time to ask for help.

How to collect and store breast milk

Wash your hands well.

First wash all the parts of the breast pump that will come in contact with milk in hot soapy water or in the dishwasher, if dishwasher safe. Rinse in cold water and air dry on a clean towel or paper towels. I also boiled mine after the dishwasher to get rid of any possible residue.

If you plan on freezing, leave some space at the top of the container. Like most liquids, breast milk expands as it freezes.

If you are storing it in a plastic bag, roll down the top several times and place the small bag in a larger bag for further protection.

Label with the date and the amount inside.

Freeze in 2–4 oz portions as this small amount thaws quicker and you will waste less. Remember it is liquid gold.

You may continue to add to the same container throughout the day, chill in the fridge, and then freeze that night.

You can also add to already frozen breast milk after you chill the fresh milk. However, you must only add a lesser amount than the already frozen milk.

Immediate refrigeration after pumping is recommended. At room temperature (66–78 degrees), however, it will be safe for a few hours, even up to six hours is acceptable.

Fresh milk can be stored in the fridge for 72 hours. This is ideal and it can last up to five days. Frozen milk at the back of the freezer can be stored for up to 3–6 months.

If you have a deep freeze (-20 degrees), milk can be stored for up to 12 months.

Defrosted milk can be stored for up to 24 hours in fridge.

Never use a microwave to defrost your breast milk, instead, warm it in a cup of hot water.

How to increase your milk supply

Some of this is easier said than done, I know, but it is important to take care of yourself. It is important to get adequate sleep. When that baby is sleeping, try to sleep too. Reduce stress as much as possible (let the small stuff go) and drink enough fluid (an 8oz glass of fluid every four hours while awake).

Pump your breasts for 10 minutes after each feeding. You will need extra help with this, as it will be like feeding twins. Be aware that you won't see milk when you first start: You are trying to tell your body that you don't have enough and need to make more.

If you are just trying to make more milk for an extra feed, it is important to pump for at least 10 minutes after the milk has stopped flowing.

Nursing is easier the second time around. "Women produce about 1/3 more milk for the 2nd baby," say researchers at the Institute of Child Health in Bristol, England. In fact, those who had trouble producing enough milk for the first baby had the greatest increase in milk for the second, according to the institute of Child Health they also found that it takes about one hour less each day to breastfeed a second baby. So, if breastfeeding did not come easy with your first, there is still hope with subsequent pregnancies.

Breastfeeding when you are sick

If you are sick, you can continue nursing, or you can pump and have someone else feed from a bottle, as long as you are on a medication that is compatible with breastfeeding. My suggestion is to call your OB, pediatric nurse, pediatrician, or pharmacist before you take or use _anything_ that you are not 100% sure about. It never hurts to be extra careful.

Your milk will carry your antibodies, but you might want to wear a mask while nursing if you have a respiratory illness.

You should, however, use good hand-washing techniques and try not to smooch on the baby (I know this is very hard).

Vitamin D supplements for Mom and/or Baby

In 2008, the AAP Committee on Nutrition started recommending that, within the first few days of life, all breastfed babies need 400 IU per day of vitamin D or Mom can take a minimum of 6,400 IU of vitamin D3/day instead, to get enough to their infant.

Human milk only has 25 IU/liter.

If your baby is getting at least 1,000ml / 32oz of formula, there is no need for extra vitamin D.

If you are doing a combination of both, speak to your pediatrician about their recommendation on how much vitamin D your child should have.

Formula feeding

Formula comes in three main types:

Cow's milk, soy, and protein hydrolysates (non-milk / non-soy)

According to the American Academy of Pediatrics, formula based on cow's milk is closer in content to breast milk than formula based on soy. They recommend starting with a cow's milk formula when possible.

During pregnancy, the baby receives DHA and ARA (fatty acids) from the mother. Both are building blocks for the brain and eyes. When a baby is breastfed, he/she will continue to receive these via milk.

A baby can make some DHA and ARA from nutrients in infant formulas and also later in solid foods. The new formulas with DHA and ARA added are at levels similar to those found in breast milk.

Breastfeeding mothers can also increase the amount of DHA in their breast milk by eating foods like salmon, tuna, and sardines (yet many experts say to limit fish intake to 1x/week due to mercury).

In an article, Stephany Watson says, "Enhanced formulas were available in over 60 countries including the United Kingdom, Hong Kong, and China for more than five years before being introduced in the US."

Cow's milk formulas

Cow's milk formula has been around the longest and is the preferred formula to start, according to the AAP.

It contains proteins from cow's milk, fat from vegetable oils, its carbohydrate is lactose, and vitamins and iron are added.

Soymilk formulas

Soy formulas are used for babies who are "intolerant" to cow's milk or babies whose families have a strong history of cow's milk intolerance.

Some cow's milk intolerance on an "allergic" basis is due to the milk protein.

Some intolerance is related to lactose which some people have difficulty digesting.

Soy formulas are made of soy protein, vegetable oil, and sucrose or corn sweeteners as primary carbohydrate, and vitamins and iron are added.

It is possible to also be allergic to soy.

Elemental or protein hydrolysate formulas (extensively broken-down proteins)

These are partially pre-digested and are used when children have difficulty with soy and cow's milk formulas.

They are expensive and many babies do not like the taste.

They can cause relatively loose stools.

Occasionally an infant with colic on soy or cow's milk formulas gets dramatic improvement from this type of formula.

Signs of a formula intolerance

Vomiting, diarrhea, blood in stools, severe reflux, constant crying, and occasionally severe skin rash.

Formula feeding basics

Formulas also come in three different formulations:

Ready to feed: just pour and feed.

Concentrated: you need to add water first to dilute.

Powdered: again you need to mix with water.

Care of bottles

The American Academy of Pediatrics recommends you boil all new nipples, bottles, and pacifiers, etc. for two minutes before the first use.

To be extra safe, you can sterilize bottles and nipples for the first three months. By then the baby's digestive system is well colonized with bacteria. I ran my bottles and pumping equipment through the dishwasher, then rinsed everything in a pan of boiling water and set it on a drying rack to air dry, for the first three months.

Formula temperature

If your baby was previously breastfed, then they will most likely prefer formula at body temperature, however, some prefer it colder, and some warmer.

The best temperature is the one your infant prefers.

There is no health risk involved with temperature as long as it is not so hot that it burns their mouth. Once I was done breastfeeding, I tried to get my kids used to bottles straight from the fridge as soon as possible for convenience's sake.

This made it easier when going out in public, as well as keeping their bottles on ice and giving it to them without finding a place to warm it up.

Formula amount per age and weight of baby

Formula-fed newborns feed approximately every 2–3 hours and take approximately 1–3 oz per feeding the first week and gradually increase to 4 oz by the end of the first month.

On average they should take 2.5 oz per lb. So, for example, a 2-month-old weighing about 12 lbs. might take approximately 30 oz per day. Most babies take between 24–32 oz of formula by around two months of age.

Babies max out at around 32 oz a day and are typically ready for solids by around four months of age.

More to come on solids in later chapters.

Some pediatricians say to take the age in months and add three to figure out how many ounces a baby should take per feeding. So, a 3-month-old may take 6 oz per feeding, maxing out at 8 oz per feeding.

How to store formula

Most formula manufacturers recommend that you use all open, liquid ready-to-feed or mixed formula within 48 hours.

Mixed formula left at room temperature for more than one hour needs to be thrown out.

If your baby takes part of a bottle and leaves just a little bit in the bottom, throw it out as bacteria from the baby's mouth has gone back into the bottle.

Burping

Burp halfway between feeding, when Baby pauses, and at the end of the feeding.

Wet burps and slight spit-up are common as are hiccups and occasional mild choking. Repetitive forceful vomiting, however, or green or blood-tinged vomit could be a sign of a serious medical condition, so notify your doctor.

There is no need for additional water before the first six months.

Do not microwave breast milk and, if you microwave formula, always mix well and test prior to feeding.

Worrying about their baby getting enough to eat and sleeping through the night are the most common concerns for new parents.

I know breastfeeding was my biggest challenge of parenthood in the early days. Looking back, I wish the younger me had someone to tell me it was all going to be OK when I was going through those rough weeks. I hope I can be that someone for some of you. Yes, I am an advocate for breastfeeding. I do believe breast is best. I also know that it is not for everyone, and babies and mamas can do quite well on formula, if they are not able to breastfeed for one reason or another. So, give breastfeeding a try if you are on the fence and if it goes well, hooray for you! Celebrate the opportunity and benefits, but if it doesn't that is OK too. Do not beat yourself up over it and don't let it get you down. You have the tips and tools in this chapter to make sure your baby is thriving with the breast or the bottle. There will be so many more moments of motherhood to celebrate. Don't stress over this one.

CHAPTER 7

THE POSTPARTUM PERIOD

*"Everybody always tells you what an awesome
and unique experience being a parent is.
Words can never do the feeling justice."*

– Eric Church

Parenting article by Valerie Frankel entitled the *New Parents' Survival Guide*:

"It is 3:30 am and you are having a lovely dream about fitting into your pre-pregnancy clothes. Suddenly you jerk awake to the sound of a crying newborn in the bassinet next to your bed. As you stand to collect her, you realize that your maxi pad has done the work of a mini. You don't know whether you should clean yourself first or nurse. You decide to dash to the bathroom. Your stitches tug on the way. You do what you can to tidy up and quickly return to your infant. Feeding does not go smoothly. You try everything but the baby, it seems, would rather starve than take nourishment from your breast. Desperate, you give her formula. Two ounces later she spits it all over herself and the bassinet. You clean her off and redress her. You change the crib sheets. As you lay her back down, she grunts cutely and empties the contents of her bowels. Overage soils her tiny pjs. You change her into her third outfit of the night. You place her back in the bassinet. Almost compulsively you rock and imagine how susceptible you'd be to joining a cult right now. You begin to sob. Your husband, who apparently would sleep through a bombing, stirs. Groggily he asks if there is anything he can do to help. You know that you would not respond kindly, so you vow silence. You lie down. It is now 5:30 am and in only 30 minutes you get to do it all over again."

This is not intended to scare you to death. Of course, there will be wonderful moments during these first weeks, but it is also important to have a realistic view of the challenges that lie ahead.

I guarantee you that you will have at least one night like this and instead of sobbing, you can laugh and say: Monique told me there would be a night or two like this. I am not alone.

This cute little story is also realistic in the amount of time you often get to sleep between feedings.

It is no wonder we are so tired, cranky, and often feel overwhelmed. Which are all symptoms of sleep deprivation. Human adults cannot doze at half-hour intervals with any degree of satisfaction.

So, plan in advance for this time. Make meals ahead of time. Buy premade meals, or have meals delivered. Factor is a great company that sends out chef-prepared meals that you just have to put in the microwave.

In this chapter, we are going to cover what happens after delivery and I am going to tell you some things I wish I knew prior to delivery. Yes, motherhood is beautiful but there are some uncomfortable parts that we are going to talk about in this chapter.

What is the postpartum period?

Postpartum is the time immediately after delivery, up until the time when your reproductive organs return to their pre-pregnant state.

This period usually lasts 5–7 weeks.

If friends and family want to help, let them help with house cleaning, laundry, and cooking for the first couple of weeks. This is what you need. You need help, not visitors coming to see the baby. This is a time of recovery and a time for you to rest.

Your uterus

Prior to pregnancy, your uterus was about the size of a pear and is located halfway between your belly button and your pubic bone. Immediately after the baby is born, your uterus becomes firm and about the size of a large grapefruit.

You can feel it with your fingers halfway between your belly button and pubic bone. Your nurses will be coming in periodically to check to see how firm your uterus is and where it is located. This is not the most comfortable thing, especially if you have had a C-section. They will also check to see how much you are bleeding, which will be significantly more once they go pushing on your uterus 😉

Within 12 hours of delivery, your uterus should be about level with your belly button and, five days later, it should return to halfway between your belly button and pubic bone.

Six weeks later, your uterus should have returned to its normal size.

Some mothers feel painful afterbirth contractions when they nurse. You will also typically feel an increase in bleeding. These contractions usually disappear in five to seven days.

In the meantime, you can help ease the discomfort by applying heat to your abdomen (ask your nurse for a heating pad), taking a mild pain reliever like ibuprofen or acetaminophen prior to nursing, gently massaging your abdomen, and keeping your bladder empty will also help.

Lochia

Lochia is what the vaginal discharge or uterine lining after delivery is called.

Lochia usually persists for three to four weeks following a cesarean birth and six to eight weeks after a vaginal birth. Like a period, it starts out heavy and ends light. Expect bright red blood for the first 3–4 days then growing progressively paler. During the first 10 postpartum days, lochia should follow a regular pattern. For the first few days, you will see red blood and possibly small clots. It is normal for the flow to increase whenever you increase your activity, even if that means simply getting out of bed.

The flow will go from bright red blood, possibly with clots, then turn to brown or dark red blood and mucus. Use pads rather than tampons to absorb the flow. Tampons can cause infection. Wait for your OB to approve use.

If the flow turns bright red and becomes heavy after you have been discharged from the hospital, you should rest and count the pads you use. If rest does not slow the flow and you saturate a pad in less than two hours, call the doctor immediately.

Between 2–3 weeks of delivery, the discharge will turn white or yellow mixed with mucus and sometimes blood. The flow will slowly decrease to a very small amount over the next several weeks.

You can take showers or baths and no special vaginal care is necessary, except for rinsing with your peri bottle and watching for signs of infection such as odor and change in discharge.

Your menstrual cycles resume at varying times after delivery, but it may take a few months for your cycles to become regular again.

Nursing mothers often find it takes 18 weeks or longer to resume menstruation. Remember, you can become pregnant before your menstrual periods resume, and you can become pregnant even if you are nursing.

Be sure to discuss family planning with your doctor.

The perineum

The perineum is the area between your vagina and the rectum.

This area may be very tender for 2–3 weeks because of stretching that occurred at delivery. This may be particularly the case if this area tears or if you have an episiotomy. To relieve any discomfort or stinging after giving birth use your peri-wash bottle with warm water to clean the perineal area in a front-to-back direction after you go to the bathroom or when your vaginal discharge is heavy.

Continue to use the peri bottle until the bloody vaginal flow has decreased.

You may also wash the area with soap and a soft washcloth as you shower or bathe.

On the first day or two, apply ice packs to the perineum to reduce pain and swelling. And after that, you may find that soaking in a clean bathtub for 10–20 minutes several times a day helps relieve pain and discomfort.

Your doctor may prescribe creams or topical anesthetics such as sprays or jelly, hydrocortisone, or vitamin E cream to use in this area. You may even need oral painkillers.

Vaginal and episiotomy stitches

If you have had any tearing or had an episiotomy, this area is going to be sore for some time. It may take a month or so to heal. Limit your activity, especially lifting, for at least 2–3 weeks and speak to your doctor before exercising, as they may want you to postpone for several more weeks.

Vaginal and episiotomy stitches will dissolve on their own and they do not need to be removed.

Try to elevate your feet while you are sitting and when you sit, sit on cushions.

You may be more comfortable if you lie down, rather than sitting for prolonged periods of time.

Ask for ice packs and continue to put ice on and off the entire time you are in the hospital. Remember nobody can see under the covers.

Watch for signs or symptoms of infection. Call your doctor if have increasing pain, redness, a foul odor, or fever.

Cesarean section

If you have a C-section, you will likely need a little longer to recover.

The abdominal incision will be tender to touch and may be a bit red.

The incision may be covered with Steri-Strips. You may also have some numbness above or below the incision or in patches around the area.

It is alright to get the Steri-Strips wet, so you can shower as soon as you feel up to it (I was so excited to shower). You can remove the Steri-Strips if they have not come off on their own by day 10.

It is OK to lift the baby but nothing heavier for a while.

Plan not to drive a car for two weeks after birth and don't do any exercises that tense your abdominal muscles for at least 6–8 weeks, and make sure you talk to your doctor prior to returning to exercise and have his or her approval first.

Listen to your body. You will know you are overdoing it if your bleeding increases or if your incision, abdomen, or back begins to hurt when you are doing an activity.

Urinary tract

It may take a few days for your bladder to return to normal and for you to regain your normal bladder control.

This is true in both a regular delivery and a C-section.

Because your urethra may have been bruised or the bladder overstretched during delivery, you may be more susceptible than usual to urinary tract infections as well.

Drink plenty of liquids and empty your bladder at least every 3–4 hours.

Many women experience urinary incontinence during the first month after delivery so doing Kegel exercises and frequent emptying of the bladder will help regain control of those muscles as soon as possible.

I think you could all use a little humor about now. So, I will share one of the most embarrassing moments in my life:

One of my best friends came to see me after Taylor was born, and she asked me when the last time I got up to urinate was. I told her they took my catheter out several hours ago, but I did not need to go. Now this is a friend whom I have known since I was four years old and who had just had twins via a C-section. She also happens to be a nurse. She said: trust me you have to go; you just don't know you do. I thought she was nuts. I thought to myself: I think I would know if I had to pee or not, besides, it is going to hurt when I get up as my stomach was just cut open. Well, she wasn't having any of my procrastinating. She made me get up, and I was slow, and my stomach hurt. She was trying to take my mind off the pain, so she started talking about when we were kids. I cannot remember now what story she was recalling, but just as she got me to my feet and in my slippers, she hit me with the punchline, and I started to laugh. Well … that bladder that I did not think was full was apparently ready to burst and burst it did, like a dam that broke. I was mortified, but once it started, I could not stop. I realized I had no control of my bladder whatsoever.

Well, to say the least, my slippers ended up in the trash can, we had to call maintenance for a clean-up on aisle 5 (room whatever), and my friend had to wash her shoes and feet in my shower. "Yikes" is right. Thank goodness it was one of my besties, because I do not know what I would have done if it was someone else. My sweet friend with the biggest heart and best sense of humor just giggled and said: "I told you that you had to go." As embarrassing as that story is to tell, I tell it to all my classes. I hope it prevents them from having "a Monique moment" and saves their friends' and family's feet. As soon as you are able get up and try to use the restroom, do it! Then continue to go every few hours until that bladder "wakes up."

Swelling

You may experience some swelling in your legs and feet soon after you give birth.

This is common and surprisingly significant. It happens with both a vaginal delivery and a C-section. Although it can be uncomfortable, it is not dangerous, nor is it a sign of infection or circulatory problems. You may take warm baths and elevate your feet to make yourself more comfortable. Within a week the swelling should be gone.

Let the nurse or doctor know if you have pain in your leg/s or a spot is tender to touch. If you have a warm spot in your calf or leg, or it hurts to pull your toes toward you, etc., this could be an indication of thrombosis/blood clots.

Bowels and hemorrhoids

Lack of physical activity and perineal soreness may make constipation and gas that new mothers typically experience worse.

Drink plenty of fluids, eat fruits, leafy veggies, whole grain bread, and cereals.

Start walking to get things moving. Your doctor will probably prescribe a stool softener or laxative such as Colace, Senokot, Metamucil, Milk of Magnesia, or Miralax… if not, ask for it!

If you have rectal stitches, try not to strain with bowel movements. If the stool softeners are not working and the constipation is severe, rectal suppositories or enemas may help.

Most women find that going home to increased activity and private surroundings helps.

If you are already suffering from hemorrhoids, they often become tender and inflamed after a vaginal birth.

To relieve hemorrhoid discomfort on the first day after giving birth, use ice packs to help reduce swelling and ask for a donut cushion to sit on. After that, warm, moist heat, such as soaking in a clean tub may bring relief. You may want to use a topical anesthetic.

Avoid prolonged periods of sitting or standing and try to alternate periods of rest and activity.

What to expect in the first days and weeks home from the hospital

It may surprise you how much work it is to take care of one little baby or how stressful it can be, especially if your baby is fussy.

You may feel overworked and overtired. You will be chronically sleep deprived. It is normal to feel anxious, clumsy, and unsure of yourself at first, and you might even feel a bit overwhelmed at times. That feeling of being overwhelmed may be increased if you do not have a lot of support, especially from your spouse.

You need to ask for help and sleep every chance you get. Allow your close friends, husband or partner, and family to help with chores such as cooking, cleaning, and laundry. You may want to hire someone to come in for a couple of hours a day, even if it is just to let you sleep.

If you get a helper, clarify that your role is looking after the baby and the helper's role is to cook, clean, do laundry, wash dishes, etc., whatever you need done.

Do not be surprised if you have a difficult time getting things done in the first few months. Household chores can wait. Your main job is taking care of yourself and the baby.

You might find it easier to tell everyone that you will not be having any visitors for the first few weeks, so you don't worry about your house and entertaining, and others being around the baby. This way, you can nap when the baby naps, nurse in privacy, etc. Or, if that seems too restrictive for you, then you may want to limit visitors to only close friends and family during your first month at home and only if they are well.

Sometimes you feel as if you have to entertain when guests come, and you really don't need this now. If you do have guests, talk with your spouse ahead of time. Have a cue or code between the two of you, so you can cut a visit short. An example of how to cut a visit short: I don't mean to be rude, but could we cut this visit short, I think mom and baby need to take a nap now, or I am really tired, or I need to nurse the baby, etc.

Many moms, especially those who were previously working, sometimes find themselves feeling socially isolated staying home with a new baby.

These feelings are probably at their worst around 1–2 months when the novelty of the experience has worn off and when the baby is still waking at night. Help has gone home, and your baby has not really become socially responsive.

What can you do?

Again, do not be afraid to ask for help, especially from your spouse. Trade-off responsibilities. Take turns going out for diapers and being gone for an hour.

Get some exercise; hook up with some friends, perhaps with other parents of newborns, for strolls, trips to the park, etc.

Travel with your baby. Between two months and nine months is ideal for a trip to visit relatives and show off the baby (after the first set of immunizations).

Take your baby outdoors: You can take your baby outdoors at any age. As soon as you feel up to it and the weather permits, dress your baby as you would dress, avoid direct sunlight, and get some fresh air. Take a walk around the block each day or sit on the patio. Until after the first immunizations, you should avoid close, crowded areas and allow strangers to look but not touch.

Get a few hours away by one month, recruit a dependable babysitter and make a date with your spouse. This is important. My husband and I have done Friday night date night for almost 30 years now. (You will probably still spend the night talking about the baby, but it is good for your relationship and good for the baby.)

Try to make things easier on yourself. Use a laundry detergent that the whole family can use (e.g., All Free for everyone's clothes).

You do not have to answer your phone. Turn your ringer to silent.

Put a sign on the doorbell: "Baby and Mom sleeping."

Keep a big tub in the room for items that need to be put away and clear up and make one sweep at the end of the day.

If you cook or someone comes to help you cook, double the recipe, label, and freeze a meal (you can also do this several weeks before the baby arrives). You might buy a small extra freezer before the baby arrives to store breast milk and extra meals.

If you have an upstairs-downstairs, have things in both places so you are not running up and down for things.

Practice saying no.

If grandparents' or relatives' help or advice is interfering rather than helping, find a way to politely say "thank you" but then ignore them and follow your instincts and your own advice.

Dad's role

If Dad is unable to take an extended period of time off work, he should take time off for labor and delivery and the day Mom comes home from the hospital.

If you are going to have your mother stay and help, you might have your husband or partner go back to work while your mother is here, and then take time off after she leaves, or vice versa.

Dad or the partner should help and be involved right from the start with feedings, changing, bath, chores, and even calling the doctor.

Dads are often less confident about taking charge when parents first bring home a new baby and tend to step back and allow Mom to do the majority of the caregiving.

They often feel they will not be as good as Mom at doing something. Some feel as if parenting only comes naturally to moms.

If they do get involved from the start, however, they will build up confidence and, the more they do something, the more comfortable they become, and a routine develops.

Let your spouse know you feel or felt unsure at first, too.

You might ask the nurse at the hospital to show you both how to do things before you leave the hospital.

Statistics taken from *Parenting Magazine*; article entitled "Father's Time."

According to a recent study of nearly 1,800 families.

Researchers found that, on weekdays, dads spend about 65% as much time with their children as moms do and on weekends 87% as much time.

That is 2.5 hours a day during the week and 6.2 hours on the weekends.

In the early 1990s, dads only spent 43% of the time moms did directly engaged with their kids.

Parenting Magazine, "New Parents' Survival Guide", Valerie Frankel writes (tells it like it is):

Now this may not be everyone's husband, some are absolutely wonderful right from the start. This is for those whose husbands need a little nudge.

Valerie Frankel writes: "Your husband will not wait on you hand and foot: He means well. But try as he might, he will never understand the struggles of childbirth. My husband, Glen, watched every vein-popping second of Maggie's birth: the blood, and the gunk, and the screaming for the anesthesiologist. And he assumed that, because I could walk to the recovery room, I was as good as new. When we got home, he was not an aggressive diaper changer. He waited for me to ask him to do everything. We bickered. Was he doing his equal share? Why didn't he seem to love Maggie? Why was he insisting there was an emergency at work when his boss had instructed him to take time off?"

Dr. Jane Greer, Ph.D., explains saying: "Just as men can't understand our experience with pregnancy, labor, and delivery, we can't fully understand their take on new fatherhood."

The colossal change of the baby's arrival is overwhelming for a man.

Some men bond with the baby during pregnancy but most do not believe their fatherhood until it is thrust upon them. The dad cannot breastfeed, and he is often not sure where he fits in. This is why the husband may retreat to the office, a place where they understand the rules. On top of that alienation, dads sometimes feel exempt. Moms do more, so it follows that they learn more quickly about how to care for the baby. A father can fall way behind after only a few days. What can you do about it? Dr. Greer says that before a mom accuses her partner of not doing enough or caring enough, she should ask him whether he would like to do more and give him suggestions. For instance, Valerie figured out Maggie stooled with each feeding, instead of passing Maggie to Glen afterward and asking him to change her, she should have explained that Maggie had this pattern so he could anticipate it. That way he might have felt more in tune with her rhythms.

So, Frankel's advice to women is:

Tell your husband that you understand. It will be comforting for him to know that you are scared, overwhelmed, and need to flee too. Then the two of you can take turns going out for diapers and returning three hours later.

Dogs / animals

If your baby has always been your dog, there are a few things you can do to help your fur baby adjust to the new arrival.

Make any changes, such as making something off-limits, at least one month before the baby comes home.

One vet suggests you get a stunt double, a life-sized doll to rock and hold and stroll and put in the bassinet, and correct any behavior prior to the baby coming home.

When the baby is in the hospital, have your spouse bring home a receiving blanket that your baby was wrapped in and has the baby's scent on it, and let your dog smell it.

When you return from the hospital, greet your dog when you first come in the door and introduce them, yet keep a tight rein on the dog.

Do not leave the baby and dog alone and make special time to include your dog during the day.

Parenting Sept 2001

Recent research done by the University of Arizona found that, when a child spends time with cats and dogs as infants, he or she is as much as 30% less likely to develop asthma later in childhood. Being around them and all their bacteria may help tone a baby's immune system, so it won't overact by producing excessive antibodies to allergens (this is the theory).

Yet Dr. Harold Farber says those with a strong family history of asthma appear to get little benefit from having pets around, as the genetic predisposition is too strong. If a child already has asthma, pet dander can trigger asthma attacks and they recommend that you think of removing the pets if the child has asthma. They found that removing the pets relieved symptoms in 40% of asthmatics under the age of six.

You may want to get a crib tent if you have a cat and you are worried about the cat jumping in the crib, or keep the door shut and cat out.

Baby blues

Being over-tired can leave you feeling overwhelmed at times.

More than 50% of women experience postpartum blues on the third or fourth day after delivery.

Symptoms include tearfulness, tiredness, sadness, and difficulty thinking clearly.

The main cause is probably the sudden decrease in maternal hormones.

Since the symptoms most often start the day Mom comes home from hospital, the full impact of being totally responsible for a dependent newborn may contribute to these feelings.

Symptoms usually clear within 1–3 weeks as hormone levels return to normal, and you develop routines and a sense of control.

How to deal with postpartum blues

1. Acknowledge it.
2. You may want to talk to a mom who has gone through this already, a friend or family member, and/or to your husband if he is supportive.

3. Sometimes it just helps to know you are not alone: this is normal, and it will pass.

4. Get rest and lots of it.

5. Get help with the work.

6. Get out of the house at least once week, even if it is only to the store and at 3–4 weeks go out on a date.

7. If you do not feel better after one month or if you feel like you are losing control, talk to your doctor.

To help you get through this, get fresh air, as I mentioned before. Get away for a few hours. You will most likely feel refreshed and miss the baby and feel better when you get home.

Now is the time to take care of yourself. Your only jobs are to take care of your new baby and yourself. I am typing this as I sit on a plane and the oxygen mask analogy rings true for new parents. The flight attendants tell you to put your oxygen mask on first, so you will be able to take care of your child and put their mask on. If you run out of oxygen, how can you help your little one? If you do not take care of yourself, you can't be the best parent you want to be. So, it is OK to be a little selfish right now. Don't feel guilty about anything. A messy house is not a sign of a poor housekeeper, it is a sign of a parent with better things to do. Learn to let things slide or get help.

"Cleaning your house while your kids are still growing up is like shoveling the sidewalk before it stops snowing." Phyllis Diller

CHAPTER 8

POSTPARTUM DEPRESSION

"While we try to teach our children all about life, our children teach us what life is all about."

— Angela Schwindt

Statistics

One in four women suffer from depression before, during, or after pregnancy, according to a new study in the American Journal of Psychiatry, and the College of Gynecology. That is a 25% chance.

This is different from the baby blues which affects 70–80% of new moms (see the end of the previous chapter).

Patricia Dietz, an epidemiologist at the US Center for Disease Control and Prevention's Division of Reproductive Health, wrote in the American Journal of Psychiatry: "Postpartum depression affects 400,000 women in the United States. There is effective treatment, but it is often difficult to bring depression up at a time when you are supposed to be elated after just having a baby, but doctors should ask."

Dr. David L Katz, Director of Yale University School of Medicine's Prevention Research Center, says: "There are two potential explanations for depression. Either the challenges of pregnancy, from hormonal changes to psychological adjustment, induce depression, or the medical monitoring that occurs around the time of pregnancy identifies depression that otherwise would have gone undiagnosed. Of course, both factors could be at play."

My OB/GYN says she often sees a chemical imbalance that may be triggered by the sudden drop in hormones after pregnancy and some women need medication for a short period of time to get the chemical imbalance back in balance.

Symptoms

Depression can be described as two or more weeks of feeling sad, blue, unhappy, irritable overwhelmed, crying a lot, having no energy or motivation, eating too little or too much, sleeping too little or too much, having trouble focusing, remembering, or making decisions, feeling worthless or guilty, loss of interest or pleasure in activities, withdrawal from family or friends, headaches, chest palpitations, hyperventilation, restlessness, agitation or slowed movements, and some women have thoughts or ideas of suicide.

Womensheatlth.gov article/ Depression during and after pregnancy

They answer some basic questions:

How common is depression during and after pregnancy?

Depression that occurs during pregnancy or within a year after delivery is called perinatal depression.

Researchers believe that depression is one of the most common complications during and after pregnancy.

Often depression is not recognized or treated, because some normal pregnancy changes cause similar symptoms and are happening at the same time.

Tiredness, problems sleeping, stronger emotional reactions, and changes in body weight may occur during pregnancy and after pregnancy. But these symptoms can also be signs of depression.

Causes

The causes of depression can be many. Some include hormonal changes or a stressful life event can cause chemical changes in the brain that lead to depression. Depression is also an illness that runs in some families. We mentioned a couple of things above as well.

After pregnancy, depression is called postpartum depression or peripartum depression. After pregnancy, hormonal changes in a woman's body may trigger the symptoms.

During pregnancy, the amount of two female hormones, estrogen and progesterone, in a woman's body increase greatly. In the first 24 hours after childbirth, the amount of these hormones rapidly drops back down to their normal pre-pregnancy state.

Researchers think the fast change in hormone levels may lead to depression, just as smaller changes in hormones can affect a woman's moods before she gets her menstrual period.

Occasionally, levels of thyroid may also drop after giving birth. Low thyroid levels can cause symptoms of depression, including depressed mood, decreased interest in things, irritability, fatigue, difficulty concentrating, sleep problems, and weight gain. A simple blood test can tell if this condition is causing a woman's depression. A good OB/Gyn will check your thyroid first before putting you on medication for depression.

Other factors that may contribute to depression include broken sleep and being overtired; feeling overwhelmed; feeling stress from changes and trying to be Super Mom; feelings of loss of body and self; loss of free time; staying indoors for long periods of time and social isolation.

Resources

If you are struggling, here are a few more resources for online support and support groups, please reach out. You are not alone!

www.postpartum.net

www.postpartumprogress.com

www.ppdtojoy.com

CHAPTER 9

SLEEP

*"People who say they sleep like a baby
usually don't have one."*

— Leo Burke

Helping your child to learn to self-soothe and raising a child with good sleep habits is one of the best gifts you can give your child. Infant sleep issues that are not corrected can continue through childhood and beyond. To me this is one of the most important chapters in this book!

In this chapter I will be describing my approach to encouraging healthy sleep habits. Finding the right method for you and your family can be confusing. There are at least four levels of quality evidence most parents use when trying to find a sleep approach that works for them. The first is advice from family and friends, the second is advice from a trusted advisor, the third is by following national guidelines, and the fourth is turning to the internet where you might find unfiltered or unverifiable sources.

My approach has evolved over the past 25 years and comes from three of the above approaches. The first is from personal experience as a nurse and mom, the second is from trusted advisors such as Dr. Ron

Fischler and Dr. Jeffrey Siegel and other physicians I have worked with over the years and continue to work with, and finally, advice adopted from national guidelines from the American Academy of Pediatrics.

I thought that it would be fun to see a typical 24-hour day of a 1-month-old taken from *Parents Magazine*:

16.5 hours sleeping = 69% of the time.

3 hours eating = 13% of time.

1 hour wetting, stooling, and being changed = 4% of the time.

2 hours crying = 8% of the time.

2 hours staring into space = 8% of the time.

Special concerns
SIDS

SIDS is one of the greatest fears for most parents. So, I will start this chapter by talking about SIDS.

Barton Schmitt explains in his book, *Your Child's Health*, how the "Back to Sleep" campaign came to be in the United States and how it came to be recommended by the American Academy of Pediatrics (AAP).

In the 1980s, research studies done in Europe, Australia, and New Zealand showed a 20–67% decrease in SIDS with a supine (back lying) position.

The prone or stomach position had a 3–9 times greater risk of SIDS.

The side-lying position had a 2 times greater risk than the supine position. It was a better option than the stomach, yet it was still not as good as the back.

In 1992, the AAP recommended back-lying or side-lying due to 6–7,000 deaths from SIDS per year. They recommended that all healthy infants be positioned for sleep on their backs *or* side rather than the traditional tummy or prone position.

This recommendation was based on the findings from numerous studies completed abroad, which again indicated that babies who slept on their stomachs were at higher risk of dying from SIDS.

Two years later, in 1994, the AAP, along with the National Institute of Child Health and Human Development and other health experts, joined efforts to spread the word that back- *or* side-sleeping was best for babies.

As a result, thousands of US babies' lives were saved.

In Seattle alone, from 1992–1995, there was a 30–50% drop in the incidence of SIDS when people followed this advice.

In 1996, the AAP officially changed its position to recommend back- over side-lying.

As the data suggested, the back-lying position for sleep poses a lower risk of SIDS than side-lying and is therefore preferred.

A theory or possible reason the tummy position might increase SIDS is that, when a baby is on their stomach, this puts pressure on the child's jawbone. As a result, the airway in the back of the mouth becomes narrower. In addition, if the child sleeps on a soft surface, the nose and mouth may sink into the mattress, so the baby is breathing from a small pocket of stale air.

In my classes, I also bring up CPR classes. One of the first things they teach you is to place the person on their back and tilt the head back, to establish the best airway. I also tell parents to think of the airway as a straw. When you kink a straw, you are not going to get the same flow as you do when that straw is straight. So, when your baby is on their back that straw/airway is straight, and your baby has the most wide-open airway possible. This is also a good reason not to let your little one sleep slouched in a swing or infant car seat.

The original reason for the US and Canada to recommend the prone position in the 1950s was fear of aspiration if a child spits up or vomits.

Yet the AAP says they may recommend a tummy or side-lying position if there is a significant medical condition that would mandate this.

Discuss sleep positions with your doctor if there are any medical conditions (such as severe reflux). Now, if you recall, my babies had severe reflux to the point of causing apnea and my pediatricians still recommended my babies were put to sleep on their backs. We just put a wedge under the mattress to add a slight incline to the head of the bed.

SIDS prevention recommendations

Some additional recommendations from the American Academy of Pediatrics include:

Do not let infants sleep on sofas, soft mattresses like the parents' mattress, or any other soft surface.

Keep pillows, quilts, comforters, and stuffed toys out of a child's crib.

Avoid devices designed to maintain sleep positions. They have not been shown to reduce the risk of SIDS. They can entrap a baby and act as a pillow on each side of the face.

Avoid overheating a baby with excessive nightclothes, like hats, or elevated room temperature. If possible, a ceiling fan should be used.

In general, the temperature should be comfortable for you.

Instead, place your infant down to sleep on a firm, flat mattress and use a fitted sheet.

Never allow cigarette smoking around your baby.

If possible, breastfeed your baby.

Make sure your infant receives immunizations. Immunizing your infant decreases the risk of SIDS by 50%.

Notify your doctor if you see a change in behavior or signs of an illness.

A sleep space that is separate but close to a parent is ideal (more on this later in the chapter).

Consider offering a pacifier at bedtime once breastfeeding is established.

If swaddling an infant, it should be snug above the shoulders and loose at the hips, and always lay the baby on their back. It should not be done past three months of age due to the risk of the baby rolling over and breaking out of the swaddle and then having a blanket in the bed over the baby's face. It should not be so tight that the baby can't take a deep breath.

Avoid relying on products or home monitors that claim to *reduce* the risk of SIDS because most have not been tested for effectiveness and safety (more on this in a moment).

Encourage teaching of "Back to Sleep" guidelines for all secondary caregivers.

No bumpers in the crib.

I recommend reversing the direction in which you lay the baby in the crib every week. Babies tend to turn, even if slightly, toward the side where they can see people and toward the light.

This helps strengthen neck muscles on both sides and also helps prevent flat spots and neck torsion.

It is also important to give your baby time on his/her tummy during the day to allow them to push up with their arms and build upper body strength and neck support. Tummy time also helps prevent the development of flat spots on the head.

Since your baby probably won't like being on his/her tummy, you may need to entertain him/her while he/she is doing tummy time. Choose times when he/she is playful and alert, then get down to his/her level and try these diversions: make silly faces and sounds, play peek-a-boo, or sing. Stop when they get fussy. If your baby falls asleep, this is not productive tummy time. Before a baby is able to lie flat, you may use a bolster roll to help prop the upper body.

Mattresses

There are also now new, breathable mattresses. Again, these cannot be counted on to prevent SIDS and I would not put my baby to sleep on their tummy thinking they were safe due to the breathable mattress, but it is one more thing you could do to decrease the risk.

SafeSleep mattress is one brand of breathable mattress with an open box spring and not a fiber filling. It has an air-permeable mesh surface with no sheets and fits a standard crib. This mattress can be found at safesleeptech.com

This is just one of many types of breathable mattresses available.

Swaddling

SIDS and swaddling, *Arizona Parenting Magazine*, December 2006, p. 39

Swaddling decreases the startle response in infants, and it often allows babies to sleep longer through the night and will often allow them to stay on their back or side. It is important that the swaddle is not too tight. The baby needs to be able to breathe easily. He or she needs to be able to take a deep breath and expand the chest. So, make sure the swaddle isn't so tight that it prevents the chest from moving up and down. Doctors also warn against swaddling in warm blankets as this could be a risk for SIDS. There is a higher incidence of SIDS in winter months and the peak age is between two and four months. In Australia, India, and Asia, infants are commonly swaddled until four months and incidence of SIDS is almost nonexistent. Solona babywear sells breathable, lightweight muslin wraps that are great for swaddling.

A sleep suit like the Merlin Sleep Suit may help if your baby is rolling onto their stomach but cannot roll back to their back and waking themselves up crying or getting stuck on their stomach. Now AAP is opposed to weighed sleep suits or sleep wear that holds babies in one place. I need to make clear that when your baby is strong enough to roll in a weighted sleep suit or the Merlin sleep suit it is time for them to come out of it, as these could cause your baby to be stuck on their stomach. So, if your baby is strong enough to roll in the Magic Sleepsuit, it is time to take them out of it. It might be a nice transition, however, when your baby is breaking out of a swaddle but not ready to roll back and forth yet. This may keep your little one on their back longer.

Average hours of sleep

North Scottsdale Pediatrics website www.nspeds.com

As most of you already know, newborns sleep a lot during the first month of life.

Your child may sleep anywhere from 12–20 hours per day with an average of 16 hours. The duration of this sleep is variable: from 15 minutes to 5 hours.

Most newborns wake up 1–3 times during the night in the first 3 months of life.

The majority of infants can be expected to sleep through the night by 4–6 months of age. Although there are a few babies that may not acquire this skill until closer to a year. The most important skill to teach young babies is to self-soothe and put themselves back to sleep when they wake. More to come on this.

"Sleeping through the night"

The definition of sleeping through the night by age:

6–8 hours by 4 months

8–10 hours by 6 months

Just like adults there are some of us that can get by on fewer hours of sleep and those of us who need extra hours. Your baby may also need more or less than the average.

Many parents think that the reason babies wake up is because their baby is hungry. This may be part of the problem in the first two months, but there is much more to it. Infants wake up several times during the night because they have an immature sleeping pattern.

Now, the saying "sleeping though the night" is a bit misleading. All babies, and adults for that matter, wake during the night. However, we are unaware of this, as we can fall back to sleep on our own. The goal for us as parents is to not have to do anything to help our little ones fall back to sleep. We want to help them learn to self-soothe and fall back to sleep on their own.

Sleep patterns

By the 8th month of pregnancy, the baby's sleep periods consist of two distinct sleep patterns: REM sleep and non-REM sleep.

Two general patterns exist:

REM sleep (Rapid Eye Movement)

This is an active sleep pattern. Babies may have restless movements, irregular breathing, brief awakenings, and twitching. Infants may go through this pattern 2–4 times a night. Babies wake at the end of each REM pattern. Newborns spend 50% of their sleeping time in REM sleep, whereas adults only spend 25% of their time in REM sleep. It is no surprise that babies wake up so much at night. Fortunately, this pattern decreases by age 3–4 months, allowing most children to sleep through the night.

Non-REM sleep

Non-REM sleep is a quiet sleep pattern. You will notice little movement. A regular breathing pattern is noticed and deeper sleep from which it seems very difficult to awaken your baby.

Some general guidelines for waking babies at night in the first few weeks (Repeat from Breastfeeding Chapter)

Wake babies every four hours in the first two–three3 weeks. By then most babies are up to birth weight and have established a nice pattern of gaining weight. By six weeks, if a baby is sleeping let them sleep. Many pediatricians feel that once normal weight gain is established, you can trust the baby to know when to wake and feed. This happens around the six-week mark, sometimes later but sometimes earlier. Follow the above as guidelines rather than firm rules except for the first two-three weeks when we need to ensure that a baby sleeping longer is not due to dehydration or undernutrition.

Encouraging healthy sleep habits: "sleep training"

"Sleep training" or encouraging healthy sleep habits can start from day one. It is important to have a plan. If you follow this plan, many babies sleep through the night by 2 months of age and almost all babies by 4–6 months of age. Keep in mind, however, that when infants start sleeping through the night is mainly a process of maturation. If you are practicing good sleep habits, you can positively influence your baby to sleep through the night earlier but if your baby takes a bit longer that is OK too. Keep practicing healthy sleep habits and your baby will get there when he or she is developmentally ready.

Here is the plan for your newborn

If you remember from the breastfeeding / bottle feeding chapter, babies will need to take approximately 2.5 oz per lb. in 24 hours. If they sleep all day, they will be up feeding all night. The key is getting your baby to eat as many ounces during the day and waking hours as possible.

One of the best ways to do this is to not let your newborn go more than three hours during the day without eating. Wake them gently if they are sleeping longer. Now most will not go this long. Occasionally though, your little peanut has their days and nights mixed up and they will want to take their long stretch of sleep during the day instead of the night when you are sleeping. Conversely, do not let a baby graze all day long at the breast either. Keep in mind, you are not a pacifier.

Most newborns eat every 1.5 to every 2–4 hours, gradually extending the time as the baby grows (bottle-fed babies tend to go longer between feeds than breastfed babies). Remember they typically max out at 24–32 oz/day.

More frequent daytime feedings, such as hourly, lead to frequent awakenings for small feedings at night. This is called grazing. However, if they do not get enough during the day, they will need to eat more at night.

Attempt to wake your baby up during the day and keep them entertained. Provide extra playtime during the day. This way the time when your infant sleeps the longest is during the night, when you are sleeping too. This plan will hopefully give you more sleep at night. Your baby starts to learn the difference between night and day.

When you feed them at night, do it quietly and without a lot of disruption. Try to keep the middle of the night's feedings brief and boring. Don't talk or get them too excited, let them know this is nighttime and Mom and Dad are different at night than during the daytime. They will soon realize this is not the time to play.

When they wake at night for feedings, do not turn on the lights (use a flashlight or night light, not directly in their line of sight). Do not talk to them or rock them. Your job is to get them fed as quickly as possible and get them back in their bed.

Do not change diapers during the night. The exception to this rule is if they have stooled or if you are treating a diaper rash. If your baby gets used to you changing their diaper every time it is damp, they will wake every time they are damp. They are going to be in diapers at night until they are almost three. These diapers are absorbent and are meant to pull moisture away.

The next step towards sleep training is to put your baby down to sleep drowsy but awake. You do not want your baby to fall asleep nursing or being rocked or at the bottle every time. You want your baby to learn to fall asleep on their own without needing you to put them to sleep. This is key and a very important step.

The reason for not rocking your baby until they are completely asleep is that they will go through a normal sleep cycle for 1–3 hours, and then have a normal waking up period after this first cycle, but if the rocking isn't there anymore, they start to cry, as they rely on the rocking for comfort. All babies habituate to circumstances they come to associate with going to sleep. This could be sound, rocking, sucking, etc. If you teach your newborn that rocking is the way to fall asleep then you are committing yourself to doing this for a very long time and they will have to be weaned from it at some point. It is better to prevent than to have to fix a problem later. So, rock to calm but then put your baby down drowsy but awake, even if they fuss.

Also do not expect your newborn to fall asleep as soon as you lay him or her down. It often takes 20 minutes of restlessness for a baby to go to sleep. Some experts call this cradle fidgeting. Most people do not fall asleep the second their head hits the pillow; we toss and turn a bit (unless you are my husband lol).

If they are crying, rock them and cuddle them but when they settle down, try to place them in the crib before they fall asleep. This is how your child will learn to put him/herself back to sleep after normal awakenings.

Handle naps in the same way. Do not let your baby fall asleep in the swing every day for a nap, or on you for all naps.

Do not help your infant when he or she doesn't need help. So, if your baby is just fussing let them fuss. Your baby may just be trying to settle and will fall asleep. Fussing is different than crying.

Hold your baby for all hard crying during the first three months. You cannot spoil a baby under three months of age. However, even babies with sensitive tummies have a few times each day when they are drowsy and not crying. On these occasions, place the baby in their crib or bassinet and let them learn to self-comfort and fall asleep on their own.

Crying is the only form of communication newborns have. Yet crying does not always mean your newborn is hungry. Do not let feeding become a pacifier. He or she may be tired, bored, lonely, or too hot, etc. Hold your baby at these times or put them to bed if they seem tired. For every time that you nurse there should be 4–5 times that you snuggle your baby without nursing. Don't let them get into the bad habit of eating every time that you hold him or her. This is called grazing.

All new babies cry some during the day and night. Gentle rocking and cuddling seem to help the most.

If your baby cries excessively all day long or every time he or she is flat, there could be a medical reason for it, so have them checked out by the pediatrician.

Carry your baby for at least three hours each day when he or she is not crying. This will reduce fussy crying. Using a front infant carrier may help with this. It certainly saved my back.

Do not let your baby sleep in your bed. Once your baby is used to sleeping with you, a move to his/her own bed will be extremely difficult. This is a bad habit you just don't want to start and have to break.

The AAP is opposed to the family bed. They warn of the dangers of suffocation. The AAP cautions against routine co-sleeping in a family bed. Tiny infants can be smothered under bedclothes or the weight of a much larger body. In the US, people sleep on soft mattresses with bulky covers. The U.S. Consumer Product Safety Commission opposes bed sharing by infants and adults, particularly if there is more than one adult in the bed. Many cases of infant suffocation have been reported due to bed sharing. Co-sleeping may hamper the child's attempts to develop his/her own resources for getting to sleep.

For the first 2–3 months you can keep your infant in a cradle, bassinet, or crib next to your bed if you want, but I recommend the sooner you can move the baby out of your line of sight the better. If they can see and smell and hear you, they will fuss, wanting you, when they wake. In addition the further they are away from your bed the less likely you will be tempted to bring the baby into bed with you to nurse or feed.

The next thing I recommend is feeding your baby right before you go to sleep. So, we top off their tummy and allow them to sleep when you are sleeping. Give the last feeding at your bedtime at 10–11 p.m. (some sleep experts call this a dream feed).

Some babies like to be swaddled, and some do not. If you have a little one who does, keep them swaddled and keep the room at a temperature that they will be comfortable at or that you would be comfortable at if you were dressed or swaddled the same way. Do not over-bundle. Remove the swaddle at around 3–4 months when the baby is breaking out of it or rolling over.

Give them their own space. Try to move your baby to their own room by two-three months of age. You will most likely move with every movement of your baby. You may want to wait, however, until the baby is sleeping at least 4–5 hours without waking as this is less stressful for Mom.

Now the new recommendation from the AAP is to keep your baby in your room for the first six months and, if possible, a year. When I spoke to the AAP about this, they said this is because the baby won't sleep as soundly and nor will Mom or Dad, so this reduces the risk of SIDS. I worry this has the potential to create sleep issues with older infants not learning to sleep soundly through the night. It may also keep parents sleep deprived. Although the risk of SIDs is not zero until after two years of age, with most cases happening under 6–8 months of age, taking reasonable, science-based precautions lowers the risk of SIDS dramatically. Speak to your pediatrician about this first for their advice.

Background noise or music may help. Try to wean your little one from noise by four months, however, if you use it, or it will be something they always have to have. Having said this, although it is a crutch, it is one that is easily broken and much less concerning than rocking a baby to sleep or letting them fall asleep at the breast each night.

Establish a calm/soothing bedtime routine. More details to come.

Dr. Barton Schmitt feels that, with a sleep plan such as this, 50% of infants can sleep through the night by two months of age. Many experts say that a baby must weigh about 12–13 pounds before they can hold enough food in their stomach to sleep through night. Having said this, there are those babies who will wait until four months of age and a few who will not be physically ready, despite all the healthy sleep habits you are imposing, until 9–12 months. It is important that you don't blame yourself if your little one is slow to get the hang of it. The important thing is you don't give up and you don't give in to bad habits! If you continue to follow healthy sleep habits once your baby gets the hang of it, they will be a good sleeper for life.

Your 2-month-old infant

Here is a plan for your 2-month-old baby if they are not yet sleeping through the night.

By now your baby should be down to one feeding during the night if they are feeding every three hours during the day, are healthy, with no reflux, and they are an adequate weight. Many babies are taking approximately 24 oz of formula or breastmilk during the day, so they do not need extra nutrition at night and are waking up due to a habit.

At this age, never wake your baby at night to feed except at your bedtime. This is your dream feed.

You may want to move your baby's crib into their own room if you have not done it already but speak with your pediatrician about this first.

This will help parents who are light sleepers sleep better. Also, your baby may forget that his/her parents are available if he/she can't see them when he/she awakens.

Try to delay the middle-of-the-night feedings by at least 15 minutes. If your little one wakes up, make sure they are truly crying and not just fussing. If they are truly crying, try to delay the feed by 15 minutes when you go to them. This changes their little internal clock and throws it off a bit. Similar to how we feel when we travel with jet lag, our schedule is off a bit. Babies become very scheduled and wake at the same time, almost to the minute. If we delay a feeding for 15 minutes and they are getting enough to eat during the day, this may be enough to stop them from waking at night. So, in other words, if they cry out wait a few seconds. If they persist, go to them and intervene, just delay feeding for a few minutes.

Before you prepare a bottle or offer the breast, try holding your baby briefly or offer a pacifier to see if that will satisfy them.

Your 4-month-old infant

A 4-month sleep plan if your baby is not yet sleeping though the night.

By four months of age, most babies should be able to sleep at least 8 hours without being fed. Try to discontinue the 2 a.m. feedings before it becomes a habit.

By four months of age, your formula-fed infant does not need to be fed more than four times per day. (This is if they are able to take enough per feeding. Otherwise, an additional bottle may be necessary during the day.) Breast-fed babies do not need more than five nursing sessions per day. (Again this is if they are taking enough per feed. Some babies need six.)

If you do not eliminate the night feeding at this time, it will become more difficult to stop as the child gets older. Remember to give the last feeding at 10 or 11 p.m. when you go to bed. This is so the baby sleeps when you sleep. If your bedtime is 9 p.m., then your "dream feed" is 9 p.m.

If your child cries during the night, use your stall techniques to make sure they are truly awake and won't fall back to sleep. This also continues to throw off the clock. Soothe them with patting or gentle words rather than feeding. Offer a pacifier. Try to do as much soothing in bed as possible without doing too much to help. You want your baby to self-soothe.

Now, if you are satisfied that your baby is getting enough to eat during the day and waking at night out of habit, and the stalling has not been enough to eliminate that middle-of-the-night feeding, you might try another method:

When you feed, offer them 1–2 oz less of formula than you would during the day. If you are breastfeeding, nurse for slightly less time at night than you would during the day. If your baby goes back to sleep and wakes in the morning, you are on the right path to your little one sleeping though the night and they are showing you they are getting ready to drop that feeding.

If, however, your baby wakes up hungry an hour later, they are not quite ready for less formula or breast milk. So, give a full feeding at that next wakening and you might wait a few more weeks and try this method again.

Do not allow your baby to hold his/her own bottle or to take it to bed with him/her. Babies should think that the bottle belongs to the parents. A bottle in bed leads to middle-of-the-night crying when your baby reaches for the bottle in the middle of the night, and it is empty or on the floor. (Not to mention it can cause cavities.) Later it is OK to put a sippy cup of only water in the crib, as my belief is children should stay in a crib until the age of three when they are developmentally ready to be alone and unsupervised in their bedroom.

Continue to make middle-of-the-night contacts brief and boring and comfort your child as little as possible between 10 p.m. and 6 a.m.

Remember all children have four or five partial awakenings each night. They need to learn how to go back to sleep on their own.

This is the age babies can developmentally learn to fall asleep on their own and can start practicing going to sleep when awake and falling back to sleep on their own, and brief periods of crying is part of that process.

If your baby cries for more than 10 minutes, visit them but do not turn on the lights, don't play with them and try not to take them out of their crib. Comfort them with a few soothing words and stay less than one minute. This brief contact usually will be enough to discourage your baby from waking you up every night. If the crying continues you can check on your baby every 15–20 minutes but do not take them out of the crib or stay in the room until they fall asleep.

The exception to the rule is when your child is ill.

If this technique does not work, try rocking until your baby is drowsy but not fully asleep and then put them back down again.

If you don't give in to bad habits, like bringing your baby back to sleep in your bed, or allowing them to sleep in a swing, or nursing them to sleep every night, or allowing them to graze all day so they don't learn to take enough to stretch their tummy etc., healthy sleep habits will follow.

If you want to start working on a nap schedule this would be the appropriate age as well. I typically say wait until your baby is sleeping through the night before you start working on naps though.

Your newborn will be taking several naps per day with no set schedule. Eventually, at around 4 months of age, many babies will be at 3 naps and then 2 at around 6–7 months of age. At 1.5 to 2 years of age is when most children usually give up their morning naps. They don't give up the afternoon nap until between 4 and 6 years.

I feel you can follow your baby's cues and then adjust to fit your schedule. Look at their daily routine to keep a time log, and you will see a pattern emerge. If your little one is still taking three naps, they should be about an hour each. When they are ready to drop a nap, they will still nap a total of three hours, but each nap will then stretch to about an hour and a half. This will be the same when your little one drops down to one nap at around one year of age. This will be one nap lasting approximately three hours. It typically takes about three days to change sleep habits, so once nighttime sleep is established, you can start working on naps. If your baby is not yet sleeping through the night concentrate on this first, then work on naps. The key is consistency. If your baby typically goes down for example from 10–11 a.m. but fusses and stays awake in their crib from 10:30–11 a.m., do not let them sleep from 11–11:30 a.m. Get your baby up at 11 a.m. Try to keep them up until the next scheduled nap time by keeping them entertained. When trying to work on naps, don't go for a stroller ride or car ride as your little one will take a cat nap, recharge their battery and mess up the sleep schedule. So, when you are working on a nap schedule, plan on being at home.

Your 6-month-old infant

If your baby is still not sleeping through the night, do not worry, just keep doing everything above and be consistent. Remember, babies cannot sleep through the night until they are able to take enough ounces during the day that they don't need them at night. So, make sure they are getting enough formula or breastmilk during the day.

At this age, if your baby is developing "normally" (eating well and no health issues) and is still waking out of habit, this would be an appropriate age to safely use the traditional "cry it out" method, if you so desire. If your baby is crying for longer than an hour, which would be very unusual, or not sleeping after three days, speak with your pediatrician.

I had two completely different kiddos and had to sleep-train them completely differently. Both were sleeping through the night on their own by four months of age even though they were preemies. But after an illness or life event, I would have to sleep train again. My daughter just needed to know that I was there or close by. I could go in and offer her a pacifier, rub her head, and slip back out if she woke up in the middle of the night. My son was in a completely different situation. When he was nine months old, he had his first of many bouts of pneumonia. We were up doing breathing treatments all night for several nights. He got into this habit and, once he was well, he was still waking up at night. I would let him cry for 20 minutes then go in to soothe him like I did with my daughter. But, unlike her, instead of him calming down with my presence and a gentle head rub when I went to him, this just confused him and made him cry harder. He was reaching out to me confused as to why I was not picking him up. So, I learned with him it was better to not go in at all. I asked our pediatrician who reassured me it was emotionally safe to allow my son to cry himself to sleep. In Dylan's case, it was actually less confusing for him and easier on him in the long run to not go in.

Now I am not saying this was easy. I cried outside my son's door with him. I had to keep telling myself I was doing this to help him. He needed sleep for his health. The first night he cried for almost a full hour then fell asleep, waking several times during the night. The second night he cried for about 20–30 minutes and by the third night he was sleeping through the night.

Now I have to repeat that this type of sleep training should only be done if your child is in good health and taking in enough calories during the day and if going in to soothe them does not work for your little one. Again, I know this is not for everyone. It would certainly not have been the method for my first child, but it was actually easier and less confusing for my second.

Sometimes you will have a baby that was previously sleeping well start to wake up in the night. This could be due to a couple of reasons.

Separation anxiety

At the age of six months, children may start to be anxious about separation from their parents. Separation anxiety normally occurs between six months and two years of age, and some have trouble even later than that. Separation anxiety can be seen during the day when your child loses sight of you. These fears are often accentuated at bedtime and during the night. Separation fears can be the main component of nightmares.

Dr. Robert Dahl, director of the Children's Sleep Evaluation Center in Pittsburgh, says:

"We are genetically wired to fall asleep when we feel safe and, for a lot of kids, safety means being in close contact with a parent, which is why children who wake up in the middle of the night cry out. Provide lots of cuddling during the day. Children of moms that work outside the home may need extra cuddle time in the evening before bed. Play separation games like hide-and-seek to encourage alone playtime."

During the day, respond to separation fears by holding and reassuring your child. This lessens nighttime fears and is especially important for mothers working outside the home. Play games that help with separation anxiety like peek-a-boo and hide-and-seek with toys, so kids understand people and items still exist even when out of sight.

For middle-of-the-night fears, make contact prompt and reassuring. For mild nighttime fears, check on your child promptly and be reassuring but keep interaction as brief as possible.

If your child panics when you leave or vomits while crying, stay in your child's room until they are either calm or go to sleep. Do not take them out of the crib if possible but provide whatever else they need for comfort.

Leave the door open to your child's room. Children can become frightened when they are in a closed space and are not sure their parents are still nearby. Keep the light off and do not talk too much. You can sit next to the crib with your hand on them. These measures will calm even a severely upset infant.

Waking at night hungry after previously sleeping through the night

The next reason could be that if you have not started solid foods yet, your little one may have an extra need for more calories. We often see this with larger babies between 4 and 6 months that have not yet started solids and are maxing out past 32 oz of formula or breastmilk. Some call it a sleep regression. If this is occurring, it might be time to start solids. I see this sometimes as well when babies start solid foods and are eating too much in the way of solids, and not keeping their breastmilk or formula up to where it was prior to starting solid foods. Their intake should not decrease just because they started solids. More about how to introduce solids in the coming chapter on infant nutrition.

Bedtime routine

I am a huge advocate for establishing a bedtime routine as soon as possible. Establishing a regular bedtime is extremely valuable. By following a routine, infants and children are much more likely to fall asleep easily.

The younger the baby is, the shorter the bedtime routine should be. A bedtime routine could be as simple as the same song before bed, with a bottle or nursing, or the same book. Try to carry out as much of the bedtime routine in the child's room as possible to associate their room with sleep.

Bedtime routines can be feeding, brushing teeth, cuddling, rocking, a bedtime story, singing or prayers. The key is repetition each night.

Dr. Robert Dahl from the University of Pittsburg says babies often learn to associate certain rituals with the process of going to sleep, such as cuddling, rocking, and singing. Again, we are all genetically wired to fall asleep only when we feel safe.

As I mentioned before, there is also a biological clock inside all of us that controls when we get drowsy, when we secrete hormones, when our body temperature rises and falls, a whole symphony of physiological regulations. If you stretch your normal 24-hour pattern one way or another, like I mentioned with jet lag, sleep disturbances can occur.

There is a fine balance with sleep. If your infant is overtired, it may be difficult to get them to sleep. If they have had too much sleep during the day, you may also find that it is difficult for them to fall asleep.

Once your baby is sleeping through the night, you can try to drop the dream feed. If your baby wakes too early in the morning, they are not quite ready to drop it. This is a bit of trial and error. I am not a morning person, so I did the dream feed a bit longer to allow for a later wake-up time in the a.m.

Blackout shades were also a great investment. My ultimate goal was 8 p.m. bedtime / 8 a.m. wake-up with a 3-hour nap from 1–4 p.m. Before one nap they took two 1.5-hour naps. I achieved this with both kids.

Some sleep experts say to try to follow a pattern of: eat, activity, and sleep. I personally feel this is more for an older baby when you are working towards creating set nap times. Newborns do not have set nap times and sleep most of the day with little activity. Four months is a good time to start keeping a log of when your baby tends to fall asleep each day and looking at patterns to emerge for a nap schedule that you can follow.

Flipping on their tummy

New skills, such as rolling over, may cause your little one to wake up crying in the middle of the night. There is no perfect solution. The good news is this is short-lived. Teach your baby how to get back over the other way. Work on this skill during the day, each day. Extra tummy time will help.

What do you do if your baby keeps flipping onto their stomach? If you find them on their tummy, flip them on their back. You might try the Merlin's Magic Sleepsuit, but if your baby is strong enough to keep flipping, the sleepsuit might hold them on their tummy. So, if they can flip in the Merlin suit, it is no longer appropriate. The good news is if they are strong enough to keep flipping, we allow them to remain that way. Otherwise, you would not get any sleep yourself.

Again, like I said, if you find them this way flip them, if they flip again after, you leave them be. Typically, this starts occurring after six months when the risk of SIDS has decreased by more than 50% and the baby is obviously strong enough to pick up his or her head.

Anything that disturbs your little one's routine can change the sleep pattern, and you may have to sleep train again. Examples of this include travel, illness, teething, and visitors.

Go back to the days of early infancy and practice all your old maneuvers.

If he or she is sick, it is fine to relax your normal routines but try to get back on schedule as soon as they feel better. You may need to sleep train all over again with each new illness or trip.

Nighttime separation anxiety

As I mentioned before, some babies start to develop separation anxiety around six months of age. Separation anxiety may exacerbate nighttime crying. Parents can offer comfort, and this may lessen the crying. Unfortunately, it is up to the child as to when they will get past this, but parents can help. As mentioned above, games like peek-a-boo provide practice with the idea that mom and dad leave but they come back. Parents should really emphasize the reunion, and this can be done by saying, "I will see you in the morning", the night before. Creating a safe, comforting, dependable bedtime routine is the other way to help. If separation anxiety is severe, talk to your pediatrician about introducing a transition or comfort/love object at around 8–9 months. A small stuffed animal, blanket, or other security object or love object can be introduced to give comfort and allow your baby to fall asleep without you and help put them back to sleep if they wake at night or early in the morning. It is a source of reassurance and it helps with nighttime separation fears. It should be something as safe as possible and, if you can hold it so it has your scent, that will also help.

Ask your pediatrician about this first, however, before you ever put anything in the crib and make sure the baby is at least eight months old. Use this as a last resort. Even though the AAP talks about the use of comfort objects/love objects at 8–12 months of age and above for severe nighttime separation anxiety, they also say not to have any stuffed animals or toys in bed until after a year, so make sure your baby is developmentally ready for this first. So again, speak to your pediatrician first before introducing anything into the crib.

The other question I get often is about a pacifier. When babies are very attached to their pacifiers they will wake at night and cry wanting it. Until they can find it and put it in on their own, you may be tempted to rush over and "re-bink" (we called the pacifier a "binky") them, as I used to say. You will drive yourself insane doing this all night. I wish I had a good answer for this one as well. One thing you can do if this is happening, which I found has worked with many babies, is when they fall asleep carefully slip the pacifier out of their mouth.

This too is very short-lived as they will either learn to put it back in their mouth on their own or, if you do not want it to become a comfort object, remove it before six months.

Additional sleep safety

Watch for items that have ties or strings that could wind around them.

Be on the lookout for things they might be able to reach for from the crib. This could be curtains, blinds, and blind cords, pictures and wall hangings, and the mobile.

Do not leave a lot of toys in your older child's crib that could get piled on as steps. Remember, unless you have already discussed it with your pediatrician, nothing in the crib besides the baby before 12 months of age.

Comfort objects if you use them, never before eight months and again with the doctor's permission, need to be looked at carefully to make sure they have no removable pieces, such as beans for stuffing, button eyes, and pieces that can come off or out, or a ribbon that might come loose etc.

Do not put your baby to bed in clothing that has buttons that may be removed or tie strings that could be pulled out. Remember pajamas are typically designed for safe sleep. Some of the cute outfits we have them in during the day are not meant to sleep in, so keep that in mind at nap-time.

Do not hang things over the crib.

Nightmares

<u>Overstimulation</u>

Keep the hour before bedtime as calm and quiet as possible. Overstimulation can cause restlessness. Calm and relaxation help prevent nightmares. If your little one is having nightmares, try to establish a calm, relaxing bedtime routine and look for the book "Tell Me Something Happy Before I Go To Sleep." It is a book for a slightly older child but a wonderful book that helps prevent nightmares by talking about positive, happy things before your child falls asleep.

Dr. Barton Schmitt describes nightmares as vivid, scary dreams from which the child usually wakes up and may have trouble going back to sleep.

Occasional bad dreams are normal at all ages after about six months of age. It is important to realize that everyone dreams approximately 4–5 times per night. As adults, however, we have learned to put ourselves back to sleep and often do not wake up or remember our dreams.

Dreams help the mind process complicated events or information. The content of nightmares usually relates to developmental challenges. A recent study done on nightmares in children found that in infancy, nightmares are about loud noises, falling, separation from parents, strange faces, and sensory overload. In the preschool age group, nightmares were about animals, darkness, separation from parents, imaginary monsters, change, school, and fear of the unknown.

The AAP says nightmares usually happen during the second half of the night when dreaming is most intense.

If your little one is waking up at night frightened, unlike sleep training, go to them right away to let them know you are there. Try to soothe them without picking them up. Try to allow them to calm down as much as possible on their own with your offering of reassurance. Once they have calmed, go back to your own room and try not to stay any longer than you have to. If your child is extremely upset, try sitting next to them in a chair with a hand on them, rather than picking them up. Pick them up as a last resort.

You might leave the door open if it was shut previously and use a nightlight, although not directly in their line of vision.

Some other common sleep problems parents face

1. If your child is overtired, they might have a hard time getting to sleep at night. Try to keep the hour before bedtime relaxing. You might try a warm bath and a quiet book or rocking.

2. If your child is falling asleep and taking cat naps while you are driving around during the day, they will not take solid naps. You may need to stay home until a nap schedule is in place.

3. If your child is sleeping too many hours during the day, they may not want to sleep at night.

4. If your baby is waking when the sun comes out, get blackout shades.

5. If your little one wakes up in the middle of the night and wants to be entertained, you might use something like the Fisher Price Sights and Sounds monitor that attaches to the side of the crib to get your child to sleep without needing you.

If you are looking for a book solely on sleep, I have several resources for you below that I have read and recommend. I wish I could tell you there was one perfect sleep book out there. This chapter and my lecture are from many sources. You must do what feels right for you and look at your child's own unique temperament. Both of my children were so different I could not sleep-train them both the same.

I like *parts* of all the books below. Which book is best for your baby depends on your baby's temperament and yours.

I believe that helping your child develop good, healthy sleep habits is one of your biggest jobs as a parent. It comes with a tremendous lifelong reward. However, it is not easy, and it takes work from all parties involved. So be consistent, follow through, and don't give up! If at first you don't succeed, try, try again…. a different sleep method 😉

Here are a few books to read if you are still struggling:

Solve Your Child's Sleep Problems by Dr. Richard Ferber

AAP Guide to Your Child's Sleep

Your Child's Health by Dr. Barton Schmitt

On Becoming Babywise by Gary Ezzo

Touchpoints by T. Berry Brazelton

Happiest Baby on the Block by Harvey Karp

Healthy Sleep Habits, Happy Child by Marc Weissbluth

The No-Cry Sleep Solution by Elizabeth Pantley

CHAPTER 10

GROWTH AND DEVELOPMENT

"His little hands stole my heart. His little feet ran away with it."

— Unknown

Typical growth

The American Academy of Pediatrics says that the average newborn gains weight at a rate of 2–3 oz or 20–30 grams per day. By 1 month of age the average newborn weighs about 9 lbs. He/she will grow between 1 and 1½ inches during the first month.

Between 1 and 4 months of age, your baby will gain between 1 ½ and 2 lbs. per month and grow 1- 1½ inches.

He or she will grow faster in the first four months of their life than at any other time in their development.

A newborn head may gain an inch in circumference in the first month and about half an inch per month the rest of the year.

In the second year, their head circumference will only grow about one inch. This makes the toddler's head almost the size of their adult head size.

Between 4 and 7 months of age, your baby will continue to gain approximately 1–1 ¼ lbs. per month. By 8 months of age, your baby will probably weigh about 2 ½ times their birth weight.

The typical weight of an 8-month-old boy is 14 ½ –17 ½ lbs.

The typical weight of an 8-month-old girl is approximately 1 lb. less at this age, at 13 ½ lbs. to 16 ½ lbs.

As previously mentioned in the breastfeeding chapter, growth spurts are most often noticed by nursing moms at 7–10 days of age, 2–3 weeks of age, 4–6 weeks of age, 3 months of age, 4 months of age, 6 months of age, and 9 months of age.

After 12 months of age, there are no large growth spurts that are standard. Your child may have mini growth spurts which are individual to each child, or your baby may go weeks or months with no growth at all.

Normal weight gain between ages 1 and 5 is 4–5 lbs. per year and a child can go 3–4 months without any weight gain.

Dr. Barton Schmitt gives the average weights at different ages:

5 months = double birthweight

8 months = 2 ½ times birthweight

12 months = triple birthweight (average length is 28–32")

2 years = quadruple birthweight

The average 15-month-old girl weighs about 22 lbs. and is approximately 31 inches tall. Boys tend to be a bit heavier but about the same height. By age 2 both boys and girls weigh between 27 and 28 lbs. on average and are approximately 34 inches tall.

Babies do not typically double their birth length until they are four years of age.

Preemies

Dr. Judith Groner, a professor at Ohio State University School of Medicine in Columbus, says studies show that by age 8, preemies typically completely catch up in height and weight to children born full term.

An exception is those born before 32 weeks, who sometimes remain slightly smaller.

Vision

Within the first week or two after birth, your baby will follow your face with their eyes and notice and pay attention to your voice.

The AAP says that newborns see best at a distance of 8–15 inches away. But by 1 month of age, your baby can focus briefly on things as far away as 3 ft. By the time your baby is 2 months old, he or she will be able to see you clearly from across the room.

He or she will begin to see more accurately as the retina develops and the eye muscles become strong enough to hold the eyes in alignment.

1 month

At birth, babies sometimes have a difficult time using their eyes together, so they wander a bit. But by the time they are one or two months old, the muscles have become stronger, and your little one is able to focus both eyes better. However, they may still wander or cross occasionally.

He or she will be able to track a moving object (though they may already have been able to do this for brief periods since birth). They prefer black and white or highly contrasting patterns. They prefer the human face to all other patterns.

2 months

Starting at two months and continuing through to four months of age, colors start to become clearer to your baby. As a result, he or she will probably begin to show a preference for bright primary colors, and more detailed and complicated designs and shapes.

4 months

Sometime around four months, your baby will begin to develop depth perception. They will also be gaining better control over their arms, so this new visual development milestone comes at just the right time to help them grab for things such as your hair, glasses, earrings, etc., with much more accuracy.

The AAP says only now can your baby distinguish subtle shades of reds, blues, and yellows. Yet favorites among many infants are red and blue.

5 months

At this age, your baby will be getting better at spotting very small objects and tracking moving things. So, if you drop something on the floor, you had better find it, or the baby will.

He or she may even be able to recognize an object, after seeing only part of it. We will talk more about this in the social and emotional chapter, but this is the basis for hide-and-seek.

Most five-month-olds have already learned to distinguish between similar bold colors, and now they will begin to sort out subtle differences in pastels.

8 months

At 8 months, your baby will see the world almost as well as an adult does.

Your little one has developed full-color vision. Distance vision has matured, as has the ability to track a moving object. Your baby's vision is almost as good as an adult, in clarity and depth perception.

Though their short-range sight will still be better than their long-range sight at 8 months of age, their vision will be good enough to recognize people and objects across the room.

Developmental milestones

Below I will describe the average milestones at each age. It is important that you watch your child for one full month. This allows you to take into account any days when your child may be acting differently, sick, or upset. Sometimes children will be so focused on one area of development that they lose focus on another for a short period of time. For example, when working on a new large motor skill, they may not be as verbal and vice versa. It is also important to keep in mind that *milestones are only guidelines*. Every child develops at his/her own pace.

Some babies may develop more slowly in certain areas than children of the same age and, conversely, some may be ahead in other areas. There is a great deal of normal variation in developmental milestones in healthy babies.

Do not be overly concerned if your child is not meeting all the milestones at each age.

Jot things down and bring them up at your next well visit. Your pediatrician will help you decide if there is something to worry about, or something you need to work on.

Your newborn

During the first week or two, your newborn's movements will be jerky and uncoordinated. As their nervous system matures and muscle control improves, the shakes and quivers will become smoother movements.

Your newborn will make jerking-like, arm-thrusting movements. He or she will bring their hands within range of their eyes and mouth. Since their movements are not controlled, it is important to keep their nails short.

Your baby will move his or her head from side to side while lying on their stomach.

Their head flops back if unsupported. They hold their hands in tight fists. They have strong reflex movements.

Hearing is fully mature at birth and they recognize sounds. They may even turn toward a familiar voice or sound.

Your baby is very particular about tastes and smells. They will actually breathe deeply and turn towards smells like vanilla, banana, and sugary smells, especially breast milk. Yet your baby does not like unpleasant odors like vinegar or alcohol and will turn their head away and may even cry. By the end of the first week, babies will turn toward their own mother's breast pad and will ignore breast pads from other nursing mothers.

Newborns are also particular about sensations on their skin and, like most of us, prefer soft over coarse fabrics.

Warning signs

Notify the doctor if, during the 2–4th week:

1. Your baby seems to be feeding slowly or sucking poorly.
2. Your baby does not blink or seem bothered by bright light or doesn't focus on a nearby object or face.
3. Your baby rarely moves his or her arms or legs.
4. They seem very stiff or excessively floppy or loose.
5. Their lower jaw trembles constantly even when not crying or excited and this does not stop with sucking.
6. Your baby is not bothered or does not respond to loud noises.

Your 1-month-old:

By the end of the fourth week of life, your baby should be able to lift their head briefly when lying on their stomach, or on your chest.

They should be very interested in your face, and stare fascinated for periods of time.

He or she should calm down when you speak to him/her gently and hold him/her upright against your shoulder.

It is possible that your baby may make an "ah" sound when he or she sees your face, or hears you speak.

The chin may still quiver and the hands may still tremble, but by the end of the first month, the nervous system is starting to mature, and this happens less and less each day.

During the first month, your baby starts to smile while sleeping. By the end of the first month, your baby may smile when awake.

Your 2-month-old:

By the end of 8 weeks, your baby is starting to settle into recognizable eating and sleeping patterns.

At two months of age, your baby may be cooing, grunting, and gurgling, and making humming sounds, to express their feelings. He or she may even be able to make vowel sounds, such as "ah" and "oh".

He or she may be able to smile when you smile.

They should be able to lift their head at a 45-degree angle when lying on their stomach, for short periods of time.

Your baby recognizes the breast or bottle and gets very excited when they are hungry.

Your baby should be able to keep his or her head up when held in a sitting position, with only occasional head bobs.

Your baby stays awake for longer periods during the day and is more alert.

Your little one is learning to self soothe, and quiets down on their own. They soothe themselves by sucking on fingers, or a pacifier.

Your 3-month-old:

Your baby can raise their chest and head when on their tummy.

They can support their upper body with their arms when they are lying on their stomach. They stretch out their legs and kick when they are on their back or tummy.

Your baby is beginning to gain more control over their limbs. This is so exciting for them, and they spend much of their time waving their arms and pumping their legs.

Your baby will push down on their legs when they are held up, and their feet are placed on a firm surface.

Your baby can now bring their hands to their mouth with ease and may swipe at a dangling object like an activity gym, as they start using hands and eyes in coordination.

They have the ability to grasp and shake hand toys. Your baby can bring their hands together and is challenged by how their hands work. They use a closed fist to bat at a toy or object. Baby's hands should open frequently.

Your baby continues to watch your face intently. They can follow moving objects with their eyes. Your baby is able to recognize familiar objects, and people, at a distance.

They will begin to babble and may begin to imitate sounds. They will start to turn their head in the direction of a sound.

Your baby begins to develop a social smile, and smiles at the sound of your voice. He or she enjoys playing with other people and may cry when the playing stops.

Your baby is becoming more communicative and expressive, with facial expressions and body language, and may imitate some movements and facial expressions.

A three-month-old can lift their head with ease. By the end of this month, they may be able to lift their head up 90 degrees when they are on their stomach. When holding your baby in an upright position, they can support their head for more than a moment.

Your baby may laugh and chuckle. They should make sounds, such as gurgling, cooing, babbling, or other noises, besides crying.

Warning signs: 2–3 months of age

Notify the doctor if, by 2–3 months of age:

1. Your baby is exhibiting the Moro / startle reflex often.
2. Your baby does not respond to loud sounds.
3. Your baby does not notice their hands by two months of age.
4. Your baby does not smile at the sound of your voice by two months.
5. Your baby does not follow moving objects with their eyes by 2–3 months of age.
6. Your baby does not smile at people by three months of age.
7. Your baby cannot support their head well at three months of age.

8. Your baby has trouble moving both eyes or one eye in all directions.

9. Their eyes cross most of the time (occasional crossing of the eyes is normal in the first few months as the muscles are getting stronger).

10. Your baby does not pay attention to new faces or seems very frightened by new faces and/or surroundings.

When your baby is lying on their back, they should move they arms or legs equally well. They should not make jerky or uncoordinated movements with one or both arms or legs. They should also not use one arm all the time.

Your baby should respond to your voice.

Your 4-month-old:

By four months of age, your baby should be able to hold their head steady, in all directions, when you pull your baby up by their arms.

Your baby is beginning to realize that they influence the world around them, and will try to figure out how actions affect each other.

By the end of this month, they may be able to roll from stomach to back and may even be able to roll from back to stomach.

Your baby explores by putting all objects within reach in their mouth.

Your baby is very oral, and they will drool almost constantly. However, they may not be "teething" yet.

Your baby is developing hand-eye coordination and will attempt to reach and bat at objects, but often misses their target.

Your baby is endlessly fascinated by their hands and possibly feet too.

Warning signs: 4 months of age

Notify the doctor if, by 4 months of age:

1. Your baby does not reach for objects or toys.
2. Your baby cannot grasp hold of an object or toy.
3. Your baby does not babble.
4. Your baby does not bring objects to their mouth.
5. Your baby begins babbling but does not try to imitate any of your sounds.
6. Your baby does not push down with their legs when their feet are placed on a flat surface, like a tabletop, while holding the baby upright.
7. Your baby does not turn to look for a sound.

Your 5-month-old:

Your baby's large motor skills are improving, and the large muscle groups are getting them ready for sitting and crawling.

Even more than just a month ago, due to increased hand-eye coordination, your five-month-old will use their mouth to explore everything. They can easily bring objects to their mouth for exploration.

By the end of this month, they may be able to lift both arms and legs while they are on their stomach. I call this the "Superman" pose.

They love to make sounds. One new trick many babies learn is how to make or blow raspberries with their mouth (if you have started solids this can be particularly fun at mealtimes, LOL).

They can now roll over in one direction, usually front to back first.

They continue to be endlessly amused by playing with their hands and feet.

Warning signs: 5 months of age

Notify the doctor if, by 5 months of age:

1. Your baby does not roll in either direction.
2. Your baby seems inconsolable at night.
3. Your baby does not smile spontaneously.

Your 6-month-old:

Your baby can now roll from front to back and back to front.

When you hold your baby under their arms, they are not only able to push down on their feet, but they can bear some weight on their legs, readying the muscles for standing on their own. When your baby is on their stomach, they can support their weight on outstretched hands.

Your baby's visual acuity is improving, and they can see small objects. So, pick up those dropped items, as your little one will see them and investigate by putting them in their mouth.

Your baby is increasingly able to express their feelings, especially positive ones about you. Your little one may snuggle up against you in your lap, or they may raise their arms to be picked up. The best part is that they reserve the best smiles for you alone.

Sitting up gives them a whole new view of the world.

By the end of this month, they may be able to sit independently, and they may fuss when bored and want to be moved to a new activity. They may fuss wanting to be moved to various activities (or "stations", as I call them).

Your baby has the ability to hold their own bottle. Now you notice I say "ability", this is because, even though they can, many won't. They would prefer to just let Mom or Dad do it. Remember though, that the bottle belongs to you. Don't allow them to take it to bed with them, even if they can hold it themselves.

Your little one may begin to pass objects from one hand to the other.

Your baby continues to babble and imitate sounds and you might hear word-like sounds such as "ba", "ma", "ga" and other consonant-vowel combinations.

Your baby may start to show their strong attachment to you when you leave the room (separation anxiety may start).

Your baby turns towards sounds and voices, even those that originate out of their immediate area.

Your baby continues to make fun noises with their mouth and may start to blow spit bubbles.

Warning signs: 6 months of age

Notify the doctor if, by 6 months of age:

1. Your baby cannot sit with help or being propped up.

2. Your baby does not laugh / giggle or make squealing noises.

3. Your baby does not actively try to reach for objects.

Your 7-month-old:

If your baby has not begun already, teething begins in earnest.

Now, drooling excessively and putting things in their mouth may have started as early as four months of age, but most babies get their first teeth at six months of age and "teething" truly begins in earnest.

Teeth typically come in two at a time. Expect the two front bottom teeth first. Not all babies find the experience painful.

When your baby gets their first teeth is genetic. If you or your spouse were "late" getting your teeth, then your child may be "late" too. My kiddos were "late." My kids got their first tooth at 10 ½ months and 11 ½ months respectively. More on teeth in the dental chapter.

By the end of this month, they may be able to stand with support. Usually this is standing at the couch, coffee table, or in the crib. * As soon as your child is able to stand while holding onto something like the crib or couch your crib should be lowered to the lowest position if it isn't already.

Your baby should be able to push up onto their hands and knees readying them for crawling, if they are not doing it yet. Many babies use rolling over to move about the room.

Your baby should be able to sip from a two-handled cup with your assistance. (I like the Nuby brand and the Munchkin brand Miracle 360° Trainer Cup.)

Your baby should be able to sit without support.

Your little one reaches for things with a sweeping motion. This is different from the pincer grasp that will come later. This is more of a raking motion, sweeping food into the palm of the hand.

Your baby is imitating more and more speech-like sounds in their babble. When you hear any babble that sounds like a word, repeat it and, if possible, show your baby that object. For example, "ba" may be "ball" or "bottle". Let them know that sounds are words with meaning.

Warning signs: 7 months of age

Notify the doctor if, by 7 months of age:

1. Your baby seems very stiff with very tight muscles.
2. Your baby does not cuddle or relax.
3. Your baby seems very floppy like a rag doll and their muscles do not seem tight or strong enough.
4. Your baby's head still flops back when you pull your baby up to a sitting position by their arms.
5. Your baby only reaches with one hand all the time.
6. Your baby does not show affection for the person who cares for them.
7. Your baby does not seem to enjoy being around people and this is not a new behavior.
8. One or both eyes consistently turn in or out. One or both eyes are persistently tearing or constantly have eye discharge.
9. Your baby seems to have light sensitivity.
10. Your baby does not respond to sounds around them.

11. Your baby does not follow objects with both eyes at near (1 ft) and far (6 ft) ranges.

Your 8-month-old:

By the end of this month, they are getting more proficient at finger feeding and drop less and get more in their mouth.

Your baby is very interested in how and why things happen, so they may look for dropped objects. Your little one will often repeat this behavior over and over again.

They can pull themselves up to a standing position.

They may use their index finger to point to things.

They use a combination of a pincer grasp and a raking motion to pick up food. For example: Your baby may use a finger to rake a piece of cereal and then pick it up with their fist.

Your baby ventures away from you, becoming more independent, but because they do not quite realize they are separate beings, they get upset when you are not visible or following behind them.

Your baby can find a partially hidden object, and this can be the basis of new types of play.

Frustrations may emerge and may be a powerful tool, as your little one may struggle to get objects just out of reach.

Warning signs: 8 months of age

Notify the doctor if, by 8 months of age:

1. Your baby does not babble.
2. Your baby does not seem interested in games such peek-a-boo.

Your 9-month-old:

As your little one is getting closer to walking, your 9-month-old may push up on all fours, with a combo of crawling and walking (I call this the "crab walk"). At the end of this month, they may be able to crawl upstairs, not down. This is something to be mindful of from a safety standpoint.

Your baby may say "mama" or "dada".

Your baby enjoys water play.

Your baby lets their pleasures and displeasures be known and may object if you try to take a toy away.

Your little one may take a few steps with your support.

Your baby responds to whispers and turns when they sense someone is approaching.

Your baby can sit without the support of their hands to hold them up.

They creep or crawl on their hands and knees.

They continue to combine syllables into word-like sounds.

They stand while holding onto something.

Your baby may begin to play with their toys in new and creative ways or be more interested in their toys than before.

Your 10-month-old:

Your baby is becoming more mobile by the day.

Most babies will begin walking between 9 and 15 months (they are not delayed unless they are not walking by 18 months).

Typically, your 10-month-old is an expert crawler.

They will pull themselves up to a standing position and then cruise around furniture, holding on and occasionally letting go.

Your 10-month-old understands simple requests and phrases. They may say words like "mama" and "dada."

Your baby is becoming more curious about how things work and may start using toys in new ways.

Your child can use a pincer grasp to pick up objects.

Your baby can sign basic signs, if you have been teaching sign language, and waves "hi" and "bye."

Your child may shake their head to say "no."

Your baby recognizes their own name and looks when called.

They have very specific preferences.

Your 11-month-old:

Your baby is becoming increasingly mobile and may start to take a few steps on their own if they have not already. They will first start by letting go with one hand and then letting go for longer periods of time. (You can encourage walking by giving them toys to walk behind.)

Your baby has rhythm and loves to bounce to the beat. They may even babble sounds as if singing to songs.

Your little one is so curious and loves games like hide-and-seek with their toys.

Their vocabulary and comprehension are increasing every day. They use their two words frequently. It is usually "mama" and "dada" but in my house, it was "dada" and "dog".

Some advanced talkers may have an extra word or two.

They understand far more, however, than they can speak and can follow simple directions like, "Can you bring mommy the ball?"

Your 12-month-old:

Your little one enjoys imitating others in both play and everyday activities.

Your 12-month-old is a jabber box and loves to chatter.

Your baby uses gestures regularly and is helpful with dressing.

If you have taught your infant sign language, they are getting very good at signing.

Your child may take several steps unassisted.

Your child uses objects correctly.

They can drink out of a cup and brush their hair with a hairbrush.

Your child's comprehension with reading is improving and they can look and point at the correct image when stated.

Your child may imitate gestures.

Warning signs at 12 months of age

Notify the doctor if your child is not yet crawling by 12 months.

Walking

Learning to walk is related to an infant's physical maturity and not linked to intelligence, verbal skills, or fine motor skills.

Although you can encourage your child to walk by buying them push toys and toys they can pull, your child will not learn to walk until he or she is physically ready.

Most babies begin around their first birthday. Do not worry, your baby is not considered delayed unless they are not walking by 18 months.

Babies should never be put in a walker as they present serious safety risks and babies who use them are often reluctant to learn to walk. Push cars and toys, however, are great.

Shoes can make it harder for a baby who is first learning to walk. It is best for them to learn on bare feet. If walking outside, choose a pair of flexible shoes with nonskid soles. Soft Robeez are a great shoe for new walkers.

Feet at this age will seem flat because the arch is hidden by a pad of fat. You do not need to invest in shoes with arch support, as the arch will not even be evident for 2–3 more years, when the fat pad disappears.

Communication

Again, each child has great variation in all aspects of healthy development, including speech. Each baby develops at their own pace. It is important not to compare your baby with others. This is meant to be a timetable for "average norms."

It is incredibly important to remember that children generally understand far more than they are able to articulate. The fine motor skills needed for speech come after large motor skills.

Girls seem to develop the ability to communicate earlier than boys. In Jill Stamm's book, *Bright from the Start*, she explains that baby girls have denser cells in the area of the brain needed for language earlier than boys, so genetically, it makes sense that girls would have a verbal advantage earlier than boys.

Language can develop smoothly and continuously, or in jumps and spurts. Every child is unique in his or her own development and may progress at different rates than other babies the same age.

Your baby may lag behind the "average rate of communication" at some points but as long as he or she produces syllables with consonants, such as "ba" or "da," by 10 months and doesn't suddenly lose the ability to babble once he or she has gained it, experts say there is no need to worry.

Communication

Long before a baby can talk, he/she can communicate effectively. A 6-month-old's babbling is asking you to pay attention to him.

Typical milestones of speech

@ 7 days of age: An infant can distinguish their mother's voice from another woman's voice.

@ 2 weeks of age: They can distinguish their father's voice from another man's voice.

1–4 months: Smiles, frowns, laughs, and coos, vowel sounds "ooh," "aah," recognizes sound of own name.

@ 3 months of age: An infant can make vowel sounds.

@ 6–8 months of age: The infant has added a few consonant sounds to the vowel sounds and they may say "mama," "dada," and "baba" but they do not yet attach them to the individual. This will not occur until about 12 months.

"Your Little Genius" article from *Parents*, November 1999, by Kelly King Alexander

"At six months, babies are several months away from saying "mommy" and "daddy." But a new study by researchers at Johns Hopkins University suggests that they may actually understand what the words mean. Previous research showed that infants are not able to link words to objects such as "ball" and "cup" until around 9 to 12 months of age, says Peter Juscyzk, PhD, professor of psychology and cognitive science and co-author of the study. But he and other researchers wondered whether babies might be able to identify their parents, with whom they have a stronger bond than with any other object, by language at an earlier age. To find out, they tested 24 infants. Each of the six-month-olds sat on a parent's lap facing two television monitors. One screen showed a videotape of their mother and the other screen played a tape of their father in 10 second intervals. A synthesized gender-neutral voice called out either "mommy" or "daddy" and the infants looked longer at the parent being named. Since it's not uncommon for babies who are learning to talk to use one word for entire categories, like dog to refer to all four-legged creatures, the researchers did another test in which they included videos of unfamiliar men and women to make sure the infants weren't linking the word "mommy" with all women and "daddy" with all men. Once again, the babies proved how smart they are: They looked longer at the videos of their mom and dad than at those of strangers, so even if your baby's first spoken word turns out to be "ball" or "cup" remember: You came first."

How to stimulate language development and communication

<u>0–3 months</u>

Talk to your baby as much as possible.

Talk to them as you are doing routine things, such as dressing, feeding, changing, bathing, so the words can be learned in context.

Talk to your baby while you are doing things around the house.

Children must first receive language before they can repeat language. The more you talk to them, the more they will understand at an earlier age.

Imitate your baby's cooing and jabbering sounds. Let them know that words have meaning and the sounds they make can be repeated.

Let your baby hear as many different sounds as possible.

At this age, your baby is communicating his or her needs through crying. Remember, this is their only means of communication and you cannot spoil babies at this age, so respond promptly to your baby's cries and try to figure out what each different cry means. Your little one associates mom's and dad's voice with comfort, and you can calm them with talking soothingly.

Cuddle your baby and smile back when they smile at you.

Sing to your little one.

Read to your baby.

<u>3–12 months</u>

Continue to talk frequently to your baby and continue to use speech with daily activities, in the proper context.

Continue to repeat any sounds or word-like sounds your baby makes during babble. Encourage the babbling and if you hear a word-like sound in the babble, try to get them to repeat it.

Although it is important for them to hear various sounds, it is also important to provide some quiet time when there is silence in the home too.

If you hear a sound, draw attention to it and talk to your baby about what that sound was.

<u>Below are some communication milestones from the American Academy of Pediatrics you can expect by 7 months of age:</u>

Your baby responds to his or her own name.

He or she begins to respond to the word "no."

He or she can distinguish emotions by the tone of your voice.

Your baby may respond to sound by making noise of their own.

He or she may use their voice to express joy and displeasure.

Your baby babbles in chains of consonants.

Here are some language milestones from the American Academy of Pediatrics you can expect between 8 and 12 months:

Your baby is paying increased attention to speech.

He or she responds to verbal cues.

He or she understands and responds to the word "no."

Your baby uses simple gestures such as shaking his or her head for "no."

Typically says two words such as "mama" and "dada."

He or she may use a phrase or exclamation such as "uh oh."

Your baby tries to imitate words.

At 12 months your baby says 1–2 words and understands 25 or more words.

At 12 months they will attach "mama" or "dada" to the right person.

They can respond to one-step commands such as "give that to me."

Between 11 and 14 months your little one understands 50 words or more.

At 15 months your toddler will continue to string vowel and consonant sounds together. It may sound like mostly gibberish, yet you may find imbedded real words in that gibberish. They also may be able to say as many as 10 words.

Between 15 and 18 months they really begin to enjoy language games: Where is mommy? Where are your toes, your ears, etc. Sing songs like "head, shoulders, knees, and toes," "this little piggy," etc.

I like the little poem "you can see your fingers and you can see your toes; you can see your belly, but you cannot see your nose." Touching each body part as you go.

Before 18 months children learn approximately 1–2 words per week.

However, at 18 months an explosion in vocabulary occurs. Between 18 and 21 months a child may learn as many as nine words per day

They may add gestures to speech between 18 and 24 months and may be able to follow a two-step command, e.g., "go to the toy box and get your bunny."

Sometime between 18 and 24 months they may form simple sentences like "Daddy go."

They can finally have a conversation, well sort of ☺

The downside is their vocabulary will take a while to catch up with their comprehension. So, keep up the sign language, along with the verbal skills, to help decrease frustrations.

Sign language as a means of communication

Many experts feel that teaching an infant and toddler sign language can give young children verbal and cognitive advantages. Yet no one knows if these benefits are permanent. Some articles say teaching your baby sign language can increase their IQ.

I feel the best reason for teaching sign language is to make kids happier by helping them express themselves before they can speak. I feel sign language decreases frustration. The cognitive advantages and possible increase in IQ are just a bonus.

Literature says teaching infants and toddlers to sign improves behavior that is related to frustration. I truly believe this and have firsthand knowledge with Dylan. Once we taught him sign language, his tantrums almost disappeared.

The biggest concern I hear in my parenting classes is that parents are concerned that signing might delay speech.

"This is not the case. In fact, research shows that using signs with young children increases a child's verbal skills. Research has shown that using sign language does not negatively impact a child's language development and does the opposite up to about age four. " https://eiclearinghouse.org/articles/simple-signs/ There are deaf parents that have hearing children that learn both verbally and non-verbally with no delay.

From a developmental standpoint, signing is easier, as it uses large muscle control. Gross motor movements are easier to achieve. They develop long before articulation which requires fine motor skills, because babies have control over their hands long before they develop the fine motor skills required for speech. Sign language can be taught to infants as young as seven months old, while they are also learning to speak.

Babies are already signaling and signing with gestures (waving "hi" and "bye") and facial expressions (giving air kisses).

You are just modifying those gestures to a common one that everyone can understand.

I suggest using books or a website that teaches American Sign Language as it is recognized as an actual language and is universally understood.

You are actually teaching your child a second language. When we were teaching Dylan sign language, Taylor was watching and learning quickly. She picked up the signs at five years of age, just as quickly as Mom and Dad. In high school she took sign language for four semesters and was so good at signing that her teacher tried to convince her to become an ASL interpreter. Her senior year philanthropy project was teaching sign language to preschoolers at Arizona State University three times a week for a semester. To this day, she teaches sign language to her third grade class. They do the Pledge of Allegiance in sign language every day. I believe it was those early neural pathways she created when we taught Dylan sign language as an infant, and she in turn learned it too, that made sign language come so easy for her.

For information on how to teach your baby simple signs, visit the animated American Sign Language dictionary at www.handspeak.com or sign with your baby at www.sign2me.com. There is also a book, Sign with your Baby.

Your infant's memory

Dr. Carolyn Rovee-Collier, PhD, professor at Rutgers University in New Jersey, states that, despite the old belief that infants have poor memory prior to about 8 or 9 months, scientists who have spent the past decade researching infants' memory found that infants have both well-formed and specific memory.

She feels that, just because a baby cannot remember right away, it does not mean it is lost and gone forever. It is just that babies use their memory in practical ways to make sense of the world. Their memory may just need a bit of a gentle reminder.

She did an interesting experiment with 8-week-old babies. She tied a string to a baby's foot and attached it to a mobile, so when the infant kicked, the mobile would move.

When the experiment was set up identically to how it was a few days prior, the babies remembered how to play the game for several days. However, if anything was changed, even one animal on the mobile, or the crib had a different color bumper pad in it, the babies couldn't remember how to make the mobile move, even the next day.

She said it is almost as if babies take a mental snapshot of their surroundings.

She feels this may be why infants have a more difficult time with long-term memory than adults, because their perspective of the world is constantly changing as they grow. They see the world from a different perspective every time they grow. She compares this to an adult going back to your old kindergarten classroom. Even if the room was set up exactly the same as it was when you were five, it would seem smaller to you as an adult because you are larger, and your perspective has changed. This could be what is happening with your infant as they grow month to month. Even a slight change in perspective may be enough to not trigger the memory.

Another study I read about was conducted by Dr. Meltzoff in 1994. He took six-week-old babies and had them imitate him when he stuck his tongue out at them. The babies would copy him by sticking their tongue out at him, mimicking his behavior.

When Dr. Metzoff greeted the babies with an expressionless face when he returned the next day, the babies remembered him from the day before. They remembered the game and stuck their tongue out at him, but not when they saw other people who entered the room. However, after 48 hours, the sight of the man's face did not trigger the babies to stick out their tongue. Their memory seemed to be only 24 hours.

One way to help your little one remember, especially a relative that lives far away, is to offer reminders. You can show them a picture from time to time over increasingly longer time spans. This will act as a trigger for the memory. Initially you may show the photo to your little one every day. Then begin to stretch it out to every other day, then once a week, and eventually longer. By the time your baby is one year old, a short two-minute reminder is enough to keep a memory going for a few months. FaceTime can also be a helpful way to keep a loved one memorable.

Baby's age	Memory (long-term memory without a reminder)
6 weeks	24 hours
3 months	1 week
6 months	2 weeks
9 months	6 weeks
12 months	2 months
16 months	4 months

Sources used in this chapter include:

T. Berry Brazelton

www.babycenter.com

Ross Laboratories

AAP – American Academy of Pediatrics

Remember: Try not to be too anxious about "typical developmental milestones." Your baby is as unique as a snowflake. Just as no two snowflakes are identical, neither will two children develop in the exact same way, on the exact same clock. They will develop at their own pace. If you are concerned, bring it up with your pediatrician and then listen to their advice. Chances are, if they are "behind" in a skill, it is because they are mastering another one. I know it is easier said than done but it is one piece of advice I wish I had listened to more when my kids were little. It sure would have saved me a lot of needless and unnecessary worry.

CHAPTER 11

SAFETY

"I think, at a child's birth, if a mother could ask a fairy godmother to endow it with the most useful gift, that gift would be curiosity."

— *Eleanor Roosevelt*

If you haven't yet taken an infant-toddler CPR class, you should. In addition, anyone watching your child should take a CPR class.

Some accidents that may require CPR include

Drowning

Electric shock

Suffocation

Severe allergic reaction

Accidental poisoning

Choking / respiratory arrest leading to cardiac arrest

Preventable injuries are the number one killer of kids in the US.

Approximately 26 million children are injured in the home each year.

Accidents in the home are a greater cause of death to children than all childhood diseases combined.

Every day 100 children die of avoidable accidents in homes across United States.

Every month nearly 400 children under the age of four die in the US due to accidents.

Top choking hazards

Foods and objects can cause suffocation via blockage of the airway. I have listed 9 foods that are most often listed as top choking hazards:

Hot dogs and meat sticks (make sure to cut lengthwise and you may want to take the skin off).

Grapes (peel and dice and buy seedless).

Nuts (just avoid whole nuts for a while, as they are hard to chew up easily).

Raw carrots (they should be steamed and cut lengthwise, not in disks).

Hard candy and gum (they are too easy to swallow whole).

Popcorn (if you give popcorn to a young child, only give the white fluffy part and not the kernel).

Peanut butter (only give a small smear such as on a thin cracker not in a glob).

Apples (cut into pieces, peeled, and you may need to steam the pieces first).

Marshmallows are dangerous at all ages. I watched a show where a teenager died playing a game called "chubby bunny." She was putting as many marshmallows as possible in her mouth while still trying to say the words "chubby bunny." One marshmallow slipped down her throat and even though 911 was called, they could not perform the Heimlich maneuver because the marshmallow had become moist and swollen in the throat and the paramedics were not even able to intubate this child as it was too gooey and sticky to get an airway. I was so upset by this story, and it had such a profound impact on me, that I did not let my kids have marshmallows until they were much older. To this day, if you were to ask them the rules around marshmallows, they would tell you, "only one at a time."

Balls and small toys should be at least 1 ¾ inch in diameter.

The general rule is you should not give an infant or toddler anything small enough to pass through a toilet paper roll.

Some common choking hazards:

Coins, buttons, beads, balls, marbles, broken crayons, jewelry, nails, thumb tacks, pins, paper clips, pen caps, screws, hair clips, bottle caps, balloons, plastic bags, pieces of plastic, and button batteries (each year, 2,800 kids are treated in the ER for swallowing a button battery, that is one child every 3 hours [more on this to come]).

As we discussed in the sleep lecture, avoid anything in the crib, especially stuffed animals if the eyes or nose are removable.

Remove all ribbons and, if a toy has a squeaker or rattle, make sure your child cannot get it out.

There is a new product on the market that I think every parent should have with them at all times in their home or in their diaper bag. You might just buy two. It is called the LifeVac®. I bought one for my home, one for my daughter's classroom, and one for my son who is away at college. When I gave the one to my son, I said, "now I know you are probably going to think your mom is crazy, as you are an adult." He said, "no mom, there was a kid at a fraternity party choking, and someone's mom had given another kid a LifeVac. He had it in his car, so he ran out and got it and it took two depressions of the suction, but it saved that choking kid's life." He said, "thanks, I think it is a good thing to have. I know it works."

My daughter choked on raisins when she was about 18 months old. I had never given her raisins, but my grandmother bought one of those tiny little boxes and we were feeding her in her portable highchair, one at a time, watching her like a hawk, when all of a sudden you could tell she was choking. No sound was coming out and she was bright red. Now my kids, both being preemies, did not hit 20 lbs. until they were two, so luckily, she was tiny. I flipped her upside down and gave her a whack between her shoulder blades. Nothing happened. So, I did it again, this time much harder, and I swear the entire box of raisins came shooting out in one big wad. She had been storing them all up in her little chubby baby chipmunk cheeks. It was one of the scariest moments of my life.

The LifeVac has two sizes, child size and adult size. If you use the device, they will replace the mask for free. Now that is customer service! It does not have to be a child that chokes. One of my friends from high school recently passed away after choking on a shrimp while out at a restaurant. If someone had had a LifeVac, which I believe every restaurant should have, she would still be here today.

Poisonings

There are more than one million reported poisonings each year affecting children less than five years of age.

Remember that kids investigate their world through their senses, one being taste.

They will put anything and everything in their mouth!

Some common household poisons:

Cosmetics: nail polish / remover, and lipstick

All cleaning products

Medicines

Topical lotions, menthol rubs, etc.

Dishwasher detergent / pods

Laundry detergent / pods (in a year, 700 children under the age of five are hospitalized or experience serious effects from liquid laundry or detergent packets, averaging one per day).

Pesticides

Vitamins

Baby powder (don't keep baby powder on your changing table or within the baby's reach. Baby powder can get into your baby's lungs and is very toxic when inhaled as it coats the inside of the lungs).

Air fresheners

Alcohol both in products and drinking form (children can get alcohol poisoning from things other than alcoholic beverages, such as cologne, liquid baking extracts, mouthwash, hair products, etc.).

Batteries (small button batteries are the worst).

Fertilizers and lawn products

Gas

Lighter fluid

Plants (inside and out)

Here are just a few dangerous plants:

House:

Caladium, dumbcane, elephant ear, holly, philodendron, pathos

Flower / garden:

Azalea, crocus, lily of the valley, larkspur, oleander, daffodils, foxgloves, and many wild mushrooms can be fatal.

Veg / garden:

Tomato leaves, rhubarb leaves, potato sprouts.

Others include:

Cherry tree

Dieffenbachia

Hemlock

Ivy

Jimson Weed

Amaryllis

Teach your children never to put any plants, leaves, berries, mushrooms, or flowers in their mouth.

What to do in the event of a poisoning?
Poison helpline

If you suspect your child has ingested something, look for spilled medication, any potential burns around the mouth, or a funny odor to their breath.

1. Locate the substance and remove any that might be left in child's mouth with your finger, making sure not to push it further into their mouth.
2. Call Poison Control.
3. Don't give anything by mouth until you speak with Poison Control.
4. Give them a description of the ingested toxin, the age and weight of the child and the approximate time it was ingested.

Poison Control number – poison helpline 1800 222-1222

In most cases, Poison Control will tell you a glass of milk or water is enough to dilute the poisonous substance and soothe an irritated stomach but, again, wait for Poison Control to give you that advice before giving your child anything to eat or drink if you suspect an ingestion of something toxic or foreign.

One in six ingestions involve a grandparent's meds.

There are five types of medications that necessitate an immediate ER visit if your child ingests this category of medication:

1. Coumadin or blood thinners
2. Heart medication
3. Blood pressure medication
4. Medication to regulate blood sugar such as metformin/insulin
5. Pills containing iron

A good friend of mine's child ingested her grandmother's insulin pill. When she called Poison Control, they told her to take her to the hospital immediately, where she was admitted to the ICU to monitor her blood sugar. They came in every 30 minutes through the night to check her blood sugar. They told Mom that when it dropped, it would literally drop to almost nothing, and if the baby was not in the hospital to correct the blood sugar, she would have just slipped away in her sleep. The fix was simply juice when it did drop. The baby was OK and had no long-term side effects from the event.

We had a child in our practice years ago when I was a new RN, who ingested the dog's heart medication that the dog didn't swallow. The family gave the dog daily medicine wrapped in cheese. One day the dog ate the cheese and left the pill, and the baby picked it up and ate it. They rushed the infant into the office, and we had this baby on oxygen and rushed her to the ER next door. It was a very scary situation. Every time I gave my dog a pill from that day on, I made sure she took it. It was a valuable lesson for me, and I share the story with my parents, so this doesn't happen to them.

Inhaled poisons

Such as gases or vapors. Immediately get the child out in fresh air and ventilate the house by opening doors and windows. Call poison control.

Poison on the skin

Remove all clothing and anything else that may be contaminated from contact. Flood the skin for at least 15 minutes with lukewarm water, then wash the skin with soap and water. The best way to do this is to bring your child into the shower and undress them in there with the water running. Call Poison Control.

Poison in the eye

Flood the eye with lukewarm water for 15 minutes. Do not force the eye/s open. It is best if your baby continues to blink under the water. Again, with young children, it is easiest to put your child under the shower. Call Poison Control.

Nobody expects an accident to happen. I teach these classes every year and I had to call Poison Control once for each child. My daughter got into toothpaste when she was a toddler when I was in the shower and my son ate lip balm he got out of my purse. Kids are cleverer and quicker than you think, especially active toddlers.

Childproofing

Here are some childproofing ways to prevent accidents from happening.

My advice is to get down on the floor and look around at their eye level.

You can also pick rooms where you might choose to go crazy childproofing and others that may remain off-limits to the child, for example, a guest room or formal dining room may remain off-limits with a shut door or a baby gate.

There are companies that will come out and childproof the entire house for you or point out things that they think should be done. Then you can pick and choose which things you feel you can do on your own and which things you would like a professional to do.

Now this is not an all-encompassing list. Everyone's home is different. This is just meant to get you started and thinking.

Install latches on the cupboards and drawers in the bathroom, as well as in the kitchen. My husband did our cabinets on his own. He is pretty handy, and this saved us quite a bit of money. We used the magnetic, TotLok brand by Safety 1st. I personally would recommend only using the magnetic type of child locks, as the others are subpar and children can figure them out. This lock does require drilling into the back of your cabinet, but you cannot see it from the outside and the lock can be engaged or disengaged at any time.

Do not store razors, medicines, cosmetics, or anything that could be a danger to your child in the medicine cabinet unless you can lock it, as your child can climb up on the counter and open it up.

Put your trash cans up and out of reach or locked in a cabinet. Many people throw dangerous things in their garbage, like used razors and open cans etc., so, lock the can up.

Install toilet locks that stay on the toilet. If you purchase the kind that has to be taken off and put on each time, you will eventually get lazy and forget to put it back on.

Get a cushion to cover the faucet in the bathtub to protect against injury and burns.

Keep all makeup out of reach and locked in your drawer or cabinet.

Keep toothpaste out of reach and locked in your drawer or cabinet.

Unplug all household appliances in the kitchen and bathroom when not in use. Many burns occur with curling irons.

Turn panhandles in all the time. Children will climb and often use oven drawers and doors to climb on. If your oven door does not have a lock, buy an oven door lock.

Your oven should be secured to the wall with a no-tip bracket.

Putting window locks on all upstairs and even downstairs windows would not be a bad idea.

Make sure your water heater is set no higher than 120 degrees.

Make sure all bottles have safety caps and put all medication in a locked cabinet.

Appliance latches on all appliance doors, such as the oven, fridge, dishwasher, and trash compactor.

Put away fridge magnets.

Use electrical wire covers or cord-aways for dangerous cords.

Use a power strip cover and switch blockers.

If you have a climber you may want to look into a crib tent to help prevent your child from climbing out of the crib, or pets (like cats) climbing in. My son started crawling out of his crib around 10 months of age even with the crib in the lowest position. I should have known he was going to be a gymnast. I had to get a crib tent for him to prevent him from falling out on his head or running around unsupervised when we were sleeping.

Replace any of your doorstops that have rubber ends with one-piece doorstops. You may also want to use hinged doorstops for heavy doors to prevent fingers from being trapped.

Get a valve cover for your gas fireplace if you do not already have one.

Use straps for your washer and dryer to attach them to the wall so they will not tip (no-tip brackets or straps).

No-tip furniture brackets or straps for bookcases and heavy furniture in rooms your child will be in.

If you have a piano in the room your child will be in, make sure you have a lid support for the piano bench.

Do not buy imported wooden toys or games, as there is a risk of the use of lead paint.

Batteries are a choking hazard and dangerous if ingested. Make sure the batteries are in the compartment and that you would need a screwdriver to get it open.

Keep remote controls up and out of reach.

Plastic bags are a big suffocation hazard. Be careful with dry cleaning bags on clothes. Children love to crawl around in the closet so remove dry cleaning bags prior to putting them in the closet.

For your baby's bedding, if the sheet comes off easily when you pull on the sides or corners, do not use it! It does not fit properly.

Lock up kitchen knives and put silverware like forks and knives and other sharp objects down in the dishwasher. This way, if your child were to pull themselves up to the dishwasher and fall, they would not fall into something sharp.

Dump out the wading pool after each use.

Dump out the ice chest after a party.

Cell phone charging cables

When you unplug your phone from your charging cable, make sure to unplug the charging cable itself as well. This cable, if put in the mouth, can cause a small shock and cause some burning on the tongue or mouth. The cables are supposed to be protected and are not supposed to do this, but if they are damaged in any way this can cause a problem, so unplug them!

Button batteries

Let's talk more about button batteries.

When a coin lithium battery gets stuck in the throat it can severely burn the esophagus in as little as two hours due to saliva triggering a chemical reaction. It is essential if you think your child has swallowed a button battery to go to the ER as soon as possible. Time is of the essence. There are so many places where button batteries can be found. Musical greeting cards, small remotes, car key fobs, garage door openers, flameless candles, calculators, bathroom scales, toys, reading lights, watches, thermometers, hearing aids, flashing jewelry, holiday ornaments, portable video games, pedometers, talking and singing books, plus many more items we may not even think about. I stress this in my class every year and, one year, I had a mom come up to me years after taking my class after she had a second baby. She told me how she had taken her baby to the ER over the weekend, and he had emergency surgery to remove a button battery. She told me he was carrying around a greeting card that played music and the next thing she noticed it was chewed on and the battery was missing. She panicked, remembering my lecture, and told her husband they needed to go to the ER right away. Her husband thought she was overreacting and that they would find the battery. She told me my voice was in the back of her head and she trusted her mama gut (it rarely lets you down) and she insisted they go to the ER. The x-ray showed it was lodged in his esophagus and he had to have an emergency endoscopy to remove it. I do this lecture not to scare parents, although that inevitably happens when we talk about all the things that can happen. Knowledge, however, is power and if you know what to do in an emergency then I have done my job as your teacher.

Remove hood cords and drawstrings on all children's clothing before putting them down for a nap in that item. No buttons or ties on bedclothes, including for naps. Sleepwear is made safe for sleep, however, we often put our kids down for naps in clothes that were not meant for sleep.

Additional safety numbers

One child a month is strangled to death on a looped window cord. Take another look at window cords and make sure they are out of your child's reach. If your child climbs on a piece of furniture and grabs that window cord it should break apart easily.

To order free tassels or tie-backs for your window shades or blinds, call the Window Covering Safety Council on 1(800)506-4636 or at www.windowcoverings.org

4,700 change to 5,100 kids are treated in the ER each year for injuries sustained after falling out of a window. Move furniture away from the window and always keep windows locked. The data were extracted and analyzed by public health researchers at the Center for Injury Research and Policy at Nationwide Children's Hospital in Columbus, Ohio, and their report published in the current issue of *Pediatrics*.

You can go to the Consumer Product Safety Commission on 1(800)638-2772 or at www.cpsc.gov to find out if a product in your home has been recalled.

Another great website is www.safekids.org. This website is dedicated to child safety and has great tips on safety.

Exercise equipment

Nearly 12,000 children are treated each year in the ER for injuries related to exercise equipment. Two thirds of these kids are under five.

Most children hurt their fingers or toes as they were caught in equipment.

70% of those hurt are boys.

Never let a child play with the gears, pulleys, or wheels.

Make sure treadmills have locks and automatic stop mechanisms.

Shopping carts

25,000 children are injured each year by shopping carts. Never let your child ride in the basket. Use the seatbelt when possible, yet this will not help if the cart flips over. Don't push your child near the aisles, as they can grab items off the shelves that are breakable. In addition, grabbing onto the shelves and holding on can cause the cart to tip. Never let a child climb or hang on the grocery cart.

Toy box

Choose a toy box with a support lid that will keep the lid open in any position. Strangulation can occur as well as head trauma and finger injury when a lid slams shut. You also want one that does not close tightly and is easy for toddlers to open, so your infant or toddler does not get trapped inside.

Holiday dangers

During holidays and parties, it is easy to become distracted and it is easier for a child to go unnoticed, get injured, and for an accident to occur.

During the holidays, many children pick up scissors resulting in cuts.

Children are drawn to sparkling lights, brightly colored bulbs, garlands, and ribbons. All these items can be dangerous for a baby or toddler. Ornaments on low branches are dangerous. If you have a tree that is within a child's reach, you might put an eye hook in the ceiling or wall and attach the tree to it with a fishing line, so your child cannot pull the tree on him or herself. Never place strings of lights behind drapes or under or on a carpet.

Many holiday plants are toxic: Holly berries, mistletoe, Christmas cactus, also poinsettias can cause gastrointestinal upset if ingested.

Be careful of holiday tablecloths as infants and toddlers may pull themselves up with it, bringing down hot or heavy dishes.

A hot oven is always a danger during the holidays.

Out in a crowd

When out in public, as soon as your child is able to talk, teach them if someone other than their parent takes them, to yell "help this is not my mommy or daddy!"

Use a safety strap if in a crowded place. Some of you may not agree with me on this one, but I had a rule with the kids. They could ride in the stroller, or if we were in a crowded place, they had to wear their backpack that had a strap attached to my wrist. I did get looks and comments, but my husband and I said we will never regret being overprotective, but we would never forgive ourselves if something happened to our kids that we could have prevented. In crowded spaces like Disney® and SeaWorld, kids can get separated in a matter of seconds.

Pin your cell phone number to your child with your name on it and carry your phone.

Highchairs

Keep your child's highchair far enough back from the table that your child cannot kick off the table and tip the chair backward. *Always* use the straps *and* the tray.

Fire escape plan

If you do not already have a fire escape plan, create one. If you have a two-story house, get some escape ladders. You need fire extinguishers, at least one in the kitchen or a fire blanket. You should also have multiple smoke detectors, carbon monoxide detectors and check the batteries regularly. When your kids are older, do fire drills, so they know what to do in case of an emergency.

Environmental threats
Smoke

Don't smoke. Don't let others smoke in your house or car. Smoke exhaled from a cigarette, pipe, or cigar contains over 4,000 irritants. Even if a person only smokes in one room, those particulates will contaminate the entire house.

Those exposed to secondhand smoke are more likely to suffer from pneumonia, asthma, bronchitis, ear infections, and other respiratory infections.

Lead

If your home or a family member's home was built before 1978, test your home for lead paint hazards. Exposure to lead can have an adverse effect on the brain, central nervous system, blood cells, and kidneys. Leads effects on unborn babies and young children can be severe and include both physical and mental delays, increased behavioral problems, decreased attention spans, and lower IQs. Children are particularly vulnerable because they are crawling around and constantly putting their hands in their mouths and lead is absorbed easily into their system. Even small amounts can have dramatic effects on a developing brain.

For information on lead testing call 1(800)424-lead.

Plumbing that was installed before the 1930s will likely contain lead pipes, which can contaminate drinking water. If you are worried about possible lead in your pipes, call the Safe Drinking Water Hotline on 1(800)426-4791. Hot water tends to build up more lead from pipes than cold water, so let your water run for two minutes until it is cold. You may want to talk to your pediatrician to test your child for lead in their blood if you suspect high risk factors.

Carbon monoxide

Protect against carbon monoxide poisoning by installing a carbon monoxide detector in all sleeping areas. Try to find one that alerts at 15 ppm. Some alarms won't register until they are at 70 ppm for 3 ½ hrs. 15–20 is the first level of carbon monoxide that can affect us.

"Children are more vulnerable to carbon monoxide poisoning than adults," says Sophie Bulk MD, chair of the AAP Committee on Environmental Health, "because young children breathe faster and take in more oxygen per pound of body weight."

So, if children are exposed to carbon monoxide, they will breathe in more per pound of body weight as well. Carbon monoxide is the byproduct of any type of combustion from a fuel-burning source: Gas-fired heating systems and appliances such as dryers or water heaters, charcoal grills, wood-burning furnaces, fireplaces, or anything with an engine, including cars and boats.

In small doses, carbon monoxide can mimic a viral illness like the flu or can mimic seasickness or a hangover. Symptoms of carbon monoxide poisoning may include headache, dizziness, fatigue, nausea, vomiting, chest pain, confusion, irritability, disorientation and impaired judgment, weakness and, in large doses, loss of consciousness, shortness of breath, heart palpitations, coma, and even death.

Check all fuel-burning appliances once per year or as recommended by the manufacturer.

Keep your chimney clean and open the flue.

Never leave your car running in the garage, even if the door is open.

If you are sitting in traffic, do not vent your car into the outside air or keep windows down.

Emergency room doctors treat thousands of patients who fall ill from breathing carbon monoxide fumes every year.

Twenty-five years ago, when I was pregnant with Taylor, my mom bought us a carbon monoxide detector. Our house did not have one, even though we had gas appliances and a wood-burning fireplace. I put it in our laundry room right inside the garage door and right next to the soon-to-be nursery. My husband installed it and the crazy thing kept going off. Not constantly but every now and then, it would alarm. So, I called Mom and asked her to bring the receipt, as I told her we had a broken detector and I wanted to take it back and get a new one. So, she brought over the receipt, and I took it back and exchanged it for a new unit, and would you believe that new one did the same thing. Well, the unit was not faulty. The house was new. I called the gas company just to be safe, and sure enough there was a very small leak from the gas dryer. Thank goodness my mom bought us that detector and we installed it before the baby arrived. We have never been without them since.

Allergens / molds and mildew

Change your air filters each month to prevent mold and dust. Since most people spend most of their time indoors, it is important to minimize exposure to allergens inside as well. You might invest in a HEPA-style air purifier. Humidifiers can build up mold and mildew. High humidity in the air promotes the growth of dust mites and mildew and can exacerbate asthma and allergies. Rinse the basin regularly with a splash of bleach or vinegar. Also, do not add anything to your humidifier such as menthol. There is no proof it works any better than plain water. Also, use only a cool mist humidifier and only during times of illness.

Don't burn candles in the house. Candles will leave a black residue in the air and in your air ducts. I found this out the hard way when I had my ducts cleaned and the kitchen duct where I burned candles had this black residue in it and the man said it is from candles, he sees it all the time. Gross! I now use diffusers with pure essential oils.

Bathrooms can be a breeding ground for allergens, especially mold and mildew. Clean with bleach or vinegar products and keep the bathroom well-lit if possible. Ventilate when cleaning and try to avoid cleaning around your kids.

Change air filters regularly.

Try to prevent mold and dust.

Limit outdoor activity on a day where air pollution is high or on ozone alert days.

Dogs

One million children per year need medical treatment because of dog bites. 75% of bites are to the head or neck.

Bites are often from a dog owned by family or friends. Large dogs cause most bites. Dogs generally bite when threatened, to protect their food, toys, or territory, excited, in pain or irritated. Call your pediatrician if a dog bite breaks the skin. They will probably treat your child with antibiotics. Wash the area well with soap and water and watch for signs and symptoms of infection.

Scorpions

In Arizona, scorpions are a big deal. There are 32 species of scorpion in AZ. All species can sting, causing some pain with little or no swelling or redness. Only one will cause further medical problems though and that is the bark scorpion. The bark scorpion is one of the smaller species of scorpion. The color may vary from light tan to darker brown. It is usually between 1 and 1 ½ inches in length. It lives outside in woodpiles, palm trees, decorative bark, or any cool, dark place, which could be inside your home. (If you are stripping palms expect more scorpions as they often live in the bark.) The bark scorpion is a climber and can climb walls and walk across ceilings. The best indication of the type of scorpion you have been stung by is by the symptoms.

Symptoms that might occur (not all these symptoms will occur in every person):

Immediate local pain, no swelling.

Hypersensitivity to touch at the site of the sting.

Numbness and tingling moving to parts of the body distant from the sting.

Visual disturbances and/or uncoordinated eye movements.

Difficulty swallowing and "swollen tongue" sensation, excessive drooling, slurred speech (seek immediate medical help).

Young children may constantly rub their nose and face: This may be an indication of facial numbness or tingling.

Muscle twitching.

Restlessness and irritability: Children may appear hyperactive with rapid and uncontrolled body movements.

These symptoms usually occur within the first 2–3 hours after the sting.

Children under the age of 10 are more likely to develop severe symptoms.

Treatment:

Call Poison Control immediately.

Wash the sting site with soap and water.

Apply a cool wet compress (not ice) to the sting site.

Acetaminophen can be taken for pain.

Numbness and tingling may persist for several weeks.

Cooperative Extensions and the U.S. Department of Agriculture and University of Arizona say:

Bark scorpions are a maximum of two inches long. They are pale gold or translucent. The pincers are long and slender and not greatly swollen at the bases (those are a different species).

They can crawl and can be found in trees, on walls, and on ceilings (my exterminator says they can fit through a slit the width of a credit card). Scorpions are normally active at night and during the summer months. Always wear shoes when walking outside at night. Never swat, always brush away if they are crawling on you. Look inside shoes prior to putting them on and shake things that were on the floor. Shake off your throw pillows before you put them back on your bed. This is how I got stung. One crawled from my throw pillow in college into my bed. That was a painful lesson to learn ☹

Prevention:

Do not leave shoes, clothing, or wet towels outside.

Shake all clothing and tip over all shoes before putting them on.

Wear shoes outside, especially in the evening hours, as scorpions are night feeders.

They are attracted to swimming pools and irrigation areas.

Pull back bed sheets before getting into bed.

You may want to use a crib tent if you have a large scorpion problem.

Use weather stripping around doors and windows, seal up or place a fine screen where air conditioning or exhaust fans enter the house.

Use a black light if you want to look for them, as this will make them glow in the dark.

Keep up with pest control. If you can keep crickets under control, this will decrease the scorpion's food source.

Each year over 4,800 scorpion stings are reported to Poison Control.

Black widow spider

In Arizona, black widows are also of concern. A mature female spider has a large, black, shiny body and measures approximately ⅜ of an inch long with 1-inch legs. An hourglass shape in bright red or orange-red can be found on the abdomen.

Black widow webs are very strong, white webs. They are most often found in areas where water and insects are readily available. Around the house they can be found under outdoor furniture, barbeque grills, pool pumps and in storage areas, garages, woodpiles, and corners of porches and patios.

The female black widow is shy. She hides near the web by day and is most active at night, and she waits in her web. She produces hundreds of babies hatched from egg sacks that look like mothballs. The young black widows are white in color and spread quickly after hatching.

The male black widow is much smaller and brown and white in color. Because of its size the bite cannot pierce the skin and is therefore not dangerous to humans.

To control the widow population, it is necessary to directly hit the adult spider with a strong insecticide and destroy the egg sacs. Use a flashlight at night to find them hiding in their webs.

Signs and symptoms of a bite:

The initial bite may feel like a pin prick and may go unnoticed.

At first there are no visible signs. There is not initial swelling but about six hours after the bite, a red circular mark may appear.

The initial symptoms may be a progressive aching sensation with muscle pain at the bite site, spreading to the lower back and limbs.

Symptoms often last up to 36 hours and lingering effects for several weeks.

Watch for signs and symptoms of infection or blood poisoning.

Call Poison Control if you suspect a bite.

Approximately 350 calls are received each year about black widow bites.

Safety / car seats

Here are some important phone numbers and websites:

Car seat locator: https://www.nhtsa.gov/campaign/right-seat

This site will allow you to go to the inspection locator for inspection sites all over the US. This website also has other helpful information including car seat recalls.

www.nhtsa.gov is the website of the National Highway Traffic Safety Administration. Once at this site, click on Vehicle Safety and this will bring you to car seat information.

To report unrestrained children, call the "Buckle Up, Baby" hotline:

1800 505-BABY

You will need the vehicle license plate number and the state, where you were when you witnessed the event, and where the child was sitting in the vehicle.

Call General Motors on 1(800) 247-9168 to receive a free 32-page booklet on safety belts and child restraints.

Check with your local state for child restraint laws and restrictions.

Arizona passenger restraint law states that all children under 5 years and less than 40 lbs. need to be in a child passenger restraint device while in a moving vehicle.

Motor vehicle crashes account for nearly 42% of all unintentional injury-related deaths of children under the age of 15 years.

Proper use of a child safety seat proves to be 71% effective in reducing deaths of infants in passenger cars and 54% effective in reducing toddler deaths.

Child safety seats also reduce the need for hospitalization by almost 70%.

Motor vehicle crashes are the leading cause of injury and death for children in the US. There is not one car seat that is "the best" or "the safest." The best car seat is the one that fits your child the best. You have to take into account your child's individual height and weight and which car seat can be installed correctly in your vehicle. Not all car seats fit all cars equally. You also need to look at your car manual to see the safest spot to put a car seat in your vehicle.

Send in the registration card when you purchase the car seat, so you will be notified immediately should your seat be recalled.

<u>Birth to one year</u>

Babies from birth to 1 years of age and 20-22 lbs. should use a rear-facing infant seat.

The AAP prefers kids to stay rear facing until at least 2 years of age.

In 2011 the AAP revised its policy, as they found that children under the age of 2 are 75% *less* likely to be injured in a car crash if they are rear facing.

Both the AAP and the National Highway Traffic Safety Administration recommend rear-facing until kids outgrow the car seat around 4 years of age.

<u>Infant rear-facing seats</u>

Babies should stay rear facing as long as possible!

Keep harness clips at armpit level.

Position harness straps in lower harness slots at or below shoulder level. (The straps come up and over the shoulder.)

Do not recline more by than a 45-degree angle.

<u>Forward-facing car seats</u>

Fasten harness clips at armpit level.

Position harness straps in upper slots at or above shoulder level. (The straps come straight down over the shoulders.)

If possible, use a tether strap to anchor the top of the seat to the vehicle. This helps prevent your child's head from moving too far forward in a crash.

Booster seats – 4/5 – 8 years

Booster seats are for kids weighing 40 – 80 lbs. and less than 4' 9" tall.

Belts should fit low over the upper thighs / hips and snug over the shoulder. You need to use both the shoulder and lap belts.

4–7-year-olds should be in a harness-type booster seat.

8–12-year-olds can be in a shoulder-strap booster seat using the regular seat belt.

Britax Regent brand holds up to 80 lbs. in a 5-point harness.

Washington passed the first law in the country in 2002 that required the use of booster seats. The law states children must ride in a booster seat from 4 years or 40 lbs. until they are 6 years or 60 lbs. Experts recommend children use booster seats until they are at least 8 years old and weigh 80 lbs. The chance of a child surviving a car crash is 36% better when they are in a booster seat. Research showed that over 50% of all kids aged 4–8 years old are using seat belts too early. The booster raises the child up so the lap and shoulder belt fit properly. Approximately 2,000 children are killed and 325,000 injured each year in road accidents. 4 out of 5 children are riding in improperly installed child safety seats.

Parenting, September 2000

"A Boost for Safety"

"Thanks to the increase in use of car seats, the number of crash-related deaths among babies and toddlers has declined in the past five years. But a recent study by the National Center for Injury Prevention and Control shows that, every year, 500 children aged 4–8 are killed, making car crashes the leading cause of death in this age group. The problem is a shoulder belt can ride up over the stomach causing serious, even fatal, injuries in an accident. Booster seats can eliminate this problem."

If you have a passenger-side airbag, no child under the age of 12 years can ride in that seat. The back seat is the safest place for a child.

Some parents remove their child from the seat while the vehicle is in motion to feed or change, or burp them.

Crash tests show that, at a speed of 30 miles per hour, a 10-pound child will be ripped from your arms with a force of 200 lbs., making it a near certainty that the child would hit the dashboard or windshield, or seat in front of them, with tragic consequences.

By strapping the baby with you in the seat belt, the weight of your body thrown against them would severely injure them. So, pull over if you need to take your baby out of their seat and stop in a safe, secure location.

Used car seats

Don't use a used car seat, as you don't know if it has been in a crash, recalled, or if any parts are missing. Evenflow says the life of a car seat is 6 years and you should never buy a used car seat.

Evenflow 1(800) 233-5921.

Car seats in the heat

Phoenix Children's Hospital recommends only using a car seat for five years, as our extreme heat may decrease the safety of the car seat.

The car seat, when in place, should move no more than one inch from side to side or toward the front of the vehicle.

Cars parked in direct sunlight can reach an internal temperature of 131°F – 172°F even after only 15 minutes in the sun.

Belt and harness buckles can cause serious burns, so you may want to cover the seat. (I used to put a gel ice pack over the buckle and then a beach towel over the seat.)

You can also buy items called Noggle that will bring cool air to the back seat when driving to make sure cool air or even heat will get to them.

The car gets hotter than you realize.

On a 70-degree day (in Arizona we rarely get days this cool):

After 10 minutes = 89°F

After 20 minutes = 99°F

After 30 minutes = 104°F

After 60 minutes = 113°F

After 2 hours = 120°F

Hot car deaths

Another huge fear and troubling problem when talking about car safety is parents forgetting their little one in the car. Nobody means to do this. It is an accident but below are seven ways to prevent it from happening.

Here are seven ways not to forget your child in the car:

1. Be extra careful when you have a routine change. This is when you are at the highest risk of unintentionally leaving your child in the car.
2. Put something of your child's in the front seat of the car, on top of your stuff.
3. Leave an item you will need in the backseat with the baby. It should be something you will need like a shoe, purse, briefcase, or cell phone.
4. Place the car seat in the middle of the back seat, if appropriate, so you can see it from your rear-view mirror better.
5. Set up a system with your childcare provider so that they will call you if you do not show up. Tell them you will always call if your baby is not going that day.
6. Discuss the topic of hot car deaths with every person that drives your child anywhere. Tell them to follow the steps above each and every time they drive your child.
7. Always look before you lock! Make that a mantra.

Always call 911 if you see a child alone in a car!

This chapter was not meant to scare you to death or keep you up at night. I am sorry if I created some anxiety. It was not my intent. I teach this lecture every year because I know I have saved babies' lives over the years. None of us are perfect parents. We all make mistakes, and they call these accidents for a reason. I just wanted you to have the information on what to do in case something was to happen. Better yet, this may prevent an accident from happening. It is my opinion that knowledge is power and now you are all empowered.

CHAPTER 12

HEALTH LECTURE

"Mothers don't sleep, they just worry with their eyes closed."

- Author Unknown

Colds

Colds are a childhood rite of passage. No matter what you do to try to prevent illness, your child will have cold-like symptoms at some point in their childhood. A cold is a virus and is usually mild. Symptoms include a runny and/or stuffy nose, sometimes a fever, and sometimes a cough.

Nasal discharge is usually clear, yet sometimes it is yellow or green. Color does not always mean infection. Nasal discharge is often thick and yellow or green in the morning after secretions have pooled or at the tail end of a cold. If the discharge stays thick green or yellow throughout the day for longer than five days, see your child's doctor as your child might have a sinus infection.

With a cold the greatest concern with little ones is respiratory distress. Signs and symptoms of respiratory distress include:

Increased respiratory rate, for example:

For children under 2 months >60 breaths/min is too fast

Aged 2–12 months >50 breaths/min is too fast

Aged 1–5 >40 breaths/min is too fast.

If your child is showing signs or symptoms of a rapid respiratory rate, contact your doctor.

A fever can increase a person's respiratory rate. Respiratory rate rises by three for every degree of elevation in temperature (Fahrenheit) above normal.

Another symptom of respiratory distress is something called retractions. Retractions are when the chest or stomach is sucking in hard with inspiration. Retractions mean a child is working too hard to get air. If your child is having retractions when breathing, contact the doctor.

Noisy breathing is also an indication of respiratory distress. Any audible wheezing or stridor-like breathing is concerning and should warrant a call to the doctor.

More severe signs of respiratory distress include a bluish or grey color to the skin or lips and excessive lethargy. Depending on the severity, this may be an ER visit or 911 call.

Treatment for minor colds includes the use of a cool mist humidifier. Bring your little one into a steamy bathroom for approximately 15 minutes. Saline nose drops in the nose accompanied by a bulb syringe or NoseFrida. You do not always need to get discharge out of the nose. Since the nasal passages in infants are very delicate, if you are not getting secretions out, just put the saline drops in and leave them be. The saline will still help. You might want to elevate the head of the bed by putting a wedge under the mattress if your little one is extremely stuffy.

Unless recommended by your doctor, the new FDA recommendations suggest no over-the-counter cough and cold medicines under the age of two and they warn about careful use under the age of six.

The average baby, toddler and preschooler will catch 6-8 colds per year. If your child attends a daycare setting, you can assume your child will catch their first cold earlier than a child who is not. That is not necessarily a bad thing, however, as kids who were in daycare are often healthier when they attend school than kids who were not in a daycare setting prior.

It is important to say that the only scientifically proven way to catch a cold is by contracting a cold virus from a person who has it or by coming into contact with something that person has touched, or the virus itself, on droplets of air or surfaces. (You cannot catch a cold by going outside with wet hair or no shoes. Sorry, Mom, that's an old wife's tale.)

Coughs

Coughs are often associated with colds. Most are minor and improve without any treatment needed.

Please have your child seen by a physician if the cough sounds like it is deep in the chest, your child is experiencing pain with the cough, or crying with each cough, or if they have a cough with fever, cough with a rash or, again, wheezing or stridor.

What is croup?

Croup is a virus. A croupy cough is a distinctive, barky-like sound associated with a cough. Your child often has a hoarse voice along with the cough and it is usually worse at night. The croupy, barky noise is due to the constriction of the vocal cords.

Croup is most common between the ages of three months and five years, in the fall and winter months.

Danger signs that require immediate attention include pale or blue color to the skin or lips or if your child is leaning forward and drooling as if unable to swallow.

If the croupy cough is associated with stridor, rapid respirations, or retractions, have your child seen immediately as he or she will probably need oral steroids such as Prelone or a shot such as Decedron.

You can treat mild croup symptoms with home comfort measures if there are no signs or symptoms of respiratory distress.

Comfort measures include those similar to those above for a cold. Sitting in a steamy bathroom, or a cool mist humidifier. One thing that works for croup is a rush of cold air. If it is cold enough outside, bundle your little one and let them breathe the cold night air. If you do not want to go outside or it is not cold outside, you can open the freezer and let your child breathe in the cold freezer air, while you look at the frozen peas.

RSV

Respiratory syncytial virus is the most frequent cause of serious respiratory tract infections in infants and children under the age of four. It is so common that virtually all children have been infected by the age of three. In most young children and adults, it results in a mild respiratory infection that is not distinguishable from the common cold. Diagnosis of RSV is through a nasal swab. RSV occurs throughout the year, but it is most prevalent during the winter months. Symptoms of RSV include nasal stuffiness, runny nose, cough, and sometimes ear infections. Your child might have a low-grade temperature as well. A child can get a second RSV infection. However, if your child is unlucky enough to get RSV twice, it is likely that the symptoms will be much milder than the first time. In 2023 a new RSV vaccine became available for infants as well as pregnant moms during the 32–36th week of pregnancy.

Ear infections

In small children, ear infections often follow colds. It is most common to see an ear infection with a cold, or after a cold. Fluid pools in the ear from the cold and then bacteria settle in that fluid, causing an infection. Some children are more prone than others to ear infections and they are largely genetic. It has to do with the shape and length of their Eustachian tube.

Signs and symptoms of an ear infection can include pulling or batting at the ears, and not wanting to suck from a bottle, breast, or sippy cup, as sucking causes pressure on the eardrum. Not wanting to lie flat, as again lying flat puts pressure on the eardrum.

Waking frequently during the night with a painful cry is a good sign your baby has an ear infection. Increased fussiness / irritability. Sometimes fever, but not always. If your baby has a cold and has yellow or green drainage from the eyes, have your little one checked for an ear infection as well, as this is often an indication. Ear infections themselves are not contagious unless your child comes into contact with infected fluid from the ear (which would be very unlikely). The viral illness that usually precedes the ear infection is contagious.

Dr. David Darrow, an associate professor of otolaryngology and pediatrics at Virginia Medical School, says, "Every year ear infections account for 25 million visits to the pediatrician's office and nearly half of all children will experience three or more before their third birthday. Ear infections are most common in children under five because they have shorter, wider, and more horizontal Eustachian tubes, making it more likely for bacteria from the back of the nose and throat to infect the ears."

"The tubes are also less mature and don't function as efficiently as they do in adults, and more babies and young children are more likely to develop frequent viral upper respiratory infections, which in turn predisposes them to ear infections."

Teething

It is a myth that teething can cause a high fever, vomiting, or diarrhea.

A temperature of 101°F or higher is *not* caused by teething. Since the immunity Mom passes on to Baby starts to wane at six months of age, this is the age most children will contract their first illness. Since this is also the time the first teeth typically make their appearance, it would make sense that many first illnesses are blamed on teething.

Many parents find it difficult to determine if increased fussiness is from new teeth popping through or another illness, such as an ear infection. If in doubt, make a quick trip to the pediatrician.

To help with teething, offer cold items to chew on: teething rings, chilled bananas in your baby-safe feeder or other frozen fruit, and popsicles (Pedialyte pops or 100% juice, although not too much juice as you do not want to cause loose stools). Be careful with teething biscuits as they can be a choking hazard. Offer teething biscuits in a baby-safe feeder. Textured BPA-free silicone teething toys are a great natural alternative option to medication. Since your child will be teething for the next two years, use acetaminophen or ibuprofen sparingly. You do not want to mask symptoms of illness. Pain should not be severe. Ibuprofen should not be used in infants under six months of age.

Fevers

The definition of a fever is:

A rectal temp >100.4°F (insert thermometer about ½ inch just past the metal tip using KY jelly or Vaseline for two minutes or until it beeps).

An oral temp >99.5°F (includes pacifier thermometer).

An axillary temp >99.0°F.

Ear thermometers are not accurate, and I would avoid using them.

A temperature of 100–102°F is considered low grade and beneficial.

A temperature of 102–104°F is considered moderate and still considered beneficial.

A temperature >104°F is considered a high fever and will cause your child discomfort.

A fever of 104°F by itself, however, will not cause damage.

A temperature >105°F presents a higher risk of a bacterial infection and your child always needs to be seen if they have a fever this high.

Temperatures of 107°F or greater are when the fever itself can be harmful and can cause brain damage.

You need to seek medical attention if your child has a fever for longer than 24 hours with no other symptoms.

If your baby has a rectal temperature >100.4°F and is younger than 12 weeks of age, you need to seek medical attention.

A temperature of 105°F or greater at any age, a bulging soft spot, purplish or blood-colored rash, or a rash with a fever at any time needs to be seen immediately.

If your little one cries when touched or moved, has excessive lethargy, any difficulty breathing, as mentioned above, or joint swelling, you also need to seek medical attention immediately.

Even though your child may have a fever, they should still be making eye contact, appear alert, continue to take fluids, and have plenty of wet diapers.

If your child is holding their neck stiffly or will not turn their head easily or appears to have pain in their neck with movement, especially when looking down, they also need to be seen immediately.

If your baby is over 12 weeks and acting as if they are uncomfortable from the fever itself, you can administer a fever-reducing medication such as acetaminophen or ibuprofen (if over six months of age). You can also put your little one in a lukewarm bath at 85–90 degrees. The fever should come down at least one degree with acetaminophen or ibuprofen and the child should perk up when the fever is down. If the fever does not respond after an hour the child needs to be seen.

If your baby becomes active and playful it is typically not a serious illness. If not, call your doctor's office immediately. Your child's appearance rather than the reading on the thermometer is the best indicator of the seriousness of the illness.

If the fever continues, however, and you do not see a reason for that fever after 24 hours, like cold symptoms or a gastrointestinal bug, etc., have your child seen.

Vomiting

Vomiting is usually caused by a viral illness.

The biggest concern with little bodies is the risk of dehydration.

Signs and symptoms of dehydration include fewer than six wet diapers in 24 hours. A dry mouth with dry lips, sometimes cracked. More severe symptoms of dehydration include no tears, your child being limp and lethargic, and the eyes appearing sunken in.

If vomiting has been occurring for >24 hours, it is a good idea to have them evaluated for dehydration.

Symptoms of potentially serious conditions include severe abdominal pain or constant pain, high fever >104°F, blood in stool or vomit, green vomit or >10 episodes of vomiting or diarrhea in 24 hours.

Treatment for vomiting includes withholding solid foods until your little one is first able to keep down liquids. Under the age of one, I suggest withholding solids for 24 hours as they don't really need the solids. They only need the fluids. If there has been no vomiting for at least 30 minutes, offer small amounts of breast milk or formula (1 tbsp). A syringe works well for this. If that is kept down for 10 minutes, you can offer another tablespoon. Repeat this 3x in a row every 10 minutes. If tolerated, you can increase to 1 oz. If your baby vomits the formula or breast milk, you can try 1 tbsp of Pedialyte or Gerber

LiquiLytes instead. Following the plan of waiting for 30 minutes since the last vomiting and then every 10 minutes if tolerated, offer 1 tbsp x3 for 30 minutes to 1 hour. Gradually increase to about an ounce and increase gradually from there to a couple of ounces at a time. If your baby is keeping down Pedialyte but not full-strength formula or breast milk, and it has been several hours with no vomiting, try mixing the formula or breast milk half and half with plain Pedialyte. Start gradually again with a tablespoon and work your way back up. If that is going well and after increasing for several hours, you can try to go back to full-strength breast milk or formula again. Remember, small amounts. Do not give large amounts at any time as you are likely to lose all the progress you have made.

*If your baby is not keeping down even small amounts, it is time to go to the ER for something to stop the vomiting and replace the fluids. Their little bodies just do not have the reserves we have. The good news is vomiting typically does not last long. The worst of it is usually over in 24 hours, with the occasional vomiting here and there for the next several days.

If there has been no vomiting for more than 24 hours, you may begin small amounts of bland foods. No dairy products for 24 hours. Follow the "BRAT" diet: bananas, rice, applesauce, toast (cereals). Anything lacking color is usually a safe bet. No juices of any kind and stay away from non-constipating fruits.

Diarrhea

It is not uncommon for diarrhea to follow vomiting. The good news is it is the lesser of the evils. With diarrhea, you can at least push the fluids and offer constipating foods.

The reason for avoiding juices and non-constipating fruits is because, after vomiting, you can assume diarrhea is around the corner and we do not want to lose even more fluid or electrolytes through stool. Diarrhea is a watery stool and often green or yellow as it moves through the digestive tract faster. Color, however, is not a concern if your child has a green or yellow stool that is not watery. This is not diarrhea, it just means the stool did not hang around long enough in the intestines to pick up dead red blood cells that give stool a darker color.

Again, offer the "BRAT" diet. Bananas are wonderful because they are not only binding, but they are also a good source of potassium which is often lost with diarrhea. Other food suggestions include crackers, toast, cereals, mashed potatoes, sweet potatoes, squash, apple sauce, carrots, high-fiber foods, noodles, and lean meats.

Avoid all dairy products. The lactose in dairy is very hard to digest on an upset tummy. For infants less than one year of age, most doctors usually do not recommend stopping formula. If the diarrhea is severe and happens after each milk-based bottle, your pediatrician may have you try a soy formula as it does not have lactose. They usually have your little one stay on the soy formula for 5–7 days after the diarrhea subsides. Continue to monitor for signs and symptoms of dehydration. Call if you notice blood in the stool or if your child is experiencing severe abdominal pain. Viral diarrhea can last 5–7 days. It is always worse on days 1 and 2. Call your doctor if your little one is stooling >10 times per day or if this has been going on for more than 10 days.

After a GI bug, your baby will have lost some of his or her good GI flora. Since approximately 80% of your immune system is in the gut, it is very important to keep good gut health. You can purchase infant probiotic drops to replace what was lost with loose stools. One brand is Culturelle for kids as it is lactobacillus GG and has sprinkles which make it easy for little ones to take. A couple of other brands are Gerber Soothe probiotic drops and Florajen. My pediatric immunologist recommends probiotics with each tummy bug and with each course of antibiotics. Both events wipe out the good gut flora. My pediatric immunologist also says to mix it up a bit and not continually use the same probiotic brand. He suggests when you complete one, switch to another, as you get different strains of probiotics.

Diaper rash

Often with diarrhea you end up with diaper rash, no matter how often or how fast you change them after a bowel movement. Call your doctor if you notice a peeling rash, or the rash is associated with a fever, or your baby has open weepy or yellow sores, which may be a staph or strep infection. A regular diaper rash is pink to red and sometimes looks very raw as though it might bleed in some areas.

Treatment for diaper rash, if not yeast, includes stopping using your regular diaper wipes. You can either use a soft paper towel or rinse out your wipes and put them in a Ziplock bag. This will still be convenient yet won't irritate delicate skin. Even fragrance-free can irritate skin. Or use a soft washcloth, however, this can lead to a lot of laundry and mess. You can also use your peri bottle from the hospital with warm water and just rinse the bottom off and pat it dry.

Air exposure is the best thing (I know you're saying sure, Monique, I am going to do this with a baby having diarrhea, but a waterproof pad in the crib at nap time works well or just outside for a bit if it is warm enough).

Sitz baths are great too. A warm bath in the tub or sink a couple of times per day with two tablespoons of baking soda to a small tub of water. ¼ cup in a full tub.

Your typical other-the-counter diaper rash creams are fine to use as a barrier if the skin has not broken down and is only pink. But if the rash is very bad, you might call your doctor for a prescription medication. There is a medication that needs to be compounded. It is a mixture of Questran in Aquaphor. If your doctor has not heard of it, let them know the mixture is 56g of Aquaphor and 4g of Questran to make a 60g tube or container, and apply with every diaper change. This works wonderfully and will clear the worst of rashes quickly. Some compounding pharmacies may also just mix it as 5% Questran in Aquaphor.

If the rash is not responding to the typical diaper rash treatment as I just described after three days, or it is getting worse rather than better, it may be yeast. Yeast diaper rash is bright red, sometimes with raised bumps, and often has what we call "satellite" spots. This is a small area of rash or spots off from the main rash. Treatment is similar to regular diaper rash. Again, air exposure is recommended more so even with yeast, since moisture makes it worse. Sitz baths with baking soda, no diaper wipes, the same as above. The difference, however, is you need an antifungal cream such as Lotrimin cream. You can find this over the counter, and it needs to be applied times per day. The cream needs to be applied an inch past the borders of the rash and used for 7 days past the clearing of rash, typically for a total of 10 days. Or you can ask your doctor to see if they will call in nystatin cream or another antifungal cream for you.

If there is still no change after three days of antifungal treatment or if symptoms increase or a fever develops, you need to make an office visit.

Constipation

Since we are on the subject of poops, let's talk about constipation too.

Constipation is hard pellet-like stools, or no stool in more than 7 days, your child is trying to go and unable to, or pushing for >10 minutes with no results, or in pain with a stool.

Warm baths often help to relax the muscles, as well as a change in diet if your little one is on solids.

Decrease constipating foods such as dairy, especially cheese which can be very constipating. Yellow veggies such as cooked carrots, yellow squash, and sweet potatoes also tend to be constipating. Increase fruit juice and fruits such as prunes, peaches, and grapes, etc. To help keep your baby regular add foods high in fiber like green veggies, peas, beans, and broccoli. Other foods include apricots, peaches, pears, figs, and prunes. I typically recommend when starting new foods to offer a constipating food and then a non-constipating food, so you can fix a problem one way or the other with food.

It may take one week on a diet to see a change.

Fruit juice at one ounce for every month of age works well too, especially if your little one has not started solids yet. If your baby has not started solids yet, however, you want to try to figure out why they are constipated as this is not typical. Make sure they are drinking enough breast milk or formula. Remember, after a month, breastfed babies have very little waste and may not stool for up to 10 days. Try taking a rectal temperature and if the stool is a normal breastfed stool, the baby was not constipated.

You can also try an infant glycerin suppository if the fruit juice does not work and your little one is miserable.

If this is a long-term problem, speak with your doctor. Your physician may have you try a medication like MiraLAX or Milk of Magnesia but never use it without the doctor's advice.

Pink eye or conjunctivitis

Pink eye and ear infections often go hand and hand. So, if your child has a cold and drainage from the eye, have their ears checked out.

There are two types of conjunctivitis: viral and bacterial.

The incubation period if your child is exposed to pink eye is 24–72 hours.

With viral conjunctivitis

You may see redness, or pink color to the sclera (the white of the eye). The eyes are usually watery, yet no discharge is present. With viral conjunctivitis no treatment is necessary, just monitor.

With bacterial conjunctivitis

There is discharge: either yellow or green. With bacterial conjunctivitis, the sclera is not always pink or red and the eyelids are often puffy but should not be swollen like a boxer after a match. The lashes may be matted shut, particularly in the morning upon waking and after naps. Bacterial conjunctivitis should be treated with antibiotic drops. Have your child evaluated in the pediatrician's office or urgent care. Call your doctor right away if the eye orbit / socket becomes swollen, especially if the eye is swollen shut or there is a fever associated with it.

A clogged tear duct as we discussed in a previous chapter may look similar and, if there are copious amounts of discharge, it is treated the same as bacterial conjunctivitis.

Illnesses with a rash

It is very important for me to say that, if your child has a fever at the same time as a rash, they need to be seen! It is not uncommon with many viral illnesses in childhood, however, for a child to develop a rash after a fever.

Roseola

Roseola is a viral illness that most children will get at some point. The typical age that kids catch roseola is between six months and three years.

It is easy to get as it is airborne and can be transmitted from secretions from the nose, mouth, and throat, and can also be on surfaces and in infected droplets in the air.

Most parents bring their kids to the pediatrician because they have an unexplained fever lasting anywhere from 2–4 days and no other symptoms (remember, I said if your child has a fever for more than 24 hours without an obvious reason, see your doctor).

So, the baby is seen, and the doctor says, "I do not know the cause." "The ears look clear. This could just be a virus." They send you home and say to use a fever reducer and then the fever goes away. Some kids may have a slight runny nose and be a bit irritable.

Twenty-four hours later, a rash appears. Now the fever is gone but the child has a rash that typically lasts a day or two and then goes away. You usually notice it in the bathtub. It is not itchy. It is fine pink and not blood-colored or purple.

The incubation period for roseola is typically 5–15 days with an average of 9 days.

Chicken pox

We don't see chicken pox much anymore. When I first started in nursing many moons ago, we did not have the varicella or chicken pox vaccine, so we saw this quite often. I wanted to include it, however, as it is an airborne virus and can be on surfaces and droplets of air. If a child who has not been vaccinated were to get chicken pox and go into the store with even one open pock before your child has had both vaccines, there is still a chance your child could get chicken pox.

A typical case of chicken pox is 400–500 pox. Before we knew that children needed a booster of the varicella vaccine, we would see kids with chicken pox with very mild cases of just a few pox. I want to describe the chicken pox rash to you so you will be able to distinguish it if you see it.

A person or child is contagious two days before the rash appears which makes it even easier to pass along. The incubation period is also very long: 7–21 days.

Chicken pox progresses within 24 hours through all the following stages:

It starts as a small red spot. That spot then becomes a thin-walled water blister. That blister then turns into a cloudy blister. That cloudy blister becomes an open sore and then dry brown scab. This entire progression of the pox all happens within 24 hours. If you are seeing a red spot that doesn't scab by the following day, it is not chicken pox.

New pox can continue to crop up for 4–5 days.

Remember I said that the child is contagious until every pox is scabbed over, even if it is in the hair.

If your child develops chicken pox, I have listed some ways to help keep your child comfortable: Aveeno antiitch cream, or calamine lotion, oral Zyrtec, acetaminophen (<u>avoid ibuprofen- or aspirin-containing products</u>), and oatmeal baths (either Aveeno oatmeal baths that come in packets or simply take regular cooking oatmeal such as Quaker oats and put it in an old sock, tie it off, and put it in warm water. You can also use baking soda: two ounces for a tub of water).

What is Reye's syndrome?

Reye's syndrome, also known as Reye syndrome, is a rare but serious condition that causes swelling in the liver and brain. Reye's syndrome can occur at any age but usually affects children and teenagers after a viral infection, most commonly the flu or chickenpox. Symptoms such as confusion, seizures, and loss of consciousness need emergency treatment. Early diagnosis and treatment of Reye's syndrome can save a child's life. Aspirin has been linked with Reye's syndrome.

Children and teenagers recovering from chickenpox or flu-like symptoms should never take aspirin. https://www.mayoclinic.org/diseases-conditions/reyes-syndrome/symptoms-causes/syc-20377255

Fifth disease

Although this is a mild illness for the child affected, it can be dangerous for expectant mothers. Although rare, fifth disease has been associated with miscarriages and stillbirths. If your child has been exposed or has fifth disease, stay away from expectant mothers if possible.

Since the virus is contagious the week prior to the rash, it is easily transmitted without you knowing you have been exposed. Once your child has symptoms, they are no longer contagious.

This viral illness has a very distinct rash that has a lace-like or net-like appearance to it. One mom described it to me as looking like her child had doilies on her.

The rash begins as bright red cheeks. It looks like your child has been out in the cold or the heat. The red cheeks last 1–3 days and a lacey or net-like rash follows it on extremities, mainly on the thighs, upper arms, and shoulders.

The rash is not itchy or painful. There is no fever or a low-grade fever under 101°F.

The rash on the body may come and go for 1–3 weeks and extreme temperatures, hot or cold, as well as a bath, make the rash more distinct.

Fifth disease typically occurs most often in late winter / early spring and the normal incubation period is 4–14 days. This virus is transmitted via contact or is airborne.

Coxsackie or hand-foot-and-mouth disease

This is a terrible childhood illness from the standpoint of misery for your little one. We primarily see hand-foot-and-mouth disease in the summer months and early fall. The incubation period from exposure to illness is fairly short, about 3–6 days, and typically kids get this viral illness between the ages of six months and four years.

Most kids present with small, painful ulcers in their mouth. These are typically seen on the tongue and the insides of the cheeks and sides of the throat. These mouth ulcers are present in 99% of kids with coxsackie.

70% of kids also experience small, thick-walled water blisters or red spots on the palms and soles of their hands and feet and also between the webs of the fingers and toes. Most children develop approximately 1–5 blisters per hand or foot. 30% of kids also develop blisters on their buttocks as well. Children often develop a low-grade fever up to 102 degrees with blisters as well.

The fever lasts 2–3 days and mouth ulcers last up to 7 days. The blisters or rash on the body can last up to 10 days. Children can go back to daycare and be around other children when they are fever free, and their mouth ulcers are gone, as children pass it back and forth by contact with mouth secretions from chewing on toys. Good hand-washing procedures need to be followed as the virus is still shed in the stool for several weeks.

The greatest concern with coxsackie is dehydration. Since the ulcers are so painful, children do not want to eat or drink. Offer acetaminophen for pain, lots of fluids, cold drinks, and popsicles like Pedialyte pops. Avoid citrus or salty foods.

Impetigo

Impetigo is a staph infection of the skin.

Impetigo starts out as small red bumps which rapidly change to cloudy blisters, then pimples that open up and weep.

Sores are often covered by a soft brown or yellow scab or crust that intermittently drains pus. These sores are usually found around the mouth and nose. These sores can be spread if they are picked at.

Impetigo needs to be treated with a topical antibiotic ointment or cream and, if the impetigo infection is severe, the child may need an oral antibiotic. Schedule an office visit if your child has a fever above 100 degrees with the sores.

Call your pediatrician's office first, prior to scheduling an office visit. If it is just a small spot, your physician may call in an antibiotic cream such as Bactroban and save you a visit.

Hives

There are multiple reasons your child might develop hives.

Hives are raised, itchy pink spots with pale centers.

The shape and size may vary greatly, as well as location. They can range from half an inch to several inches. They may also merge together, making it difficult to tell one spot from the next. They change rapidly and repeatedly.

Give an antihistamine such as Zyrtec right away and watch for signs and symptoms of difficulty breathing or swallowing / anaphylaxis.

Hives are usually associated with an allergen, so try to find the cause. If the hives go away with an antihistamine, you need to become a detective, so you do not keep introducing that allergen to your child. Zyrtec is one dose every 24 hours and can be given to children as young as six months of age. If you see any sign or symptoms of breathing difficulty, go to the ER or call 911.

When my cousin's baby was little, they called me saying the baby was covered in hives and was drooling. He had had a new food. I told them to give him Benadryl immediately and I gave them the dose based on his weight. This was prior to the new recommendation to give Zyrtec for allergic reactions. They said they didn't have any in the home and had him in the tub. I suggested they pull him out of the tub and go to the corner drugstore and give him Benadryl in the store. I called to check on them 10 minutes later and they said they had called 911 as the drooling became more severe. I said, "Great it's better to be safe than sorry." My cousin called me about an hour later and said he wished he had listened to me. I asked him what had happened. He said, "Well we now have a bill for the ER and an ambulance, and they gave him Benadryl and sent us home to see our pediatrician." I often tell parents to give an antihistamine and drive towards the ER then, if you need to go in, you are already there. If the meds kick in and your child seems OK, you can turn around and go home.

If your child ever has a severe allergic reaction like that, however, going to the ER is always a safe thing to do. You will probably then want to speak with your pediatrician or see a pediatric allergist so you can have a pediatric epinephrine pen on hand. It is not uncommon to have future exposures that are worse than the first.

You can also see hives in some forms of pneumonia, such as mycoplasma. This is usually accompanied by fever. Remember, fever and a rash, appointment.

You may also see hives in some cases of strep throat, although not a typical symptom, but again, your child would have a fever, so again fever and rash, appointment.

Some children also develop viral hives. So, if the hives do not go away with Zyrtec have your child seen.

Some other rashes not associated with illness are eczema and contact dermatitis.

Eczema

Presents as dry or red scaly skin, bumpy skin, or rough patches.

Most children improve before the age of two.

It is important to moisturize daily, at least two times a day, with a dye-free, fragrance-free, lanolin-free, paraben-free, formaldehyde-free cream such as Eucerin cream or Vanicream (my new favorite product on the market).

Keep bath time brief. Apply the cream when skin is still damp out of the bath. You may want to decrease the frequency of baths and use a mild baby soap or unscented soap like Vanicream. You can also bathe without soap.

Anti-inflammatory cream such as .5% or 1% hydrocortisone cream or ointment can be applied to bad areas for very short periods of time, or you can see your physician for a prescription cream. However, steroidal creams should not be used more than 2x per day or for longer than 1–2 weeks because they can cause skin thinning and discoloration. If this is a long-term problem, speak to your physician about a non-steroidal option. Make sure there is nothing in your child's diet or environment causing eczema, e.g., diary or detergent.

Contact dermatitis

Is a localized rash that may or may not be itchy.

Try to find the irritant. Contact dermatitis is caused by coming into contact with an irritant.

Contact dermatitis can be caused by things like new detergent, soap, new clothes, or even snaps on pajamas, i.e., a nickel allergy.

Wash the affected area with mild soap and you can apply hydrocortisone cream twice a day.

Strep throat

Most children under the age of two do not get strep throat. A sore throat and fever, however, without cold symptoms, should always be screened for strep, especially if there has been known exposure and the child is over two years of age. If strep throat is also associated with a rash, it is called scarlet fever. The rash is a small pinpoint rash that almost looks solid red until you look closer, and it feels rough like sandpaper.

Injuries

Bites

For a human bite: Wash the area well with antibacterial soap and water. If the bite broke the skin, call your doctor, as they may want to put child on an oral prophylactic antibiotic for three days or antibiotic cream or ointment.

Watch for signs or symptoms of infection, including redness at or around the site, warmth around the area, fever, streaks from the area, or discharge.

For an animal bite: If the animal is a household pet, follow the human bite protocol.

Other animals, such as mice, rats, moles, gophers, chipmunks, prairie dogs, and rabbits, are considered rabies-free so yet again follow the human bite protocol.

Squirrels can carry rabies but have not been known to transmit it to humans.

Other wild animals like bats, skunks, foxes, and coyotes are especially dangerous and, if your child is bitten by an animal that cannot be located, your child may need rabies shots and possibly an immune globulin injection.

Bee sting or yellow jacket sting

Watch for signs and symptoms of an allergic reaction or anaphylaxis.

If the stinger remains in the skin, use tweezers to pull it straight out or use a credit card or the edge of your fingernail to scrape it out.

A cool pack can help alleviate pain.

Baking soda with water on a cotton ball held to the area or a meat tenderizer with water on a cotton ball will help pull out the toxin and the stinger if it is still embedded. This neutralizes the venom and decreases pain and swelling.

Watch for difficulty breathing or swallowing for up to two hours after the sting.

Call your physician if the swelling is severe or it begins to look infected.

You can also give Zyrtec to decrease itching or if you suspect an allergic reaction.

Cuts and scrapes

Again, wash well with antibacterial soap.

Tetanus is not an issue if your child is up to date on his or her shots.

Apply Neosporin or Neosporin Pain Relief or other antibiotic ointment. Watch for signs and symptoms of infection. If you suspect there is a possible need for sutures, don't wait until the next day, seek medical advice as soon as possible—optimal is fewer than six hours from injury. If you wait too long, they will not suture due to risk of infection.

Head trauma

If your little one hits their head, you need to watch them closely for three full days. (If your child falls from a height of four feet or more, they need to be evaluated by a physician right away.)

Monitor your child for any loss of consciousness, any altered mental status (is your child acting appropriately?) vomiting, or blurred vision (I know this is difficult to assess in an infant). If your baby is walking or crawling, are they still able to walk and crawl normally? Make sure there is no clear fluid running from the nose when they are not crying for a time period of greater than 20 minutes.

Most head injuries are usually minor and just look bad. It is not uncommon for them to develop a goose egg or black and blue mark. Treat the area with a cool pack or ice and monitor for the signs and symptoms of a serious head trauma above.

It never fails that your child will have this sort of head injury when it is nap time or bedtime. If your child is acting sleepy and it is not their normal nap time, have them seen by your provider, but if it is around their normal nap time and, especially if they just cried for quite some time and wore themselves out, let your child fall asleep. If it is nap time, wake your child at the normal time they would wake up, if they are not yet awake, and check on their mental status. So, for example, if your child typically takes an hour-long nap, wake them at an hour, if your child takes a 2-hour nap, wake them at two hours. As long as your child seems to be acting appropriately, don't worry.

If the event happens near bedtime, wake your child after two hours of sleep. If your little one is acting normally for a child that was just woken up, let them go back to sleep. If your child's symptoms change, or they act confused, vomit, or seem excessively sleepy, call your doctor.

Mouth trauma

Mouth traumas always look worse than they are because blood mixed with saliva looks like a significant amount of blood. Children often cut the inside of their mouth with falls, especially when they have a toy in their mouth and fall on it, cutting the frenulum. The frenulum is the skin that holds the lip to the gum. You can feel it with your tongue when you run it between your lip and gum. This area bleeds a lot and can look very scary.

Give the child a cold popsicle like a Pedialyte popsicle or ice cube to chew on and clean up the area to assess it. Like I said prior, it is usually that the child cuts the frenulum or bites the tongue. The mouth heals on its own and does not typically require sutures. The only exception to this is if a tooth has gone through the lip, or the tongue has been severed. Otherwise, there is nothing much you can do but love and cuddle your little one. This will heal on its own. If bleeding continues >10 minutes with pressure or cold, call your doctor.

Thermal (heat) burns

There are three degrees of burns. I have personally seen a child with a third-degree burn from just turning on the outside water hose in Arizona.

1st degree: reddened skin without blisters, does not need to be seen.

2nd degree: reddened skin with blisters, usually takes 2–3 weeks to heal.

3rd degree: deep burns with white, charred skin. Skin sensitivity is absent. If the area is larger than a quarter, it usually needs a skin graft to prevent bad scarring.

Put the burned area in cold water until it stops burning or pour cold water over the area for 10 minutes. This lessens the depth of the burn and relieves pain. For little ones, the most common place for a burn is their little hands as they grab a curling iron or a hot object. So, if possible, put their little hand in a bowl of cold water all the way to the doctor if it is a blistered burn, as it needs to be treated.

For first degree or mild second degree burns, wash the area gently with an antibacterial soap twice per day. Don't open blisters.

You can apply antibiotic ointment.

Pain medication such as ibuprofen (anti-inflammatory) and cold compresses will usually help.

First- and second-degree burns do not typically leave scars.

Burns can become infected easily, so watch for signs and symptoms of infection.

With sunburns, replace fluids and give cool baths.

Most pediatricians like to see most second-degree burns recommend Bacitracin on all burns, regardless of severity, due to the high risk of infection.

Cactus / foreign body

Cactus spines are not poisonous, yet some can cause skin irritation, contact dermatitis, and infection. Try to use tweezers and pull the thorn out at the same angle as it went in, if possible. Elmer's glue or paraffin wax left on for 15 minutes to dry and then peeled away may remove those fine hair-like slivers that some cactuses leave. You may try tape or even a mask that forms a peel. Soak in warm water for 20 minutes. A bathtub is the easiest way to do this for young children. Baking soda may help soothe skin and help bring the thorns to the surface. Clean with soap and water after removal. Watch for signs and symptoms of infection. One of my best friend's little boys ran into a barrel cactus when he was little. These have very long thorns, and it broke off in his skin. She had him soak trying to get it to come to the surface, but it was not visible by the naked eye. She asked me what to do. I said if you cannot easily pull it out, leave it be. I told her organic material like a cactus thorn will work its way out. She decided to go to the ER instead. She sat and waited for hours to be seen and when the ER doctor saw him, he said almost word for word what I said, "It is organic and will eventually work its way out." She was pretty frustrated at this point after waiting so long and now paying for an ER visit, so she said, "No, I want you to try to get it out." So, he did try but due to natural swelling of the tissue, he was unable to get the thorn out, so her little boy ended up with it still in his skin, a laceration, and Steri-Strips. She called me so I could share with my parenting classes to leave organic material alone and let it work its way out. If the material is non-organic, such as glass or metal, it does need to be seen.

Information from this chapter was adapted from Dr. Barton Schmitt's triage protocol.

1. A recent big change involves using Zyrtec instead of diphenhydramine for allergic reactions. Most pediatricians and allergists have moved away from diphenhydramine and are using Zyrtec for all allergy situations. After much review, data suggested that Zyrtec is safer than diphenhydramine. Many practices have changed triage advice to recommend Zyrtec which is approved down to six months age.

* Zyrtec can be given every 24 HOURS ** Under age 12 MONTHS, PLEASE CONSULT YOUR PROVIDER *

Dosing: ¼ tsp=1.25ml ½ tsp=2.5ml 1 tsp=5ml

ZYRTEC	Children's 24hr suspension	Children's chewables	Children's chewables	Tablets	May be given every
Concentration	(5mg/5ml) 1 tsp	5mg/5ml	10mg/10ml	10mg/10ml	

WEIGHT	AGE						
14-17 lbs.	6-11 mos	1.25ml daily	---	---	---	---	
18-23 lbs.	12-23 mos	2.5ml daily	---	---	---	---	24 hours
24-35 lbs.	2-3 yrs	2.5ml daily	---	---	---	---	24 hours
36-47 lbs.	4-5 yrs	2.5ml daily	1/2 tablet daily	---	---	---	24 hours
48-59 lbs.	6-8 yrs	5-10ml daily	1-2 tablets daily	1 tablet daily	1 tablet daily		24 hours
60-85 lbs.	9-11 yrs	5-10ml daily	1-2 tablets daily	1 tablet daily	1 tablet daily		24 hours
85+ lbs.	12+ yrs	10ml daily	1-2 tablets daily	1 tablet daily	1 tablet daily		24 hours

CETIRIZINE DOSING (ZYRTEC)

AAP: estimated oral fluid and electrolyte requirements:

Body weight in lbs.	Minimum daily fluid req	Electrolyte solution for Mild diarrhea 24hrs
6-7lbs	10 oz	16oz
11 lbs.	15 oz	23oz
22 lbs.	25 oz	40oz
26 lbs.	28 oz	44 oz

Parenting, August 2002

How clean is too clean? Why some germs may be good for your child's health.

"The modern war on germs may have gone too far, wiping out too many of the good guys along with the culprits that cause disease. Exposure to certain types of bacteria in the first year of life is crucial for teaching the developing immune system to recognize friend from foe. Without this early training, the imbalance within the body's immune cells may predispose them to attacking a host of harmless substances such as cat dander and pollen, etc. Immune system immaturity may be a major contributor to one of the most perplexing public health problems our country faces: increasing numbers of kids with allergies, asthma, and eczema. The hypothesis is a leading theory to explain the rising rates of these illnesses, says Dr. Richard Johnston. Experts are also investigating possible links in adult autoimmune diseases such as diabetes, multiple sclerosis, and lupus. Numerous studies have shown that allergies and asthma occur less frequently among children who:

Have older siblings.

Spend time in daycare in the first 1–2 years of life or are in playgroups.

Have early exposure to pets or farm animals.

Live in rural parts of the country or in areas of the world that lack modern sanitation.

The good news: The organisms that babies and toddlers need to encounter to develop healthy immune systems are not the kind that make us sick, rather harmless bacteria found in dirt, mud, puddles, and ponds.

The hundreds of antibacterial products flooding the market each year may be making the problem worse. Dr. Stuart Levy, microbiologist, says these products are likely to encourage bacterial resistance. Researchers discovered that triclosan, an active ingredient in most antibacterial cleansers, works more like an antibiotic drug than a disinfectant. Instead of obliterating the bacteria and then evaporating like bleach, triclosan blocks a specific enzyme that germs need to survive. The problem is that microbes can mutate and find a way to change and grow. Triclosan also lingers on surfaces such as counters, toys, tubs, etc. for days to weeks, which gives bacteria plenty of time to develop resistance. There is also another antibacterial used that poses the same danger called triclocarban, which is a close relative."

Use a bleach cleanser for countertops. Wash your hands with soap and water for 30–60 seconds. It is still not a bad idea to wipe the grocery cart handle or put a baby cover over it.

We went from one scary chapter to the next. I am sorry about that. I wish I could tell you that, by reading this book, you could protect your kids from all things dangerous and all illnesses, but I would not be telling you the truth. Kids are going to get sick, and it is the most helpless feeling a parent can have. Yet, just like with the safety lecture in the previous chapter, you are now armed with tools on how to help your little one when they do get sick. You will know what to do to keep them comfortable and when to seek medical care. You've got this!

CHAPTER 13

DENTAL

"It is a smile of a baby that makes life worth living."

— *Debasish Mridha*

Your baby's teeth

Your baby is born with all his or her teeth, but they are buried beneath the gum line. Most children sprout their first tooth at about six months of age. Timing, however, is mainly determined by genetics. If you or your baby's father got your teeth late or early, your children will most likely be similar.

Teeth usually come in two at a time. They usually erupt in the following order:

1. Two lower incisors
2. Four upper incisors
3. Two lower incisors and all four first molars
4. Four canines
5. Four second molars

The typical timeline of how and when the teeth come in is as follows:

Between 6 and 10 months: The first two teeth to appear are the two lower front teeth.

Between 8 and 13 months: The top four incisors are typically the next teeth to come in.

Between 10 and 16 months: Two more incisors will appear in the lower front and then the first back teeth or first year molars will come in.

Between 16 and 23 months: The canines will come in

Between 23 and 33 months: The last remaining teeth come in. These are the back molars (second year molars). By the time your child is three years of age, they will have all their primary teeth (20).

Don't worry if your child's baby teeth don't all come in straight or evenly spaced. The placement of permanent teeth won't necessarily follow the same pattern.

Even though your child will eventually lose all his or her baby teeth, they are still very important.

Baby teeth will preserve spacing for the permanent teeth, help maintain proper alignment of the jawbones and allow your baby to learn to chew and speak clearly.

Cavity prevention

As soon as your baby has teeth or even a tooth, parents should begin cavity prevention. You can use a soft washcloth or piece of gauze to wipe teeth off, or a finger brush or baby toothbrush. I love the little banana toothbrush. You do not need toothpaste or, if you want, to you can use kid toothpaste that is non-fluorinated.

At around one year, use a smear of regular toothpaste.

At the age of two, use a pea-sized amount.

Decayed baby teeth can cause gum infections and the only treatment for a severely decayed tooth is extraction. This may affect spacing of permanent teeth.

The first sign of a cavity is discoloration or minor pitting of the tooth.

Cavities in infants are most often caused by milk or juice that pools around baby teeth when infants fall asleep with a bottle in their mouth. During sleep, saliva production, which normally rinses teeth of sugar, slows down. So never let your baby go to sleep with a bottle.

Permanent teeth do not start sprouting until age 5–6 years. Again, this is genetically determined.

The American Academy of Pediatrics suggests the first dental visit to be at age three. My pediatric dentist suggests two and a half for the first cleaning when all the baby teeth are in.

However, call your dentist if your child breaks or chips their tooth or if one is knocked out. Although the dentist won't re-implant a baby tooth, they can check for retained fragments and determine if there is any root damage to the permanent tooth.

Fluoride

Fluoride has recently become a concern but not in the way you may be thinking.

In the 1950s, fluoride was found to prevent tooth decay if given in small amounts. Since fluoride was introduced, tooth decay has fallen. But today's parents are not giving as much sugar, they are brushing regularly with fluoride toothpaste, most states in the US have fluorinated water as their public water, many canned foods contain fluoride, infant formulas contain fluoride, so the risk of too much fluoride could actually outweigh the risk of not enough fluoride.

Now there is a worrisome increase in cases of fluorosis. This is an unsightly brown staining of the teeth from too much fluoride. So, physicians are not recommending routine fluoride supplements anymore unless the child is having significant cavities.

Instead, many pediatricians and dentists are applying fluoride varnish to the teeth as early as six months of age, two to four times per year. However, some pediatric practices and dentists do not do this until the age of 18 months. If your pediatric practice is not applying the varnish at six months and if you are solely breastfeeding, offer a sippy cup a day of fluorinated or nursery water starting at six months of age.

The ideal amount of fluoride in water is 0.7 – 1.0 parts per million which means 1 quart of water provides 1mg of fluoride per day.

A pea-sized amount of toothpaste that is swallowed is estimated to be about 0.3mg of fluoride, which is approximately ⅓ of the daily allowance.

Reverse osmosis filters out fluoride.

Teething

Parents always ask me what they can give their baby to help with teething.

I typically say stick with natural things like teething rings and frozen fruit, as your baby is going to be teething for the next two years. You don't want to be giving them medication all the time. My general rule is, when the first two teeth are actually breaking through and if your infant seems uncomfortable, give some acetaminophen or ibuprofen if your baby is over six months of age. But this may be just one or two times to get them through the roughest time. As teeth typically come in around the age of six months and this is also the time that Mom's immunity from birth wears off, this might also be the first illness. So, if your child seems unusually uncomfortable, you don't want to mask something like an earache with pain reliever. Have them checked out by the pediatrician, especially if they have a fever or other symptoms.

Teething rings and toys are a baby's way to massage sore gums. You can massage sore areas with your finger for about two minutes. Popsicles like Pedialyte pops, frozen banana, or other fruit in a baby-safe feeder, or frozen bagel in a Baby Safe Feeder can all be natural ways to help a teething baby.

Be careful with teething gel as there is the possibility of a drug reaction with some medications and it may numb the throat and can pose a choking hazard. It really does not last long enough that I feel it is beneficial.

The ZoLi Teether and Zoli Bunny Dual Nub Teether are great for teething infants. The banana toothbrush and Chubby Gummy gum massager on Amazon are a few of my parenting families' favorite items for teething babies as well.

Start good dental habits early and your child will have good dental habits for life. Even though the baby teeth are not permanent, they are very important. Children need healthy baby teeth for speech and to maintain the spacing and development of adult teeth. Cavities can lead to infection and a healthy smile helps kids feel more self-assured, leading to more positive self-esteem. So, take good care of those pearly whites as soon as they come in and show your child how you practice good oral hygiene. They are always watching you, so set a good example.

CHAPTER 14

SOCIAL AND EMOTIONAL DEVELOPMENT

*"Just like a plant needs light and space to grow,
a child needs love and freedom to unfold."*

— Sigrid Leo

Barton Schmitt says, "From birth *the main determinant* of an infant's social, emotional, and language development is the amount of positive contact he has with his parents."

Wow! No pressure, right? It is not like we do not put enough pressure on ourselves already. But it does make sense. We are our baby's first friends. We are the ones to first teach them that even though their behavior may be developmentally appropriate, it may not be socially appropriate. Your baby's strong attachment to you will make him/her eager to learn from you.

Warren Umansky, PhD, says, "From birth through age one, *security leads to autonomy and independence.*" I feel this carries over all through a child's life.

A full-term baby starts to show his or her own unique temperament around 3–4 weeks of age. This is due to a maturing nervous system.

Babies at this age show they have predictable physical responses to negative and positive stimuli. A baby's heart rate will speed up with negative stimuli and will slow down with positive stimuli. You may even see your baby's unique temperament emerging as early as three weeks.

One of my favorite developmental pediatricians, Dr. T. Berry Brazelton, as well as the American Academy of Pediatrics say parents can start to see their baby's emerging temperament by how they transition through six different states or stages of consciousness throughout the day, at as early as three weeks. The style or manner in which they move or transition from one state to another, either *rapidly* or *gradually with warning*, is an indication of his/her emerging temperament.

The six states or stages of consciousness are as follows:

1. Deep sleep

This stage of consciousness can be described as sleeping deeply. Your baby lies quietly without moving. His or her breathing is deep and regular.

2. Light or REM sleep

This stage of consciousness can be described as light or restless sleep. Your baby is on the verge of waking up. He or she startles at noise and moves in his or her sleep. If your baby has a pacifier in his or her mouth, you may see him or her sucking from time to time. Breathing is not as deep as deep sleep and not as regular.

3. Indeterminate state

This is the stage I say to put your baby down at. Drowsy but still awake. Their eyes are just beginning to close, and they are dosing off. You might notice some cradle fidgeting and fussiness but not full-blown crying.

4. Wide-awake alert state

This stage of consciousness is the best time to play and interact with your baby. They are quiet, attentive, and alert. They are wide awake. Their eyes are open wide, their face is bright, and they are receptive to play or communication. His or her body is quiet, and their breathing is calm and regular.

5. Fussy alert state

This stage of consciousness often follows the wide-awake alert state after a baby has had enough play or is getting to the point of too much stimulation. This state is an active state where the body and face are moving actively. The baby may become fussy and turn away. The baby's movements become uncoordinated or jerky and the breathing becomes irregular.

6. Crying state

This stage is very disorganized. It is typically seen when your infant is hungry, tired, uncomfortable, wet, etc. Your baby may simply be crying or full-on screaming.

Dr. T. Berry Brazelton says:

"Most parents put most of the emphasis in the first few weeks on feeding yet <u>getting them fed is only half the job. Learning to</u>

communicate with Baby through touching, holding, rocking, talking and learning to synchronize with Baby's behavior are just as important as getting him fed."

Dr. Barton Schmitt says to use feedings to emphasize warm, personal contact, make eye contact, keep your baby close, and smile at them often.

Because of this jump in brain development and neurological maturity, your baby is ready to pay more attention to their parents and this leads to smiling and cooing.

Around 3–4 weeks, the baby is able to go a bit longer in between feeds which gives you more time for play during the wide-awake state.

Keep in mind babies can become overstimulated and will let you know when they have had enough. Some babies are more sensitive to stimulation than others.

The end of the day fussy time – the "bewitching hour"

Somewhere between 2 and 12 weeks of age, most babies will develop a fussy period toward the end of the day. In my house we called this the "bewitching hour".

Dr. Ronald Barr calls this the "Period of PURPLE Crying." No, not because the baby cries so hard they turn purple, but because each letter stands for something. More about this in a minute.

Dr. Brazelton also describes this developmental stage in his book *Touchpoints*.

Both doctors agree that understanding this normal developmental stage is the key to getting through it with confidence and your sanity.

Dr. Brazelton did a study with 80 moms in his practice and found that almost all had a predictable fussy period that began at the end of each day. Most would stop for a short time if nursed or picked up, yet the fussing would inevitably resume shortly thereafter.

Dr. Brazelton believes that the reason for this fussy period is that, even though the nervous system is maturing, it is still immature. He feels that the immature nervous system can take in and utilize only so much stimuli as the day proceeds. After that there is always a bit of overload. As the day proceeds the increasingly overloaded nervous system begins to cycle in shorter sleep, active, and feeding periods / cycles. Finally, your baby needs to blow off steam in the form of an active fussy period. Remember your stages of consciousness: Your baby is cycling through these stages quicker as the day progresses.

He says there are often warning signs before this happens. You might notice your baby becomes jerky or has disorganized movements prior to this fussy time. You can often begin to predict it and, once you learn to predict it, you can try to prevent it or shorten the duration.

The good news is that, after this period is over, the nervous system is ready to recognize information for another 24 hours. More good news is that Dr. Brazelton found that most babies slept better and longer after this fussy period.

He feels, unfortunately, that parents usually feel helpless during this period and want to fix it. Yet sometimes parents' well-meaning efforts to "fix it" by rocking, singing, etc. may actually add extra stimulation to your baby's already overloaded, overstimulated nervous system.

So, what do you do? Do you just let them cry? Well, yes and no.

Dr. Brazelton suggests you first go to your baby and try all your parental maneuvers. Make sure they are not hungry, they are dry, see if cuddling or picking them up helps. It may stop for a short time as a distraction usually works short term, but if the crying resumes...

Once you have reassured yourself and used all your comfort measures with no avail, let him or her be for 10–15 minutes in a quiet, possibly darkened room, and let him or her blow off steam.

After 10–15 minutes try some soothing again. If the same thing happens, you may need to repeat this cycle a few times.

Dr. Brazelton says the routine is rarely needed more than 3–4 times.

This cycle can go on for hours if parents become too anxious or if your baby is over stimulated.

If this fussy time is increasing in intensity and time, despite your restraint and low-key efforts, you need to talk with your doctor. This may be a medical condition such as reflux or other source of pain.

Dr. Brazelton feels that if parents can understand the need for their infants' fussiness, they will not feel so responsible for it.

He states that many in pediatrics call this inconsolable fussy period colic and try to stop it with medication, carrying them around constantly, nursing constantly, etc. Yet if this is only happening at the end of the day and not all day long, this is not colic.

Back to the "Period of PURPLE Crying": Dr. Ronald Barr, a developmental pediatrician, says he needed to explain this phase to parents so that they would understand that what they are experiencing is indeed normal and, although frustrating, it is simply a phase in their child's development, and it will pass. It is temporary and will come to an end. He also found through his studies that all mammals go through this same developmental stage of crying more in the first months of life.

Each letter stands for a way to describe it:

P- Peak of crying: Your baby may start as early as 2 weeks and cry more each week with the most crying at 2 months of age and then decrease each week for the next 2–3 months.

U- Unexpected: The crying can come and go with no rhyme or reason.

R- Resists soothing: Your baby may not stop crying no matter what you try.

P- Pain-like face: A crying baby may look like they are in pain even when they are not.

L- Long-lasting: The crying can go on for hours.

E- Evening: Your baby may cry more in the late afternoon or evening.

Period means it will come to an end.

What I like about Dr. Brazelton's method is that it does give you something to do so you do not feel so helpless, and it has been proven to shorten this period of time as well.

I have also found that if you can help the baby calm down prior to this "bewitching hour," it also shortened the length of time it went on.

I figured out in the NICU that my kids calmed down with warm water run over their head. Now as preemies, a full bath freaked them out. This is common with many newborns, but as they grew, the bath with warm water, quiet and soothing calmed them. So, about an hour before this bewitching hour, which for us was about 5 pm every single day, I would do one of my calming maneuvers. Sometimes it was just a little lotion on the feet, not the whole body. Sometimes it was a warm bath, or just washing hair in a darkened bathroom. This gentle, quiet time helped soothe them. It did not stop this altogether but certainly shortened the length of time it went on.

Sources for the information below came from sources including: www.pbs.org /Sassy /AAP/Ross Laboratories, and T. Berry Brazelton

Social and emotional milestones by month
3 months

Your baby can be comforted by a familiar adult.

Your infant responds positively to gentle touch.

They are interested in people, especially faces. They can watch their parents' faces for long periods of time. The more your baby studies you, the more interested in watching you he or she becomes, and they may break into a big smile. If the parents smile back, the baby may wiggle and coo.

The best time to interact with your baby is during the wide-awake alert state (this is from birth on.)

Your baby has a short attention span and gets over-stimulated easily. He or she benefits from short, frequent interactions rather than long, infrequent ones.

You are beginning to adapt to your baby's patterns of eating, sleeping, and wakefulness (they begin to develop a pattern).

Some ways parents can help in developing personal and social skills include:

When a baby is fussy, try to find and fix the cause. Respond right away when your baby cries. Crying is a baby's only way of telling you something is wrong and of communicating.

Babies show the majority of their emotions through crying. They have distinct cries for different needs. Hunger is a basic cry. They have a distinct cry for anger, and a different one for pain. You will start to know what each cry means. By responding right away to cries during the first year, you establish a strong sense of trust with your little one. By responding promptly to your baby, he or she realizes you understand their wants and needs.

Carry your baby around with you often. Talk to him/her in happy soothing tones. You cannot spoil a baby this age. While carrying your baby in a cuddled sitting position show him/her lights and/or brightly colored objects and point out sounds that you hear.

Smile often at your baby, especially when your baby smiles back at you.

Studies show that rocking a baby is both soothing for the baby and relaxing for the parent. So, snuggle up in that rocking chair.

Start a very basic bedtime routine (the younger the baby, the shorter the routine). Sing quietly or read to your baby before bed.

Between 6 and 8 weeks of age, Dr. Brazelton recommends waking your baby when you are ready to start your day and waking your baby when you want to establish their bedtime for a feeding to help them get attuned to your family schedule.

Your baby is beginning to perfect a pattern of self-comforting. Continue to put your baby down drowsy yet awake. If you have a sensitive baby and you are having a difficult time putting them down drowsy but awake, and your baby is waking when you put them down, you might try a more gradual transition from your arms to the crib. You might stay in the darkened room and rub on the baby, possibly singing, or talking softly if needed. Remember, however, the less you do for them and the more they do on their own to fall asleep, the better. Self-comforting is the key!

A schedule should develop yet should not be too rigid. You should still be following his or her cues / demands as your baby's nervous system and digestive system are still maturing.

By 8 weeks your baby's temperament should be more apparent. You should be able to tell if you have an easy-going baby vs. a more intense or sensitive baby. Does your baby roll with the flow, or does change throw them off?

Some hypersensitive babies may stiffen, startle, and gaze avert with too much stimulation. This can occur during play, or with introduction of a new person. If you have a sensitive baby, you may need to allow him or her to relax before trying to talk or play with them again. Approach slowly and touch them gently without talking or making eye contact.

Your goal is to have your baby grow up with a feeling that people respect their quiet shyness for what it is, an easily overloaded nervous system.

If I am describing your little one, the good news is that, following these kids through school years later, many of them turn out to be intellectuals and have artistic pursuits.

4 months

A four-month-old has a more predictable schedule. If you do not have a schedule yet, don't worry. Just start writing nap times down each day and you will see a schedule naturally emerge. Then try to pick times that are most commonly occurring and then pick a time and be consistent.

The "fussy" period at the end of the day, the "bewitching hour" as I called it, is being replaced by a period of alertness and play.

The American Academy of Pediatrics recommends 4–6 months to be a good age to start solids. This further involves your baby in the family routine.

One major developmental achievement is that your 4-month-old is learning how to sit up. They learn first propped up, then later to sit all on their own.

Once they have discovered how much they can see from a sitting position, many babies will fuss until parents sit them up or move them around. They fuss out of boredom. You can keep your baby stimulated by moving them around to what I call different stations. Stations are simply new activities, or a new place to move your baby to when they get bored. Examples are a bouncy seat, an Exersaucer, a swing, a highchair, an activity mat, etc.

Your baby may show a heightened interest in exploring your face with their hands. This type of exploration leads to the cognitive process of "person permanence". Dr. Brazelton describes the cognitive process called "person permanence", which is the awareness that people are real and continue to exist even when they are out of sight. This cognitive process, like most others, is just starting and will continue for the next several months.

Just as you are seeing rapid gains in their physical development, you are also seeing rapid gains in their emotional development.

Frustrations may start to emerge. But keep in mind frustration can be a powerful force for learning and can sometimes be a positive thing.

Parents can do what they can to help, yet do not feel like you have to go to your baby all the time any longer. Let them start to learn to problem-solve and self-soothe. This can be a frustrating time for both of you but allowing them to do things on their own gives them an amazing sense of accomplishment. If your baby becomes overwhelmed, step in and help.

5 months

In his book *Touchpoints*, Dr. Brazelton says, "In the 5th month babies can learn to play games with their new achievements." For example, your baby may cry and wait to see if anyone heard them and see if anyone is coming, then cry again.

Babies begin to fake cough, gag, and squeal as exploratory behaviors, to see what reactions they might get from Mom and Dad.

This is a big step in development toward the cognitive process called causality. Causality is: if I do something, I will get this result. This developmental process, like person permanence, is just beginning and will continue for months to come.

6 months

Around six months of age, many babies develop a fondness for or an attachment to a familiar object like a blanket or an animal, etc.

This is often called a love object or transition object. A love object offers comfort when Mom and Dad is not there. A love object that you hold against you while you nurse or feed, so it picks up your scent, is particularly comforting to an infant. This is the time for attachment so most doctors will tell you if you want to get rid of a pacifier before three years of age, get rid of it now before it becomes a transition object.

They may start vocal games by putting sounds together. Babbling becomes more consistent. Around this age babies may start blowing raspberries with their lips and, if you are feeding solids when this stage starts, this can add a whole new adventure to mealtime ☺

Again, they are gauging your response and the bigger deal you make of something, the more you are guaranteeing it will be repeated. This is true of both "good" and "bad" behaviors.

7 months

Your baby may start to giggle or squeal when they are happy. Oh, how I love that belly laugh!

They want all your attention.

They can play with toys more independently. They are more vocal and may say "ma" or "da" or sounds that are starting to sound like words.

Your little one's personality is becoming even more predictable. Signs of their further developing temperament are also becoming more pronounced. You are beginning to understand more what is *normal* for *your* child. You can distinguish what is their "usual self" and what is not. You will know when your child is not well based on their behavior.

Dr. Brazelton and his colleges assess temperament at this age by looking at 9 things:

1. Activity level
2. Distractibility
3. Persistence
4. Approach / withdrawal: How does he/she handle new and stressful situations?
5. Intensity
6. Adaptability: How does he/she deal with transition?
7. Regularity: How predictable is he/she in sleep, bowel habits, and rhythms of the day?
8. Sensory threshold: Is he/she hyper- or hyposensitive to stimuli around him/her, is he/she easily overstimulated?
9. Mood: Is he/she basically positive or negative in his/her reactions?

A seven-month-old can understand the word "no", yet they probably won't respond to it. They are learning that each parent is different, and they may treat him/her differently. They are also adapting to the parents' differences.

Your baby is also developing a sense of object permanence. Object permanence is knowing that an object is still there even though it may be out of sight or partially out of sight. Help develop this cognitive skill during play. Hide part of a toy and have your baby try to find it. Babies hide and seek.

Your baby may drop an object, or food from the highchair, over and over and over again, to watch it drop, to hear it hit the floor, and also to see what Mom will do each time.

This is the beginning of a period of rapid learning.

Your little one is a big explorer. It is important to let him or her continue to explore your face, and his or her surroundings.

Dr. Brazelton explains that this cognitive need to explore and their new-found mobility will lead your little one into any available trouble. Be prepared and safety proof. Provide limits and make them clear from the start.

Play games that play out separation anxieties that are common at this age, like peek-a-boo. Hide around a corner and peek around, etc. Along with the cognitive process of object permanence, they are still developing the concept of person permanence. Person permanence is grasping the fact that people exist even when they are out of sight.

Have important strangers enter their life so he/she can learn about them. This will also help with stranger and separation anxieties.

You do not need to overprotect your children but be sensitive to this stage by not letting new people scoop them up without warning.

This is a major yet demanding period of development.

Your baby is continuing to process how things work and why. "Causality:" They continue to test Mom and Dad for reactions. So, they may drop something over and over again. Will Mom pick it up every time, will it make the same noise hitting the floor. How long will they allow this game to go on?

8 months

Your baby enjoys more social play. He or she is interested in mirror play at this age. They are paying more attention to others and may respond to other people's expressions and emotions.

Your infant can express a wider range of emotions. They can show emotion through not only cries and smiles but delighted laughter, along with kicks and arm swings.

Your baby will respond when you say their name.

Those strong emotions continue, and your little one may get angry and frustrated when their needs are not met in what they consider a reasonable amount of time.

Eye contact begins to replace some of the physical contact that younger infants seek.

9 months

Your infant is expressing multiple emotions.

He or she is able to distinguish friends from strangers.

Your baby is responding more to language and may gesture wants or needs.

Your little one may show displeasure if another child takes a toy from them.

Take your baby out to places with you to increase comfort with others.

Talk to your baby while pointing to their image in the mirror and say their name and point out facial features and body parts. This will help your baby develop their sense of self.

Encourage your baby to babble / talk to themselves in front of mirror.

The cognitive process of causality is becoming more advanced. Your baby is trying to figure out how things work. At 9 months your baby may push a windup toy across the floor, curious about it, knowing it moves across the floor, but not understanding it needs to be wound up. This cognitive process will develop in the next three months so that by a year, they may be able to wind the toy and watch it move across the floor.

A baby this age wants to be on the move at all times. They are very busy.

Object permanence and person permanence are still important concepts they are trying to grasp. Continue your games of peek-a-boo and hide-and-seek to help grasp these concepts. They love rhythm and rhyme at this age. Rhythmic songs and games prepare a baby for the rhythm of a conversation later on.

10 months

Your baby is using hand movements more and more to express what they want. They may use some basic sign language if you are using it in the home. Your baby might point at objects or people. He or she may wave "hi" and "bye."

They may reach for you to pick them up.

Your baby understands and pays attention to where you are looking and pointing.

Your baby is increasingly interested in interacting with others, and he or she maintains eye contact with people during play.

11 months

Your baby is more and more interested in games. A favorite game for babies at this age is hide-and-seek with his or her toys.

Your little one loves music and rhythm and may bounce and wiggle to all types of music and may create his or her own with all types of toys that they can make into makeshift instruments.

They are becoming a bit of a thrill seeker and love to be tossed in the air, wanting it repeated over and over again.

They respond to simple 1–2 step requests: Go get your ball and bring it to Mommy.

They love to use toys in new ways, and they love to create a racket.

You might find your little one wanting to cuddle more.

They are starting to explore the world with interest in sights, sounds, and smells.

Social / emotional milestones by end of the 12th month (from the AAP)

Shy or anxious with strangers.

Cries when Mom or Dad leaves.

Enjoys imitating people in play.

Shows specific preference for certain people and toys.

Prefers mother or regular care giver over all others.

Tests parental responses to his or her behavior (what do you do when he/she cries when you leave the room?).

May be fearful in some situations where he or she was not prior.

Repeats sounds or gestures for attention.

Finger-feeds themselves with more accuracy.

Extends arm or leg to help when being dressed.

Self-image

Psychologist Michael Lewis did experiments where he put children in front of a mirror at 12 months, 15 months, and 18 months.

Without attracting attention when the child was turned away from the mirror, he dabbed the child's nose with red rouge.

At 12 months, the child studied the mirror closely.

At 15 months, the child tried to wipe off the nose in the mirror.

At 18 months, the child tried to wipe his or her own nose.

Separation anxiety

Separation anxiety is universal among infants and toddlers. Although babies can show signs of separation anxiety as early as 6 months, the crisis age is 12–18 months and can continue through 2 years.

Believe it or not, many experts feel that separation anxiety is a positive sign of a baby's healthy development. Experts agree that it is the basis of your baby's ability to form personal relationships. It is a major emotional leap when your little one realizes that Mom is a separate person, and they value her presence far more than anybody else. Separation anxiety actually marks a turning point in development. The brain is developing enough to anticipate loss.

Dr. Charles Zeanah, professor of psychology at the University of Louisiana State School of Medicine says: "Developing a secure emotional attachment early in life is one of the most important ingredients in a person's long-term emotional well-being."

Dr. Jill Stamm says: "Bonding develops healthy brains, trust, love, security, and safety. These emotions activate what are called mirror neurons in a baby's brain and actually allow them to learn empathy. There are some experts who feel that autism is the misfiring of mirror neurons."

Many children in institutions or multi foster homes with consistently changing caregivers miss the opportunity to develop close relationships early in childhood. As a result, studies have shown that, when these children enter adulthood, they often have a difficult time feeling close to other people and in some cases exhibit antisocial behavior.

It is important for a baby to develop an awareness that, although Mom cannot always be there, she will always return. If an infant gets comfort from your return, it makes further separation more tolerable. Your baby gradually realizes he or she can manage without you. It's also great cuddle time when you return.

Experts say your baby's reaction upon being reunited is a better indication of attachment than whether he or she screams bloody murder when you leave. If your baby is clearly happy when you return, then he or she is using you as a secure base and reconnecting just fine.

Now, it can also be normal if your baby falls apart and fusses upon your return. It is almost as if they are letting you know: "Oh, I am so relieved you are home. You have no idea how I missed you." Both reactions are healthy responses.

Dr. Brazelton feels it's as if the baby is saving up all his intense feelings for people who matter most to them. After a crying period, they become alert and intensely interactive with parents. If your baby ignores you and stays "mad" for more than 10 minutes, you need to spend more time together.

When my cousin's baby was 9 months old, his wife developed a brain aneurysm. I was planning on a second baby, so I had the nursery all set up. My cousin asked if I could take the baby so he could be at the hospital with his wife. Although the baby knew me, I was not his mom. To make it worse she was solely breastfeeding, he had never had formula, and he was not sleeping through the night. I cannot even imagine what this poor little baby thought. Oh, and the icing on the cake was that he developed a bilateral ear infection on top of it all. To make a long story short, he learned to take a bottle and sleep through the night without any "crying it out," as I promised her I would not let him cry at all. I grew so close to that little peanut. I am still so close to him and love him to pieces. When I brought him up to the hospital, to his mom, when she was finally going home, he clung to me and would not go to her. As you can imagine her heart was breaking. I tried to explain to her that he was mad, and this was actually a healthy sign. He was letting her know she had been away too long. He was letting her know he was not happy being left with his mean "aunt" who force-fed him formula and took him to the pediatrician for antibiotic shots. Within no time at all he was snuggling up with Mom and has had no ill effects from his short time away from her.

Separation anxiety is painful for both parents and the baby. If you look at this in evolutionary terms, it makes sense why a baby would be upset. A baby would naturally get upset at being separated from the person whom they are most bonded with because they are the person who would keep them from straying and away from predators, feed them, and keep them warm and protected.

How we deal with babies and separation is largely a cultural issue. In the United States, we stress autonomy from a very early age. But in many cultures in the world, infants are rarely separated from their mothers in the first year of life. Some cultures literally carry their child on their body for a full year.

To make it easier on them and you, allow at least 30 minutes prior to leaving, if possible, to have your babysitter or family member come and spend time with your child before you leave, while you are still there. Leave your baby with people who are familiar to him or her if possible.

If you need to leave your baby with a stranger let them get to know one another gradually. Ask your sitter to visit and play with your baby several times before leaving them alone, if possible.

Always say goodbye and that you will be back. The wise saying "short goodbyes make dryer eyes" is a great motto to follow.

Since your baby is tuned in to how you feel, show warmth and enthusiasm no matter how much you feel like crying when you leave.

Once you leave, leave! Do not go back for anything. If you forget something, leave it.

Try a practice run if possible. Leave for only an hour or less the first day.

Nighttime separation

Separation anxiety can also occur at night.

Try to keep the hour before bedtime calm. You might add a calming bath, read a book, snuggle time, whatever settles and comforts your little one.

Try to keep the bedtime routine consistent.

If your baby cries you can reassure him or her. Do not stay until he or she is asleep. They still need to learn they can do this on their own.

Give lots of extra hugs and cuddles during the day.

Playing peek-a-boo and games of hide-and-seek during the day shows your little one that if you go, you come back. Games play out anxieties during the daylight.

Stranger anxiety

Stranger anxiety can occur as early as 5 months but the typical age for it to occur is around 9 months. Around 5–6 months your baby has a new awareness of sights and sounds. They are more aware of their surroundings and the people around them. This can affect your baby's readiness to accept strangers. Unfortunately, it can come and go, and often lasts until around the age of 2.

Infants often do not want to be held by someone they do not know. Someone they do not know feels threatening to them, if they are touching them, or even looking at them. Before this stage occurs, which often seems to come out of the blue, your little one may have been happy to be passed from one person to the next.

If your baby is having a problem with strangers, have that new person talk past the baby. Ask that stranger to avoid making eye contact. Ask them to keep their voice soft and even and allow Baby to be held by Mom or keep Mom in Baby's view.

A stranger presents your baby with too much new stimuli in their comfortable world. Babies are going through a confusing time of wanting independence with learning to crawl and explore, yet they still want to stay close to those they know will take care of them. Be patient with your little one and look at it as a good sign that your child has formed a strong attachment to you. They just need time and space to handle new situations and, if you respect that, this will make this period easier for your baby and shorter, so easier also for you.

Feelings

Before a baby can talk, they are able to express emotions through their actions. They cry, smile, and kick their legs and pump their arms.

Even a newborn makes his or her likes and dislikes known. Your newborn baby expresses preferences. They will let you know how tightly they want to be held. If they want to be swaddled or not, how much noise he or she can tolerate. How long their attention span is before they look away or fuss. Minutes after birth a baby will curl up in contentment on his or her mother's chest.

"Some of this is reflex, yet some is emotion," says Dr. Steven Shilov, chairman of pediatrics at Miami Medical Center, Florida. He found that within even an hour of birth, babies will try to make the same facial expressions as they see someone else making.

Over the next few months, a baby will strive to coordinate their gestures and vocalizations as well as their expressions with those of adults around them.

A big emotional milestone is the social smile that all new parents look forward to. This is typically seen between 4 and 8 weeks of age. For many parents, the smile helps with attachment. It comes at the perfect time when you are exhausted, and the baby is still waking at night. When you go to this small little person in the middle of the night half-awake and they smile at you, it recharges your battery for another couple of months, until they are sleeping through the night. It is one of nature's miracles.

Even blind babies will smile at a familiar voice or touch.

Babies can even begin to anticipate enjoyable activities. For example, a five-month-old may wiggle in anticipation of the sight of a bottle.

Anger is also emerging, as I mentioned above. If you take a toy away from a six-month-old, they will cry a different cry than their normal hunger cry.

Copycat grief

Another sign of emotional and social development is "copycat grief." Copycat grief is when one child cries and the other follows suit. This is so cute in class when it becomes a chorus of babies.

Experts believe copycat grief may be an emotional reflex that helps "train" our nature toward a more genuine form of compassion.

At about 9 months, a baby begins to pay attention to how others feel. They will look for Mom and Dad for reassurance when they are unsure about something, as if to ask: "Is this OK?"

Experts feel the root of empathy is being able to link what an emotion feels like for you with what it feels like for others.

Another example of an early display of empathy I notice in class is if another baby gets hurt, a child looks to their own mom for help, not the baby's own mother. They know that if they needed comfort, they would feel better with their own mommy. They do not quite realize that the other child might want their own mother. It is adorable to see the way their minds are working.

Not until toddlerhood will your little one start to understand why they feel the way they do and actually name their emotions. That does not mean you cannot talk about emotions and feelings early. I love the book *Baby's Feelings*. This is a great first book of emotions for babies.

Feeling that others are tuned in to them is a vitally important part of developing their sense of emerging self. Try to resist the urge to try to protect your kids from strong emotions. No matter what you do, your children are still going to feel sad, afraid, anxious, and angry from time to time.

Your job is to help them cope with their feelings and express them in socially acceptable ways that do not harm themselves or others and are appropriate for their age and abilities. Remember there is never a feeling that is wrong or inappropriate, it is how they act on those feelings that may not be socially appropriate.

Friends

Children less than one year of age may single out another child that appeals to them and smile back and forth. A loving response to a stuffed animal is a precursor to friendship.

Parents play the biggest role in setting the stage for friendships. Parents teach first what it means to care about others. They teach the baby to learn to read others' emotions and learn social cues. Parents are the first people who have back-and-forth, give-and-take interactions with a child.

Social interactions start with watching other children and playing next to other children. Set realistic expectations according to your child's age and temperament. Provide opportunity for play dates, yet keep in mind that kids generally prefer to play with toys and other adults until about the age of two.

Begin peer contact by at least one year of age, even though the babies will not be able to play cooperatively. Teach them to take turns. Teach them what is socially acceptable. Little ones will not get sharing yet. Realize it is developmentally normal to poke, hit, and grab for a toy. Because it is age-appropriate does not mean that it is socially appropriate. Your little one will not start really sharing until about 2 ½ to 3 years of age. Sharing must be learned. You are the teacher! From 3 years of age onward, your child should be able to interact with peers without you being present.

I know this article is older, but I found it years ago and loved it, so I thought I would include it in the book: It is from *Parenting Magazine*, October 2001 "Do Caring Kids do Better in School?"

When you encourage your child to respect people's feelings, you are not just helping your child to be nice, you may also be paving the way for classroom success. Children who are tuned in to others' emotions by the end of preschool are more likely to do well academically and socially later on, according to a new study. Researchers at the University of Delaware in Newark asked five-year-olds to label pictures of facial expressions with a basic emotion such as joy, sadness, anger, fear, etc. For years later, those who did the best also got the highest grades academically and socially. Carol Izard, PhD, says: "Kids have more confidence in the classroom, they understand the teacher's moods and signals, and are better at interacting with other children.

Those less attuned to cues may have poorer relationships with peers and teachers which can lower their moral and distract them."

You can teach them sensitivity when reading to them, talk about the characters and how an event makes them react and feel, point out body language, and talk about others' feelings. Warren Umansky, PhD, says: "The first step to independence is tackling a task all by oneself. React with enthusiasm when they do something on their own."

Parents have enormous responsibility when it comes to a child's early social and emotional development. Until they are around other adults consistently, you are not only your child's caregivers, but you are their first friends. You teach them what is socially appropriate. You share your values and traditions. You show them unconditional love and support as they grow into their own identity and personality. You nurture them and let them know they are special every day. You are there to love them and guide them as they mature emotionally, cognitively, socially, and physically. You are building a strong, healthy foundation that will last a lifetime.

CHAPTER 15

INFANT NUTRITION

"All the baby books tell you that infants need to eat every 2 to 3 hours, but what they fail to mention is that this behavior continues until the child turns 18 and moves out of your house."

— *Twitter.*

Breast milk and formula

Milk (breast or formula) is the main source of nutrition for the first 12 months of life. Breast milk has all the nutrition babies need. Formula is vitamin-enriched to make sure it meets your baby's nutritional needs. All babies need a source of iron around four months of age, either in formula or added to cereal for breastfed babies. If babies are not going to be starting solids until six months of age and solely breastfeeding, a baby's iron level should be checked.

Fluorinated water

Fluoride in water should be added after six months. Mix formula with fluorinated water or nursery water or give 4 oz of fluorinated water in a sippy cup. The American Academy of Pediatrics recommends if you are not using fluorinated water and solely breastfeeding at six months of age, that you speak to your pediatrician about giving a supplement of 0.25 mg of fluoride in drop form daily, or they may apply a fluoride varnish. This may be recommended instead of offering water in a sippy cup, as babies under a year of age do not need water alone (refer back to the dental lecture).

Starting solid foods

At around 4–6 months most doctors will have you start solids as long as your infant is taking at least 24 oz of formula, and they are in good health.

Your baby will be drooling, sucking on his or her fists, and becoming very oral. He or she will begin "teething" although teeth will generally not appear until 6–12 months of age. Solid foods are a supplement to their main nutrition source of breast milk or formula and are not a requirement until 12 months.

Before four months of age, most babies do not yet have enough control over their tongues and mouth muscles to start solids. To prevent choking, make sure your baby is sitting up when you introduce solids. Always use a spoon. Do not put solids in a bottle or infant feeder with a nipple as they are choking hazards.

Babies have a tongue-thrust reflex which helps them when they are nursing or drinking from a bottle and most babies lose this reflex at around four months of age. If you start solids too early, they push their tongue against the spoon or the food instead of swallowing the food. Four months is also the average time when the energy needs of babies increase.

If intake of formula or breast milk drops dramatically with solid foods, you may need to cut back on the volume of solids you are offering or hold off a bit. First foods are intended to introduce an infant to new tastes and textures while ruling out allergies. Solids should be fun and not only provide oral stimulation, but extra iron and vitamins. If the baby does not enjoy solids, do not force-feed them. Stop and wait a few weeks before trying again. Forcing a baby to eat may create an aversion to eating and a feeding problem. I typically recommend giving formula or breastfeeding, then waiting an hour prior to giving solids.

Most doctors will have you start with rice cereal (if you don't want to start with rice, choose another iron-rich cereal). If your baby is taking formula, cereal is not as important, and you can skip it if your infant does not like it, as they are getting iron in the formula.

Start with 1–2 tablespoons of rice cereal and mix it with breast milk or formula (this can be counted in your daily fluid intake) to a consistency to feed with a spoon. It will be a bit watery at first and then you can gradually thicken it as the baby gets more comfortable eating from the spoon.

If tolerated, and there are no signs or symptoms of allergies, and the formula intake or breast milk intake does not drop below 24 oz, you can increase to twice a day.

If rice cereal constipates your baby, you can mix it with a non-constipating food or juice after three days.

Keep children's antihistamine on hand when starting solid foods, in case your child has an allergic reaction, such as children's Zyrtec or diphenhydramine.

Constipating vs. non-constipating foods

I typically recommend, when starting new foods, to alternate between constipating foods and non-constipating foods, as the addition of solids and juices will change the baby's stools.

Bananas, applesauce, and many yellow veggies, such as carrots and sweet potatoes as well as cereal, tend to be constipating, while prunes, peaches, pears, green veggies, and fruit juice tend to have more of a laxative effect.

After several days of rice cereal, if your baby's intake remains above 24 oz and he or she is enjoying feedings, you can add either a fruit or yellow veggie.

You can either make your own baby food or purchase store-bought baby food. If you are making your own, make sure you buy a book to ensure you are preparing baby food safely. Foods such as carrots can be dangerous if not prepared correctly, due to nitrates.

Gerber 1st stage foods are made without added sugar, salt, eggs, milk, wheat, or citrus.

If you are offering two tablespoons a day, you can continue one tablespoon of rice cereal and add one tablespoon of fruit or veggies. Rice cereal is more important if you are solely breastfeeding. If you are using formula with iron, rice cereal again is not as important.

It is important to wait three days between the introduction of each new food to monitor for allergies. Keep a food log. Once a new food has been tried for three days, however, you can go back to that food. For example, if you try carrots and your baby absolutely refuses them, but they loved pears, you can offer pears at that meal, but still wait three days from the start of carrots to try a new food.

It is common that a baby will push out a new food and often make a strange face. As long as they don't turn away or cry, continue to offer the food. It may just be that it is a new taste and texture rather than a dislike.

If your baby continues to turn their head, however, or cry, hold off on the food and try again later. It often takes 4–5 attempts at a new food for a child to develop a taste for it, so don't give up if the baby doesn't like it the first time. Try to make food as smooth as possible if this is occurring. Try not to bias your baby's preferences based on your own likes and dislikes.

A good rule of thumb when starting solids is: You are doing well if you get one spoonful in for every 3–4 attempts. This will improve when they get the hang of it.

Gerber suggests that you let the colors of the rainbow be your guide to ensure a good variety of flavors and nutrients throughout the day, for example:

Foods rich in vitamin A include apricots, cantaloupe, mangos, carrots, spinach / dark greens, sweet potatoes.

Foods rich in vitamin C include cantaloupe, oranges, strawberries, broccoli, potatoes, green peas, tomatoes.

Foods rich in folate include strawberries, oranges, avocados, broccoli, spinach / dark greens, green peas.

Food high in fiber includes applesauce, mangos, carrots, pears, green beans, corn.

Fruits and veggies to begin with:

Applesauce, bananas, pears, peaches, and apricots. Squash, sweet potatoes, carrots, and greens such as peas and green beans.

Avoid added sugar and salt to begin with.

Stick with only stage one foods to begin with if you are starting with jarred foods, as you want to start with only one ingredient food.

Gerber explained to me the difference between stage one and stage two as being that stage one only comes from one particular harvest, one orchard, one type of apple, for example. Whereas stage two, on the other hand, can be a mixture of orchards or harvests, i.e., stage one may be, for example, Gala apples and stage two may be Gala and Macintosh, so although this is unlikely, there is still a chance of an allergy with a stage two food even if there was no problem with stage one. (This is just an example. I do not remember which apples they said are in which products as it was years ago when I called.)

If you started at four months, your baby will probably be around six months or older once you have tried all the stage one foods and ready to move to stage two foods.

You can also start introducing table foods such as full-fat yogurt, cottage cheese (as long as there is not a dairy allergy), mashed potatoes, strawberries, and avocado, etc. I should warn you, however, that once many babies realize there is more out there than jarred foods, they often start refusing the jarred foods and only want table foods.

Somewhere around seven months most pediatricians will allow you to try meats either separately or mixed with vegetables (from personal experience most babies don't like the jarred meat alone).

Around 8 months of age most children want to feed themselves and can do so with finger foods.

Between 6 and 9 months you can also offer teething biscuits, but I recommend only giving these with a baby-safe feeder as these can break off in large chunks and pose a choking hazard.

Between 9 and 12 months most infants have four or more teeth and can handle stage three chunky or junior finger foods.

At about 12 months and over children can basically eat the same meals as you just in smaller portions.

At 12 months most doctors recommend switching to whole milk as long as there is not a milk intolerance.

Start out with one cup the first day and, if your baby does not have any signs or symptoms of allergies or stomach upset, switch over completely the following day.

Start to encourage the cup while de-emphasizing the bottle and if possible, switch to a sippy cup by 12 months of age. Offer a sippy cup with a handle by six months at mealtimes with breast milk, formula or even water. Nuby or Munchkin Miracle 360 are both great brands.

Children are not usually developmentally ready to use a spoon or fork well until about 15–18 months of age. If your child constantly tries to grab your spoon, give them one of their own to hold and play with. Teach your child to feed him or herself as early as possible. The main way to prevent feeding struggles is to teach your child how to feed him or herself as early as possible. Offer some finger food by 6–8 months of age.

Skipping a meal is harmless. Do not panic, they may eat better the next meal because they feel truly hungry. Offer a small amount of food on a small plate. They are more likely to finish it and will gain a sense of accomplishment. Often, they are more interested in textures and playing with food than eating it. A serving size is 1–2 tablespoons from infancy through toddlerhood.

Baby-led weaning

What I have just described above is considered to be traditional weaning. Baby-led weaning is infant self-feeding. The theory behind baby-led weaning is that the baby will become a more adventurous eater and learn how to control their own intake. The rule with baby-led weaning is that only the baby puts food in their mouth. You can offer soft foods that they can hold and pick up. Most parents cut the food into strips so a baby can grasp hold of the food and food is not cut into disk shapes that pose a choking hazard.

Several years ago, when many parents started to ask me about this, I honestly did not know what it was. Of course I researched it and the very first article I googled had a picture of an infant holding a pork chop. I nearly had a heart attack. I thought "Oh no way am I recommending this." Once I started to read more, however, I realized this is what I have been recommending to an extent all along. (The picture was a joke.)

I had just been recommending offering table foods in combination with pureed foods. My personal opinion is that, when kids are able to pick up food on their own, allow them to do so and monitor for choking hazards. If your child has a high gag reflex, they may need pureed foods longer. There are many foods that don't come in a jarred, pureed form, like watermelon and avocado, and these are perfect foods to offer a baby to pick up and feed themselves or help them with. Be careful that foods are steamed or soft enough to not be a choking hazard.

Foods to avoid

Avoid honey before the first year of age because of the risk of infant botulism. This includes both the raw form and honey baked into products.

No citrus before six months of age.

Foods to introduce early

The new recommendations from the American Academy of Pediatrics are early introduction of allergens, including peanuts, tree nuts, eggs (most egg allergies are to egg *whites* not the yokes, so you might want to try yolks first), cow's milk products, fish, shellfish, soy, and wheat, at around six months of age. If your child has severe eczema or you or your husband have a severe allergy to any of the above foods, talk to your pediatrician about the safest way to introduce these allergens. Keep in mind that peanuts and tree nuts are choking hazards. So, try the butter. You may want to try a smear on a cracker first. You might also try a small smear on the skin or even try peanut butter powder to eliminate a choking hazard first. Keep an antihistamine on hand prior to trying any of the above foods.

Because children often swallow without chewing, never offer a young child these foods: Spoonfuls of peanut butter, whole nuts, grapes unless they are cut, popcorn, uncooked peas, celery, hard candies, or other round foods like carrots, hot dogs, and meat sticks. Always cut them into small pieces.

Some additional food hazards for kids

Alfalfa sprouts: Warm, moist growing conditions harbor salmonella and E coli.

Safety tip: Cook before you serve.

Eggs: May be contaminated with salmonella.

Safety tip: Cook until yolks are no longer runny. Don't give kids foods with raw eggs, i.e., Caesar dressing or cookie dough.

Honey: Can contain a toxin that causes botulism (can trigger respiratory failure and paralysis).

Safety tip: Never give to a child under the age of one.

Hot dogs: Associated with listeria poisoning, which causes flu-like symptoms and, in rare cases, loss of balance or convulsions.

Safety tip: Heat hot dogs until they are steamy hot. Cut lengthwise, not in disks (caution: choking hazard)

Unpasteurized juice: May contain bacteria such as E. coli.

Safety tip: Buy only pasteurized juice and cider. Frozen and canned are safe bets.

Fluid requirements at 1 year of age: Your child needs about 32 oz of fluid per day (approximately 1,000 cc (30 cc in 1 oz)). Each year add about 100 cc, i.e., a 2-year-old needs 1,100 cc of fluid per day.

Allergies: Adapted from Dr. Barton Schmitt's *Your Child's Health* and advice from asthma / allergist / immunologist Dr. David Reeder, MD.

Depending on what study you read, 5–10% of children have a sensitization to a food vs. a true food allergy, with peak prevalence being one year of age. Only 5% have a true allergy to food.

60–70% of children develop skin symptoms first, often followed by swelling of the tongue, lips or mouth, diarrhea, or vomiting.

An anaphylactic reaction is less likely to occur in infancy due to an immature immune system. However, as children age, they develop more of a capacity to have a more serious reaction including anaphylaxis.

Symptoms of an anaphylactic reaction include rapid onset of difficulty breathing, difficulty swallowing, wheezing, turning blue, drop in blood pressure (shock) which may lead to dizziness and unconsciousness and In young children you often see excessive drooling because they are unable to swallow. Anaphylaxis generally occurs rapidly within 30 minutes to an hour though there are some instances where symptoms develop hours after the initial exposure.

If children have other allergic atopic conditions such as eczema, asthma, or hay fever, they have a higher rate of associated food allergies than non-allergic children.

Food allergies are often not inherited if siblings or parents have them but the propensity to develop atopic allergic conditions is inherited. If one parent has environmental but not food allergies, the child is 40% more likely to have the allergy and, if both parents have the allergy, the child is 75% more likely to have the allergy.

At least half of children who develop a food allergy in the first year of life will outgrow it by two to three years of age. 3–4% of infants have a milk allergy. The good news is less than 1% will have a lifelong allergy to milk. Allergies to peanuts, tree nuts, fish, and shellfish, however, often persist for life.

To diagnose a food allergy, keep a diary of symptoms for two weeks. Symptoms may vary due to the amount consumed. Food allergies may flare up more with additional environmental allergies, e.g., pollen.

Eliminate the suspected food for two weeks. If there are no symptoms, you probably eliminated the correct food. Most children improve within two days and almost all after one week of food elimination.

To treat:

If you suspect a food allergy, eliminate it while you seek care from your pediatrician or allergist. Consider avoiding other foods in that food group, if they have not been attempted yet, until you can see a specialist. For example, kids allergic to peanuts could react to soy, peas, and other beans. Provide a substitute so as not to miss any vitamins or minerals.

If under the age of three, re-challenge every six months until the age of three, under doctors' supervision. You will probably want to see a pediatric allergist to do this under a controlled setting.

Never re-challenge if an anaphylactic reaction occurs.

If your child has a severe allergic reaction, talk to your doctor for a script for EPIPEN JR and, in my opinion, go and see a pediatric allergist to see if there are any other foods that might cause the same issue, so you have no more surprises.

Cause of allergies-

Allergic children produce antibodies against certain food proteins or things in their environment.

When these antibodies come into contact with the allergic food protein the reaction releases numerous chemicals that cause the symptoms. Antihistamines block these chemicals.

The most common allergic food in older children is peanuts.

In infants milk and egg products are more common but are often outgrown. For this reason over time the most common allergic food is peanuts.

"The food group referred to as MEWS(Milk, eggs, wheat and soy) are foods that most commonly trigger anaphylactic reactions. However, the most potent type of food reaction that we most commonly know of are peanuts and fish." according to Tonia L Farmer MD ENT.

According to the American Academy of Pediatrics, 9 foods account for 90% of all food reactions in children those are the peanuts, eggs, cows milk products, soybeans, wheat, tree nuts, fish, shellfish, and sesame seed.

"The food group referred to as MEWS(Milk, eggs, wheat and soy) are foods that most commonly trigger anaphylactic reactions. However, the most potent type of food reaction that we most commonly know of are peanuts and fish." according to Tonia L Farmer MD ENT.

According to the American Academy of Pediatrics, 9 foods account for 90% of all food reactions in children those are the peanuts, eggs, cows milk products, soybeans, wheat, tree nuts, fish, shellfish, and sesame seed.

Organic foods

There is no evidence that organic foods are more nutritious than regular nonorganic foods.

The nutritional content of food varies according to when it was harvested and how it was stored and processed. Organic fruits, vegetables, and grains grown without chemical pesticides are more expensive than traditionally grown produce. I personally try to buy organic when it looks good and is not completely out of my budget. Yet there are times when the organic produce does not look as fresh, and I will opt for nonorganic. To be safe, try to buy produce grown in the US and wash it well. Wash even thick-skinned produce such as grapefruit, since a knife can carry pesticides and bacteria when you cut through it.

According to Cook's Illustrated Magazine, both conventional and organic produce are covered in surface bacteria. Many people simply rinse their produce in the kitchen sink. Recent tests, however, discovered that rinsing only removes 25% and scrubbing with a brush and antibacterial soap only removes 85%. They say the key is vinegar. Use 3 parts tap water and 1 part distilled vinegar. So, for 1 cup of fluid use ¾ cup water and ¼ cup vinegar. Rinse well under cool running tap water to remove any vinegary flavors. I bought a little 8 oz spray bottle to set next to the kitchen sink: 2 oz vinegar to 6 oz water. I also soak my produce and fruit when I first come home from the grocery store, so the kids know it is clean in the fridge.

I also try to buy meat that was raised on manual feed when possible and not given hormones or antibiotics, but again this is not always possible. Do the best you can. The good news now is that all milk I see in the stores says it is from cows that were not given growth hormone. Good change is happening.

You may want to avoid the "dirty dozen." These change every year so google to see which foods are on this year's list.

Sugar and sweets

A popular misconception is that eating sugar is harmful and many well-educated parents worry needlessly about sugar. The body needs sugar to function, and the brain needs glucose to thrive. Sweets just need to be eaten in moderation.

Infants soon after birth show a preference for sweet solutions. Breast milk is one of the sweetest things on earth. It is like sugar milk. Many humans are born with a "sweet tooth," probably on a genetic basis. Many members of the animal kingdom also show a craving for sweets.

People forget that the recommended daily amount of calories from carbohydrates, sugars, and starches is 55%. The amount of refined sugars (sucrose) should not exceed 10% of daily calories.

You will find sugar naturally in most foods, except meats. Lactose is in milk, fructose is in fruit, and maltose is in grain.

Sucrose is the sugar found in sugar cane and has no greater adverse effect on body functioning than any other sugars. It is just that refined sugar fills kids up, without added vitamins or minerals, or other health benefits.

The main risk of sugar is the ability to increase tooth decay. This is the only permanent harm that comes from ingesting too much sugar.

So as your child grows, you may want to allow sugar in moderation—do not try to forbid sugar. If a baby has a sweet tooth, it is present at birth and we have little influence over it. If you forbid it, it may be more enticing as the child grows.

You may avoid sweets during the first year of life as a child may develop a preference and not want other things that are unsweetened. Just use your best judgment. Fruit can be your alternative if your child happens to have a sweet tooth. Limit the amount at home and it won't be a temptation. Discourage sweets for snacks. Offer fruit instead as a dessert.

Brush your little one's teeth after sweets.

It may help your picky eater or a child that was primarily breastfed to sweeten their food a bit. For example, milk flavoring if your baby refuses whole milk at a year coming off breast milk. You can gradually phase it out or add a very minimal amount.

Why babies need fat

Though a diet too rich in fat can increase the risk of developing heart disease, young children need calories from fat for growth and development. Fat also helps the body absorb certain vitamins that are essential for health, such as A, D, E, and K, and adds flavor and a pleasant texture to food. These are your fat-soluble vitamins.

Children should get about half of their daily calories from fat until age two. After that fat can be cut down gradually so that by age 4–5, it makes up about ⅓ of daily calories. One of the best ways to ensure adequate fat intake is to give whole cow's milk from age 1–2. Johnson and Johnson, *Pediatric Nursing Today*, March 2000.

Iron

If you are solely breastfeeding, your baby may need extra iron. Your pediatrician will test the iron level in your baby's blood around 9 months of age. Some examples of iron-rich foods include:

Beef, prunes, apricots, creamed wheat, kidney beans, beans of all types, raisins, fortified and enriched cereals and snacks, egg yolks and spinach, peanut butter (wait on this one), prune juice, and sweet potatoes.

As I mentioned earlier, if you are not going to start solids until six months of age and only breastfeeding, your pediatrician may check the baby with a simple finger stick after four months to make sure they do not need a supplement. A baby's storage from Mom starts to diminish after three months.

Vitamins

Vitamins are not usually necessary. Most children get enough nutrients from the foods they eat so they don't need vitamin and mineral supplements. Except again, your solely breastfed infant needs 400 IU of vitamin D a day.

Yet some pediatricians recommend vitamins if the child is a strict vegetarian or vegan, or if your child has a medical condition. They may also recommend a vitamin supplement or if your child is an extremely picky eater.

Water-soluble vitamins are lost in urine and are not harmful in excess. They just cause expensive urine.

Fat-soluble vitamins A, D, E, and K can accumulate and be harmful in excess. Early Arctic explorers died of vitamin D intoxication from eating too much polar bear liver. So, do not give routine vitamins without talking to your provider.

Water

Babies under 12 months of age don't need additional water. You are better off increasing breastmilk or formula. Water fills your baby's tummy up without the benefit of calories or nutrition.

Starting solids should be fun! Solids are meant to introduce babies to new tastes and textures. Solids provide oral stimulation and aid socialization. Solids rule out allergies and develop fine motor skills. Until close to one year of age, solids are meant to be a supplement and not the main source of nutrition. So don't stress if your little one is not ready when you are. Keep things positive. If your child is not enjoying mealtimes, stop for a few weeks and start again later. Follow your baby's cues and timeline and delight in this stage.

CHAPTER 16

LEARNING PLAY

"Play is often talked about as if it were a relief from serious learning. But for children play is serious learning. Play is really the work of childhood."

— Fred Rogers

From infancy on play is the primary way children learn. Games and play are so much more than a way to keep your baby amused.

Play teaches babies important lessons about social relationships and relationships with their bodies through growth and development. Games that take turns stimulate language development. Games with actions stimulate cooperation. When the two of you take turns babbling back and forth, your baby discovers that communication requires give and take. If you mimic your baby's behavior, babies will learn that their actions can influence others.

Rhea Paul, PHD, a professor of communication disorders at Southern Connecticut State University and the Yale Child Study Center says, "Games like pat-a-cake and peek-a-boo are particularly useful. With the game pat-a-cake for example, the baby learns that after we clap a few times, we are going to throw our hands up in the air.

Through these repeated routines they learn about predictability." They understand people communicate in dependable ways.

As we discussed in the social and emotional lecture, games like peek-a-boo, where you disappear and then reappear, also help with separation anxiety. Games work out anxieties.

The American Academy of Pediatrics says the first three years are the most critical time of development. A baby's brain is twice as active as an adult's.

Mary Goodman from *Musicology*, following Jill Stamm's book *Bright from the Start*, says, "At birth the baby's brain is only 25% wired, at 1 year it is already 75% wired and, by 3 years of age, it is 90% wired." This does not mean you can't create new neural pathways

It is important from infancy through toddlerhood that lessons should be in the form of games to keep a child's interest and should be stopped at the first sign of boredom (with an infant, when they look away or get fussy, stop).

Removing the pressure from a lesson or playtime will teach your baby or toddler that learning is fun, and he or she will look forward to that activity in the future.

Enthusiasm and applause are two very powerful tools for stimulating your child to learn. Pay attention to their successes no matter how small, and your child will be encouraged to try again.

Do not expect your baby to be interested in one toy or activity for any length of time. Dr. Barton Schmitt says the attention span of your child should be on average 3–5 minutes per year of age. So don't plan long, involved activities for your little one.

Babies will fuss when they get bored with one activity. Move your little one from one activity (or what I call a "station") to the next. When they are immobile, this can be from tummy time with an activity gym, to a swing, to a bouncy seat, etc. We will talk about age-specific activities in just a bit.

Play and learning through the senses

Infants and toddlers learn through all five of their senses: seeing, touching, tasting, listening, and smelling.

The sense of smell is the sense we most often forget when thinking about play with infants. Children are born with a very developed sense of smell. Offer your baby lots of different things to smell. Allow them to smell various everyday smells like orange peel, bananas, and various foods with pleasant smells. Take a nature walk and stop to smell the roses, so to speak. Let your baby experience the smells of plants and flowers.

As I mentioned previously in the breastfeeding chapter, researchers found that newborn babies can recognize the smell of their own mother's breast milk and will turn towards their breast pad over other mothers by the end of the first week. Newborns have been known to actually turn their nose up to unpleasant smells such as vinegar and turn towards smells such as vanilla.

Because tasting and feeling are ways infants and toddlers learn, childproofing becomes increasingly important. As mentioned in the childproofing lecture, anything that is small enough to pass through the center of a toilet paper roll is a choking hazard.

<u>The following information was partially adapted from Ross Laboratories and the Denver Developmental Screening tool as well as the American Academy of Pediatrics</u>

0–3 months
Developing large muscle control

Encourage your baby to lift their head: Put your baby on his/her stomach. Dangle a bright object or enticing toy in front of your baby or make happy sounds in front of him or her so your baby will lift his or her head.

Encourage rolling over: Get him or her to look at a favorite object while you slowly move it from one side to the other further and further each time as they lean. When your baby rolls over, smile and show excitement. For safety have your infant on the floor.

Holding their head steady: Hold your baby in a sitting position often so your baby will begin to hold his or her head steady.

When he or she is awake, let your baby spend some time on his or her tummy, every day, to help strengthen the neck and shoulders and build core strength.

0–3 months
Developing small muscles and problem solving

Watching and following moving objects to develop eye muscles: Get your baby to look at your face, a picture of a face, or a colorful object, or a book of baby faces. Move your face or the object slowly in different directions to see how far your baby will watch it.

In the first few weeks you may want to introduce some simple, age-appropriate toys: rattles, textured toys, musical toys, unbreakable crib mirrors. The best options are toys and mobiles with strong contrasting colors (such as red, white, blue and black). Contrasting patterns such as curves and symmetry will also stimulate your baby's developing vision.

Feeling and touching: Allow your baby to feel various objects with different textures and fabrics such as stuffed animals, toys that make scrunchy, crunchy sounds, or smooth rubber, etc. Make sure these are large items and not a choking hazard.

Allow for quiet time. Be sure to give them quiet time to explore the world themselves.

0–3 months
Developing personal and social skills

Helping your little one feel secure and loved: Hold and carry your baby around often. Talk or sing to them in soothing tones. Newborns are endlessly fascinated by people, especially Mom and Dad and their faces, so make funny faces and smile and make close eye contact often.

Being comforted: When your baby is fussy try to find out the cause and fix it. Respond right away when your baby cries. Crying is a baby's only way of telling you something is wrong. You cannot spoil a baby at this age. So, carry and comfort your little one for fussiness but also carry your baby and snuggle them for non-fussy times as well.

Smiling: Keep a happy light voice and tone while you smile often at your baby, especially when your baby smiles back. Make lots of eye contact mixed with smiles. Let your baby touch your face and look into your eyes. Babies love to look at human faces, and even prefer facial features to other shapes or patterns.

Help your baby to observe the world around them: While carrying your baby in a cuddled, cradled sitting position, show him or her lights or brightly colored objects around the house or outside. Remember your baby can't see things far away so keep that in mind while helping them to explore.

Make funny faces: You can play this game even with a newborn who is only hours old. Put your face close to theirs and open your mouth wide and stick out your tongue. They will watch you intently and may imitate you. If they do, make another face. Keep playing until they avert their eyes, yawn, or cry. Make other facial expressions for your baby to study, learn, and imitate. The benefit of this game is taking advantage of your infant's natural instinct for mimicry. This is a terrific way to communicate and bond with them and for them to learn what it feels like to control the muscles in their face.

Rock your little one: To soothe your baby and relax yourself, rock your baby. As you hold your baby, show them love by touching and talking or singing softly. Put on some soothing music if you do not sing. Hold your baby, and gently sway and move to the music. Or rock in the stillness in a rocking chair. Sometimes peaceful calm is what your little one needs.

Enjoy bedtime: You might want to sing softly to the baby before bed. Sing the same lullaby often. The familiarity of the sound and words will have a soothing effect, particularly during fussy times. The younger the baby, the shorter the bedtime routine. This could be a song, a bath, or a book but try to do the same thing every night.

The American Academy of Pediatrics suggestions for toys and activities appropriate for your 1–3-month-old:

- Mobile with highly contrasting colors and patterns
- An unbreakable mirror attached firmly to the inside of crib

- Soft music
- Soft, brightly colored and patterned toys that make gentle sounds
- Rattles
- Sing to your baby
- Provide colorful objects of different sizes, colors, and textures
- Your face is the most interesting visual object for this age group
- If you speak a foreign language, use it in the home
- Use a favorite toy to focus on and follow, or shake a rattle for your baby to find.

Developing hand-eye coordination: Sometime after your baby turns two months of age, tie a string or ribbon to a small soft toy and hold it out in front of them. Swing it slowly from side to side. They will be able to follow it with their eyes. By about three months, your baby will have enough arm and hand control that they may take a swipe at it. The benefit of this game is that it encourages the development of important visual skills, such as focusing and tracking, and provides your baby with the opportunity to practice hand-eye coordination and develop the fine muscles in their eyes.

3–6 months

Developing large muscle control

Continue to encourage your baby to raise their head and push up with their arms to watch what is happening in the world around them. You can do this by encouraging tummy time every day. Try to get your baby to roll from stomach to back and back to stomach. You can continue to encourage with a toy and help with gentle guidance if needed.

Bearing weight: Hold your baby upright under his or her arms. Slowly lower your baby until his or her feet touch a flat, hard surface. See how much weight they can bear.

Sitting upright: Help your baby sit alone. Start by having your baby sit in a corner of a couch or chair propped safely, which can prevent them from falling over. As they get the hang of this, they will develop the muscles needed to sit unassisted.

3–6 months
Developing small muscles and problem solving

At around three months they will begin to realize that their hands and feet, which have interested them for weeks, are actually attached to their body and they will reach out and try to bat at and grab objects held in front of them. Continue to try to get your baby to follow faces and bright objects with their eyes.

Holding on and grasping: Put a rattle or other safe toy in your baby's hand and pull on it gently encouraging them to hold on. Continue to let them feel different textures. You can rub soft fabrics on their cheeks or hands.

Using both hands: Put a toy or other object in your baby's hand and see if they change it to the other hand if you offer another object. Offer two objects at the same time.

Picking up small objects: Help your baby pick up small objects. If you have started solids this is typically best done with finger foods. Be careful as this can be a choking hazard.

3–6 months

Developing personal and social skills

Talk and sing to your baby. Babies must first receive language before they are able to express language. Continue to calm and soothe your baby when they cry, smile and talk to them often. Prop your baby up so they can see what is going on around them. Use your various stations to keep your little one entertained and busy. Ideas at this age are your bouncy seat, swing, Exersaucer, activity mat, etc.

Being massaged: To relax your baby, gently stroke their arms, legs, back.

Being bathed: Run a shallow bath of warm water, hold them securely and let them splash, kick, and play.

Play peek-a-boo: Hold a magazine or book between your face and the baby and peek around. Put a light blanket over each of your heads and pull it off. Do this from the doorway when your baby is in the crib (again this helps with nighttime separation anxiety).

Working to get a toy: While holding a toy out of reach, talk and encourage your baby to get the toy.

Working to get a toy: Bounce a favorite toy just out of reach and talk to your baby so they will work to get it. Drop noisy toys and let the baby look for it.

Look at family photos and pictures of babies and people in books and magazines.

Continue to show your baby the world: Point out leaves, trees, clouds, rainbows, trains, planes, etc. Describe what they are seeing as their vision improves. Look at picture books often and point out objects in their world that correlate. Point to and name objects as your baby looks at them. Your baby may only stay interested for a few minutes at a time but try to do this every day.

Call your baby by his or her name. Repeat sounds and sing nursery rhymes.

They are showing a greater interest in people and are becoming more playful.

Look in mirrors: Show your baby him or herself in the mirror. Point out things while looking in the mirror.

Take your infant places with you to increase comfort with others.

American Academy of Pediatrics suggestions for activities between 4 and 7 months:

Read books every day, talk and sing to your baby, speak a foreign language if you know one, engage in rhythmic movements with them such as dancing with music, encourage reaching for toys, spend time on the floor playing.

6–9 months

Developing large muscle control

Continue to hold your baby in a sitting position and try to get them to bounce. Help them to sit alone. Put them into a standing position. When your baby is in the crib, encourage them to pull up to stand or pull up to stand at the side of the couch.

If you have a very active baby that likes to bounce or jump on your lap, you might look into a free-standing jumper or the ones that hang from the door frame. I love the Graco jumper that has a tray that hangs from the door frame. Make sure your baby can put his or her feet flat on the ground and, like all other devices, limit the amount of time your baby spends jumping (my son would have jumped for hours if I let him).

Walking while holding on: When your baby is standing, hold a favorite toy just out of reach. Try to get your baby to walk along the crib or furniture to get to the toy. Encourage your baby to hold on to your fingers and encourage walking.

Crawling: Place a toy out of reach and encourage your baby to try to get the toy by crawling for it.

6–9 months

Developing small muscles and problem solving

Continue to try to get your baby to use both hands to pick up objects.

During feeding: Give your baby chances to pick up and feed him or herself safe foods.

Putting objects in containers: Show your baby how to drop items into a container, then dump the items out and do it again.

Scribbling: Let your baby scribble in a highchair with a large crayon and piece of paper or an Aquadoodle. Use large chalk on the sidewalk or water on a paint brush on a brown paper bag.

Enjoy bath toys: Buy, or make floating toys. Encourage them to pick these items up. Picking items up out of the water and squeezing water out or dumping water out uses fine motor skills.

6–9 months
Developing personal and social skills

Continue to hold, cuddle, soothe, and calm your baby when they are fussy. Smile and talk to them often. Rock and love on your baby. Continue to sing and dance. Play peek-a-boo and look in the mirror with them. Play social games like pat-a-cake and how big is the baby, etc.

9–12 months
Developing large muscles

Help your baby walk with or without support. Encourage them to get toys out of their reach by crawling or walking to them. Provide push and pull toys.

Play ball: Roll a large ball to your baby and ask them to roll it or toss it back to you.

Stooping: While your baby is standing up, put a toy on the floor and encourage them to bend over and pick it up without holding on to anything (give them a basket or canvas tote bag to put it in).

9–12 months
Developing small muscles

Help your baby put items in a container, dump it out, and repeat. Encourage bathtub play again, working on those fine motor skills with multiple bath toys. Give them chances to feed themselves.

Encourage stacking objects: Show your baby how to stack large blocks. You can make your own with small shoe boxes.

Playing in the kitchen allows them to play with safe items but keep kitchen cabinets off limits. Kids who are allowed in your cabinets will not understand other peoples are off limits.

Since they are hard-wired to explore and are curious about everything, provide them with safe places to explore in rooms that are childproofed.

Let them play with other items that are not their typical toys like plastic cookie cutters, plastic containers, and things with different colors and shapes, etc. Give them Rubbermaid-type containers with lids to take off and put on, to put items in, etc. Give them a spoon and pot to bang on. Give them stackable measuring cups and measuring spoons, so they can learn the concept of inside and out.

When they hide something only to discover it later, they are learning the concept of object permanence, i.e., the idea that things continue to exist even if they are out of sight.

9–12 months

Developing personal and social skills

Continue to hug and cuddle them often. Soothe and calm them when they are upset and help them put words to their feelings. Smile and talk and sing to them often. Rock and snuggle. Love on them as much as possible with lots of hugs and kisses.

Play games like pat-a-cake.

Encourage drinking from a cup.

Have at least one meal as a family, if possible, to encourage family social time.

Encourage your child to get a toy out of reach.

Encourage toys that stimulate symbolic play, such as a play telephone, play computer, play kitchen, dolls that they can take care of, etc.

9–12 months

Developing language

Continue to:

- Talk often
- Repeat sounds
- Read
- Provide quiet time
- Sing.

AAP: Toys that are appropriate for infants 8–12 months:

- Stacking toys in different shapes, sizes, and colors
- Cups, pails, and other unbreakable containers
- Unbreakable mirrors of various sizes
- Bath toys that squirt, float, and hold water
- Large building blocks
- Busy boxes that push, open, squeak, and move
- Squeeze toys
- Large dolls and puppets
- Chunky puzzles
- Blocks
- Cars, trucks, etc.
- Balls of all sizes
- Cardboard books with large pictures
- Music push-pull toys

- Toy telephone
- Empty boxes and containers

Introduce your little one to other parents and children.

Spend time on the floor every day.

Continue to play games like peek-a-boo but vary it a bit by hiding your face with a blanket and letting the baby pull it off, hiding around the corner, and showing your baby how to cover his or her own face with your hands.

Continue to play hide-and-seek and test your child's understanding of object permanence. Let your baby watch you hide a toy — first partially hidden, then covered completely — and let him or her find it.

Teach your baby action songs like "pat-a-cake," "this little piggy," "itsy-bitsy spider," and "pop goes the weasel." Babies love to hear and learn these songs and anticipate the accompanying movements. This plays on the cognitive process of causality and stimulates memory. They learn to anticipate what is coming next.

Your little reader

It's never too early to break out the books for your baby.

Reading together gives parents and infants the opportunity to share loving cuddle moments. These positive early experiences with books can help babies grow into kids that love to read.

Dr. Jill Stamm says, "Your child loves your voice. Reading to children, beginning in infancy, stimulates pleasure centers in the brain and strengthens the parent-child bond. Snuggling next to Mom and Dad and reading helps children feel more secure and loved. The sheer volume of words spoken to a child from birth to three years also has a direct impact on IQ. Research shows that talking and reading often can actually increase your child's IQ. Reading to children provides auditory or sound stimulation when the brain particularly needs it. A child is most alert to changes in sounds in the first three years of life. Reading to young children introduces new vocabulary and reinforces familiar concepts. Sharing a book with a child gives the child a lot to think and talk about. Let your baby play with touch books and talk about what they are touching. This provides your baby with a number of sensory experiences and stimulates language development. Hearing a variety rhyming words and rhythm and repetition develops language skills."

Age-by-age guidelines for books

0–2 months

Babies this age love bold, contrasting colors. They also love to look at faces. The board books *Baby Faces*, *Baby Colors*, *Baby's Emotions* are all wonderful books for this age group.

2–5 months

Babies this age love rhythm, rhymes, and repetition. As you look through books together, try to comment on what they see in the book and in the world around them. If you come across a picture of a ball, you might say, "Look it's a red ball like yours," etc. Ham it up by using different voices for different characters.

5–9 months

Since your little one is reaching for everything at this age, give them some interesting sensory books. These books offer a variety of textures like scratchy and soft. Give them books that have activities associated with them to hold their interest. They enjoy short stories due to their short attention span. If your baby starts to chew on their books, gently take them away and offer a teether instead. As you read a story, raise and lower your voice for different parts, to demonstrate pitch. Vary your speed and emphasize tempo. You may want to bounce or clap for rhythm. A book of nursery rhymes may become your child's favorite.

9–12 months

Your almost-toddler will start to hold their own books as you read and they may even be able to turn the pages on their own. The best books for this age are the chunky board books. These are meant to fit into small hands and hold up to rough handling. They like to hear the same book over and over again.

Research shows that, if children are not good readers by third grade, there is a higher chance of dropping out. So do not give up if your little one is not interested at first, just keep trying. Dylan hated sitting in my lap to read at first. He would push off me to get down. He was just too busy to be bothered with sitting and reading but I tried every single day and suddenly, one day, he sat still and then it became a daily routine. Until he went to school, our favorite time of day was in the morning. It was our "nuggle" time as he called it. He would curl up in my lap with his sippy cup and a few good books. They are some of my best memories of his early years.

Babybug magazine is a year subscription if you are looking for material for six months to three years, made of sturdy cardboard pages with rounded corners and filled with colorful pictures and simple rhymes and stories (1800827-0027 or www.cricketmag.com/4275).

Screen time

The American Academy of Pediatrics' view on screen time:

A word about screentime for babies and toddlers

Children of all ages are constantly learning new things. The first two years of life are especially important in the growth and development of your child's brain. During this time children need positive interaction with other children and adults. Too much screen time can negatively affect early brain development. This is especially true of younger children, when learning to talk and play with others is so important. Until more research is done into the effects of screen time on very young children, the AAP does not recommend any screen time for children aged two years or younger. They don't recommend phones until 18 months unless they are FaceTiming with family and friends.

As I mentioned above, the AAP recommends completely eliminating screen time before the age of two. In fact, Dr. Jill Stamm says the amount of screen time a baby receives will actually slow language development, creating the wrong types of neural pathways in a child's brain. So do your best to avoid it. However, I am also realistic and a mom myself. In this age of electronics, it is almost impossible to eliminate all screen time completely. In class, I tell moms to try to find things to keep their child occupied other than electronics. Do not put your baby in front of an iPad, hand them your phone with a video on it, or sit them in front of the television as a way to keep them busy. Find other toys that will do the same thing that may have a positive impact on development when possible. Even having it in the background can have negative effects on speech. Now having said this, if I had told my husband he could not have sporting events on in our home prior to our kids turning two, I do not think I would still be married today. Maybe just find something else to do with the baby when the game is on or get a sitter if you want to watch too. 😊

> **As your kids grow they may forget what you said, but they won't forget how you made them feel.**
>
> *- Kevin Heath*

It doesn't matter what you do with your kids as long as you spend quality time with them each day, engaging in some sort of playful activity. Playtime is so important that the American Academy of Pediatrics (AAP) recommends pediatricians write a "prescription" for it. But the AAP doesn't recommend any specific amount of playtime—that's up to you and your baby. Babies will let you know when they want to play and when they have had enough. Every child is different and requires a unique amount of stimulation. Now I am not saying your baby needs you to entertain them every waking moment. Children need to know they are OK playing independently too. Just make those engaged moments count. As your baby grows, it is also important to remember that kids don't need elaborate activities or expensive toys. So, make messes, get down on the floor and play with toys or snuggle with a book. It doesn't matter what the activity is, it is your love and undivided attention that means the most to your kids.

CHAPTER 17

INFANT MASSAGE

"There are places in the heart you don't even know exist until you love a child."

—Anne Lamott

There are so many benefits to infant massage, not only to the baby but to the parents as well. (If practical, try to massage your baby about one hour before the fussy period begins and when they are in their active alert state.)

Benefits to Baby

*It helps regulate the digestive, respiratory, immune, and circulatory systems.

*Massage decreases stress hormones. Massage lowers hormones such as ACTH and cortisol which can suppress growth and inhibit the immune system.

*Massage increases the release of serotonin, the feel-good hormone.

*Touch also leads to the release of insulin and hormones that are important to digestion.

* Massage can help release trapped air / gas. It helps regulate the digestive system by helping to prevent constipation. Massage gently in a clockwise motion. Push the feet up to the chest and work the legs in a bicycle motion.

Developmental psychologist Tiffany Field and her colleagues have shown that massage therapy is a simple, natural, and effective way to improve the development of premature infants. In their first set of studies (1986), these researchers stroked and manipulated the limbs of premature infants in a neonatal intensive care unit for 15 minutes, 3 times a day, for 10 days. A control group of preemies did not receive touch therapy.

- The study showed that those babies who were massaged gained weight (47% more weight) far more quickly than did premature infants who received no massage.

- Not only did they show greater weight gain per day, but they were more alert, active, and showed more mature neurological development. In addition, their hospital stays were on average shortened by six days.

- Massage can help reduce the pain and stress that many premature infants endure during their hospital stay and, if continued after leaving the hospital, massage continued to show better brain development and weight gain.

In the late 1970s in South America, they found that, in areas with limited neonatal care where they used skin-to-skin contact ("kangaroo care"), babies displayed increased restful sleep, increased weight gain, decreased infections, and decreased breathing problems.

For colicky babies, in particular, a daily massage can raise a baby's stimulation threshold, helping to build a tolerance for the normal stressors of life.

Infant massage helps your baby's brain development as well. Nerves in the brain and nervous system have a myelin sheath. This is a fatty covering, similar to insulation around an electrical wire, that is not fully formed at birth. Myelin both protects the nervous system and enhances communication between the brain and the rest of the body. The natural sensory stimulation of massage speeds up myelin formation and improves your baby's brain-body communication.

Massage helps prepare their little bodies for physical activity and improves overall mobility and muscle tone.

Massage encourages muscular coordination and flexibility and helps as the baby stretches, moves, and grows. Studies have shown a decrease in growing pains and muscle tension in babies who were massaged.

Massage promotes sounder and longer sleep.

Studies have shown that gentle caressing before bedtime, such as rubbing the feet and the backs of arms and legs, helps babies fall asleep faster and stay asleep longer.

Massage promotes bonding and communication.

Massage lowers fear and excitement thresholds and increases gentleness, friendliness, and fearlessness.

Massage may relieve discomfort from teething and may also work as a natural remedy if your baby is experiencing symptoms of congestion of the gastrointestinal discomfort.

Benefits to parents

1. Provides a special focused time that helps deepen bonding and trust.
2. Helps parents to understand and respond appropriately to Baby's nonverbal cues.
3. Promotes feelings of competence and confidence in caring for Baby.
4. Improves parent–infant communication, both verbally and nonverbally, that fosters love, compassion, and respect.
5. Increases parents' ability to help their child relax in times of stress.
6. Eases stress in parents who must be separated from their child during the day.
7. It is fun and relaxing.
8. Touching and massaging can stimulate milk production and help Mom relax.
9. Dads benefit because it is a positive way to become closer to their baby.

Some additional benefits

Cross-cultural studies have shown that babies who are held, massaged, carried, rocked, and breast fed grow into adults that are less aggressive and more nonviolent, compassionate, and cooperative.

Studies show benefits for premature infants, infants with asthma, diabetes, and certain skin disorders.

Mothers with postpartum depression have shown improvement after starting infant massage.

Your baby's attention span is short so limit newborns to about 15 minutes at most. Go off your baby's cues. Babies will let you know if they are beginning to feel overstimulated. Breaking eye contact, becoming fussy, beginning to cry, or disengaging are all signs that they are done and need a break

Infant massage is not the vigorous, deep massage that adults enjoy. You will begin very softly and gently and, as the baby grows stronger, your touch can too. Strokes should be long, slow, and rhythmic. You might need to start with touch relaxation. Simply hold one leg and then gently bounce it in your hand. You might softly say relax. When you feel the leg relax, say something soft and happy like, "Wonderful, you relaxed your leg," and then move to the other leg. Then gently lay your hands on another area of the body. Massage should be something that is relaxing and that you and the baby both enjoy. The rule of thumb is to avoid a ticklish touch.

CHAPTER 18

CHOOSING A NANNY / SITTER OR DAYCARE PROVIDER

"A baby is a wishing well. Everyone puts their hopes, their fears, their pasts, their two cents in."

—Elizabeth Bard

A side note for working parents. If you plan to get an in-house nanny or hire anyone to work in your home, you may need to check with your insurance agent. Make sure you have coverage if someone is injured in your home or on your property. This also applies to adding them to your car insurance if they are going to drive your car on a regular basis (most likely the vehicle is covered but verify this).

Suggestions for getting started with the interview process

1. First, talk to each candidate briefly on the phone. Narrow down your list.
2. Set up an interview for your finalists. I suggest approximately one hour.
3. Have someone interview with you: your partner or friend. Try to have the same person interview with you each time, if possible.

4. Prepare questions and ask the same questions of each applicant and take notes.

Your question list

A few examples of questions to ask a nanny or private in-home daycare:

Start with some warmup questions by asking them about themselves.

- What are your hobbies?
- What do you like about caring for children?
- How long have you been a nanny?
- What ages of children have you worked with?
- Do you have children of your own? If so, what age are your children?
- Do you have any other jobs?
- Ask about their education and training. Safety training / CPR. Would they be willing to take CPR training? You should be prepared to pay for this.
- Why did you leave your last job? (If appropriate)
- Why are you leaving your current position?
- How might you spend your day with my child? This will give you an idea of whether or not they understand age-appropriate activities.
- What difficulties have you experienced as a nanny with parents or children? How were the difficulties resolved?
- What are your views on discipline?
- What are your views / opinions on schedules?
- How many days have you had to take off for sick days for yourself or your children, in the past 12 months?
- How will you get to work each day?
- Ask about accident history if they will be driving your child.

- If they will be driving their own car, ask about their vehicle and insurance.
- Ask if they are current on their vaccines.

Additional details to discuss

Other details you might ask about / explain:

- Explain the hours and duties of the job. Does this match up with their schedule?
- Do they object to light cleaning, laundry, cooking for the kids, or errands while watching the children?
- Discuss wage or salary.
- How would they like payment to be made: weekly, monthly Zelle, Venmo, check, cash, etc.
- When can they start?
- Ask about holidays.
- Ask if you take a vacation, how is that handled? Are still you expected to pay when you are on vacation?
- Ask about their vacation and how much notice you will get.
- Discuss the length of their probationary period.
- Ask for references.
- Do they have any questions for you?

Have them meet the baby or children. How do they interact? Are they comfortable?

A mother's intuition is a powerful and useful tool in making a decision.

If hired...

Walk through the entire house explaining exits and areas off limits for the nanny, baby, or pets.

Share a spot to hide a key in case they get locked out or give them the garage or lock key code to get in.

Explain any alarm systems and codes. Pick a separate code word for them and tell your alarm company.

Explain major appliances.

Give a list of all emergency numbers.

Leave your address and baby's information, especially your child's weight for Poison Control, and have that number posted as well as the pediatrician's number.

Show the location of circuit breakers, water shut-offs, first-aid kit, fire extinguishers.

Demonstrate the fire escape route or routes. If you have a two-story house and have escape ladders, make sure those are pointed out and demonstrated.

Introduce your babysitter to neighbors or friends in case of an emergency.

Discuss responsibilities and privileges: TV, car, food, etc.

Talk about the baby's habits and routines (you may want to type up a schedule), likes and dislikes. How they go to sleep. Talk about safe sleep.

You might provide your nanny with age-appropriate activities such as:

Baby Sparks offer age-appropriate activities.

Lovevery: age-appropriate play kits.

Choosing a daycare / preschool

The National Day Care Study found that, for children under two, the most important factors to consider are:

1. Small group sizes
2. Low staff–infant ratios
3. Strong caregiver qualifications predicted positive outcomes.

Caregivers with larger groups spent more time on management tasks and restricting behavior than on one-on-one interaction and cognitive language stimulation.

The optimum standards of the Accreditation Criteria of the National Academy of Early Childhood Programs specify:

For infants under 12 months, a maximum group size of 8 and a staff : child ratio of 1:4.

For infants of 1–2 years of age, there should be a maximum group size of 12 and a staff : child ratio of 1:4.

The lead teacher should have a baccalaureate degree in early childhood education or child development. Caregivers with little child-related formal education engaged in less frequent: : : : : " frequent positive adult–child interactions.

What to look for when choosing a preschool / daycare

Drop in and observe more than once.

A school is only as good as its staff.

- Are the teachers actively playing and involved with the kids down on the ground?

- How do the teachers seem? Are they frazzled?

- Are the staff members rocking, holding, and loving on the children?

- Does the equipment inside and out appear to be clean, in good condition, and age appropriate?

- The activities and supply boxes should be marked with words and pictures so the kids will know where things go without any help as they grow.

- For older kids, the children's artwork should be displayed. Walls should be decorated with their projects to let them know that their work is important.

- Check all bathrooms and kitchen areas for cleanliness. Check the sinks and toilets are adequate and their size.

- Look at the kids. Do the children appear happy, busy, and clean?

- Are the children able to play freely?

- Do they have set activities daily for the kids?

- What feedback is given to the parent about their child's day at the end of the day?

- Is safety demonstrated by the physical setting?

- Do you see a safe environment? Are infants able to crawl and explore safely?

- Are there toys and books within reach?

- Do the children sound happy and involved?
- Do the caregivers talk in pleasant, patient tones?
- Too much noise can mean a lack of control. Too quiet can mean not enough activity.
- Is a TV used? It should not be!
- Count the children and staff ratio in all rooms.
- Drop in and check periodically.
- The center or home should have a current license displayed, and local state, and/or national accreditation.

Questions to ask

- Ask about the background and training of the staff.
- Does the head teacher have a degree in early childhood education or development?
- Do the teachers attend workshops or continuing education courses? Do they stay up to date through training programs like CPR?
- Ask how long the staff has been there. Low staff turnover is usually a sign of a program that values good staff and works to keep them. Also, you do not want your child to finally get comfortable with a care provider and then have them leave. How much staff turnover is there? and how do they combat turnover?
- Are there health policies, and preparedness for emergencies?

- What is their policy for illness? Colds, fevers?
- Are the staff members trained in safety skills such as pediatric CPR and first aid?
- Do they do fire drills?
- What is the teacher : student ratio?
- Is their focus on learning through play? You do not want one focused on education at this age.
- Ask them some of the activities they have planned for the day or week.
- What discipline techniques do they use and when would they be enforced?
- Discipline should be non-punitive, kind and firm at the same time, designed to help children learn important life skills.
- Do they offer their teachers reimbursement for childcare classes and insurance?
- Are the diapers changed promptly or on a schedule? Also ask if they assist with potty training, if your child starts to show readiness early.
- You may want to ask for the names and numbers of other parents to ask their opinion.
- How are toys and equipment cleaned? How often?

Trust your gut instinct.

If the center or provider seems reluctant to answer your questions or to allow you to observe personnel in action, it's probably wise to look elsewhere.

Call the local licensing agency to see if they have any complaints against them.

Verify certification and length of certification.

Helping your child adjust to daycare

Your child should have previous successful experiences with a babysitter within the home to be most successful.

Separation fears are strong between the ages of 6 months and 2 ½ years and being left at a daycare can initially be stressful (for both parents and child).

Even though they are little, talk about the daycare before you go there.

Plan on staying a while or, if possible, the entire time on the first day to help your child gradually become involved with the other children and staff.

The second day, stay about 10 minutes.

Leave some items from home, i.e., blanket, toy, and pictures. Buy a child-safe photo album with pictures of people and animals they love.

Always say goodbye and tell the child you will be back later. Do Not Sneak Out!

Some children take up to 1–2 months to look forward to going to daycare. Now having said this, it should get better not worse. If it seems like it is getting worse, it may not be the right fit.

There are many choices, from a nanny to a daycare in a home with a small ratio or a larger daycare setting, to a Montessori-type setting (pre-toddlers only). Montessori allows the child to move at his/her own pace in a noncompetitive environment with both indoor and outdoor environments.

Don't be in a hurry to choose a childcare setting. Visit many different settings before making your choice.

Good childcare supports the development of healthy self-esteem and emotional well-being. At this age children need to feel loved and valued. Daycare should not be about academics. Babies and toddlers are learning to form healthy relationships with other people. Children can learn and grow in many different settings. Good childcare goes beyond simply providing a place for children to be cared for in their parent's absence.

In his book *Touchpoints*, Dr. T. Berry Brazelton says, "I would choose a preschool for the people who run it and who interact with the children, not for the learning program. If there's pressure to perform and to learn there may be too little time for children to learn about themselves. Parents should go to school and watch firsthand how much time the children have for undirected play and for learning about themselves as people. Learning about oneself and one's peers is the best learning that parents can provide in these preschool years. The one thing that children should feel about themselves at this age is, "I am important, and everyone likes me." Play is the powerful way children learn. Their most important task at this age is how to play with other children and how to handle other adults and how to learn about themselves as social people. The tasks of this age group are enormous."

Some childcare centers offer online monitoring available for parents to install to periodically monitor. Some have monitoring outside the front office so you can watch without your child seeing you.

Be involved. If there are changes that you would like to see made, bring them up, and work toward bringing them about.

Some parents do not have a choice on whether or not to stay home or go to work, they must work. Women work nearly 20 hours per month more than they did 2 decades ago. One-third of office workers routinely take work home at night. There is an arbitrary line nowadays between personal time and work time, with cell phones and smart phones with emails on them, laptops, and faxes that come over on the computer, etc.

Do not feel guilty. You are bound to have mixed emotions with whatever you decide, make choices wisely, and then trust your choice and relax.

I was reading an article from several years back from Americanbaby. magazine where the mom was conflicted about going back to work vs. staying at home. She said she made the mistake of asking others. She said that women insecure about their own decisions were more judgmental than helpful. Some working moms seemed to imply that she was lazy and unambitious or self-indulgent for wanting to stay at home and, conversely, the stay-at-home moms hinted at her being selfish for needing pursuits in addition to motherhood. One "good" friend finally told her, "Face it, either decision you make is going to feel wrong in one way or the other. You just have to do what feels best for you and your family!"

Nancy Marshall, PhD, a research scientist at the Center for Research on Women at Wellesley College says, "Research conducted over the past five decades shows that a mother's decision to work or stay home is not a good predictor of how her children will turn out, unless their care is substandard." It is not really about whether Mom is employed or not but under what circumstances and how she feels about it. Family experiences are far more important to a child's outcome than anything else. That explains why a mother's attitude to work accounts for so much. If she is unhappy, her sadness and anger can spill into her interactions with her kids. Yet most moms are surprised at how blindsided they feel after giving birth and the emotional roller coaster they experience regarding their feelings of attachment with this little human being.

According to the US Bureau of Labor and Statistics, more than 63% of mothers with children under the age of two are employed. In the year 2020, 71.2% of mothers were in the workforce. However, this was down from 72.3% in 2019.

Some parents, like me (after the first year), find a balance between work and home and choose to go back to work on a part-time basis. A research organization surveyed 2,000 workers and 51% of employees who switched from full time to part time say they are more productive now than they were when they were full time. 50% of their colleagues agreed and 40% of supervisors agreed. They said they are better able to focus and organize. It never hurts to ask if you are torn. I had no idea. I asked jokingly if they would put in a daycare for me, and the doctors I worked for said, "No we can't do that, but we can find a way for you to work from home if that will keep you with us." I was shocked and grateful.

When going back to work, do not be afraid to negotiate flexible work terms including hours, job sharing, and/or working from home. If you don't ask you won't know. You may want to take a lower position than what you had before you left if settling for less money means more flexibility. It might even work out financially in the end with gas and daycare costs.

Stay-at-home parents also need support. The frequent absence of a nearby extended family (unlike some other cultures) may create isolation for moms at home. Even if they have family nearby, moms need encouragement, social contact, and support.

In an article in *Arizona Parenting Magazine*, Dr. Domonic Barone said, "Today's working mothers try to be all things to all people, and they juggle themselves into exhaustion." He encourages a "working family" frame of mind. This takes negotiation with your partner. He thinks it is too much to expect a mom to do it all. Every member of the family needs to work together to manage the house.

I owe my OB/GYN a huge thank you for getting this message to me after Dylan was born. She said to me, "You cannot be Wonder Woman. You need help. Everyone needs help. If Dave cannot or will not, you need to learn to let things go or hire someone to do the things you cannot let go of." It was a wake-up call for me. We had to negotiate. We had to learn to budget so we could hire more help. It saved my sanity and probably our marriage. You need to negotiate duties and responsibilities. This is true on vacation too, otherwise it ends up being a vacation for one.

Moms tend to take care of everyone else before they take care of themselves, but it is crucial to find a balance between caring for your family and caring for yourself. You will not be any good to anyone if you get sick. Flight attendants instruct parents to put on their oxygen mask, so they have enough oxygen to help their child. This is a powerful analogy. You have to let some things go. A messy house is not a sign of a bad housekeeper but a mom with better things to do. Call in reinforcements: it might even be a mother's helper for an hour or two a couple times a week.

Stick to a routine. A schedule helps you get through important tasks first. This works well even with work. Prioritize your workday as you never know what will come up with kids. Get high-priority items done early in the day. Do not volunteer for extra work and learn to say no!

I want to end this chapter with a funny article I found years ago in *Parents Magazine* entitled "My Boss is a Tyrant." "Picture this: Your job demands a minimum of 18 hours a day, usually more. Your boss, although quite charming, is one of the most helpless individuals you have ever known. Each day you have a long list of tasks to complete, yet she constantly gives you more work. When she calls you, she warns in a voice that quickly becomes a howl if you do not respond immediately. Her demands do not just last through working hours: they continue past midnight. You are frequently exhausted, but she couldn't care less. She expects you to treat her with kindness and respect, regardless of her disposition. To top it all off, you work for free." This was written by Keith Shannon, a stay-at-home dad who was previously a lawyer.

This about sums up parenthood 😊

CHAPTER 19

SUMMERTIME LECTURE

"Babies are like little suns that, in a magical way, bring warmth, happiness, and light into our lives."

— Kartini Diapari-Oengider

Skin cancer

Sun is the main cause of skin cancer, which is the most common form of cancer. There are an estimated one million new cases of skin cancer each year.

Skin cancer can and does occur in children and young adults. Although most people who get skin cancer are older, we still need to protect our little ones. Current research suggests that one in every five children will develop skin cancer www.skincancer.org

Chronic sun exposure and acute blistering burns increase the risk of melanoma. Your skin remembers each sunburn and each suntan, year after year. Most of our sun exposure, approximately 80%, happens before we turn 18. This is because children spend more time outdoors than adults do, especially in the summer months.

You need to be most careful with children under the age of two, especially if your little one is fair haired, red haired, fair skinned, has blue or green eyes, has moles, or parents with moles or freckles, or have an immediate family member with a history of skin cancer.

Some medications may increase sensitivity to the sun. Antibiotics such as tetracyclines and sulfas are two antibiotics that can increase sun sensitivity. Anti-inflammatories like ibuprofen may also increase sun sensitivity. So, if you need to give your child something for pain and they are going to be in the sun choose acetaminophen instead.

Visiting a higher altitude where you are closer to ultraviolet rays can also cause a person to burn more easily. Not to mention the sun can reflect off snow or water as well.

*Research has shown that five or more sunburns doubles your risk of developing melanoma www.skincancer.org

Sunburn can also cause dehydration and fever. Too much sun exposure over the years not only can cause cancer but also wrinkles and possibly cataracts of the eyes.

The American Academy of Pediatrics suggests that babies under six months of age should be kept out of direct sunlight when possible. Try to dress your infant in light clothing that covers the body and put them in hats when possible. Move your baby to the shade or under a tree, umbrella, or the stroller canopy.

Baby sunglasses

Encourage your little one to wear UVA/UVB sunglasses as soon as possible. My daughter's pediatric eye specialist praised me when he saw Dylan in his little Thomas the Train sunglasses when he was a baby, when we went to one of her appointments. I laughed and said to him, "Oh these can't possibly offer much protection, I bought them at Target and they were not very expensive." He asked if they had a UVA/UVB sticker on them, and I told him they did. He asked to see them and took them in the back to check them with his equipment and told me they were great, and they can't say they have protection if they don't. It made me look at expensive sunglasses differently after that.

Sunscreen

Take care of yourself and be a good role model for your kiddos! Malignant melanoma is the second most common form of cancer in women 25 – 34 years old. You can best teach your kids by demonstrating. Apply sunscreen daily yourself.

For babies under six months, the risks and benefits of sunscreen use are not yet known. The American Academy of Pediatrics would prefer you keep your baby out of the sun or use clothing to protect them, but if you have to be in the sun, weigh up the pros and cons. It would be better to use sunscreen than to have your baby burn.

If you do need sunscreen, and the risk of burn outweighs the risk of skin irritation, try a small area first. The best place to test is a small area on your child's back, a few days before you need to put it on a larger area. Choose sunscreen made for children. Choose a water-resistant or waterproof version if possible. Waterproof needs to be reapplied every two hours. Avoid the eyelids. For areas around the eyes, apply with caution. Apply a non-barrier sunscreen 30 minutes prior to sun exposure.

Tighter weave clothes protect better. Hold clothes close to the light. The less light that shines through the better. Look for rash guards and bathing suits with sun protection built in. A wet T-shirt only offers an SPF of 3. Clothes have an SPF from 4–9, so you need more than clothes to protect your child from the sun's harmful rays. You can treat clothes with Rit SunGuard (you can buy it on Amazon). It has an SPF of 30 and lasts through 20 washings. This is great if you are going on a summer, sunny vacation.

You can also buy clothes with the SPF sun protection built in. Read the labels and tags, they often have an SPF of 50 in most rash guards and swim attire.

Encourage your child to wear wide-brimmed hats, such as a bucket hat or a baseball cap.

With a child's thin skin, 10–15 minutes in the sun can be enough to cause a burn. Contact your child's doctor if they get a sunburn that results in blistering or a fever. If your child is sunburned, avoid the sun until the burn is completely healed. Most experts say to avoid the sun during the hours between 11 a.m. and 3 p.m., if possible. This is when UVB rays are the strongest.

As I mentioned above, the sun's UV rays can bounce off sand, snow, water, and concrete. Most of the sun's rays can come through the clouds even on an overcast day. So, you still need to apply sunscreen even on cloudy days.

UVA/UVB

When choosing a sunscreen, look for the word *broad spectrum* on the label, this means it will screen both ultraviolet A and B rays UVA and UVB.

UVA rays do not typically cause visible skin damage as in a tan or burn but may be just as harmful in the long run. UVA rays have been linked to premature aging and mutations that result in skin cancer and cataracts of the eyes.

UVB rays cause burns and tans (B=burn).

Sunscreen types

There are two main types of sunscreen: physical and chemical. Dr. David Harvey, MD, a Piedmont dermatologist, describes the difference:

Chemical sunscreen:

Absorbs into the skin and then absorbs UV rays, converts the rays into heat, and releases them from the body. The active ingredients in chemical sunscreens include avobenzone, octinoxate, and oxybenzone. (Parsol 1789 is the most used organic sunscreen in the world right now. It is also called avobenzone and absorbs the full spectrum of UVA and UVB rays. It is currently the only approved broad spectrum organic sunscreen in the US.) https://www.ulprospector.com/en/na/PersonalCare/Detail/473/106662/PARSOL-1789

Physical sunscreen:

Sits on top of the skin and reflects the sun's rays. The minerals titanium dioxide and zinc oxide are the main active ingredients in physical sunblock.

Choose an SPF* of at least 30.

My dermatologist says anything above 30 SPF does not add much more protection, so over 30 is not really a benefit. The next best is a combination including Parsol 1789 (also called avobenzone) or titanium dioxide.

If your child is sensitive to chemicals, opt for physical blockers such as titanium dioxide or zinc oxide. Avoid sunscreen with PABA, a common skin irritant. The Environmental Working Group warns against products with oxybenzone, a chemical sunscreen, as it can be an endocrine disrupter. It can be found in some popular brands. This chemical has been linked to allergies, cell damage, breast cancer, hormone disruption, and low birth weight in baby girls when Mom used it during pregnancy. https://practicaldermatology.com/news/ewg-fda-must-ban-oxybenzone-in-sunscreen-now

Parabens are associated with infertility, abnormal testes development, obesity, asthma, breast cancer, and tumors in the digestive tract.

Here are a few of my favorites:

Thinkbaby

Badger

Vanicream

Babo Botanicals

Blue Lizard

The key to sunscreen is to apply, reapply, and apply again. Buy fresh sunscreen every year and check the expiration date.

*What is SPF?

SPF ratings indicate how much longer the sunscreen's use will allow someone to be in the sun without getting sunburn, i.e., if skin usually starts to burn in 20 minutes, an SPF of 2 protects twice as long, so about 40 minutes. An SPF of 15 protects 15 times as long, so about 5 hours.

About 15% of people with white skin have skin that never tans and only burns. Big risk factors are red hair, freckles, blonde hair, blue or green eyes. These people are at increased risk of skin cancer and need to be more diligent about using sunscreen.

It can take less than 10 minutes for a fair-skinned child to burn. Children can burn at recess or playing in the yard for just a few minutes, or riding in the car.

It is possible to get sunburn all year round, especially in my home state of Arizona. It is important to apply sunscreen every day. Clothing helps children stay cool by reflecting the heat. There are over 1.3 million new cases of skin cancer per year and Arizona leads the nation with largest number of cases.

For extremely sensitive people, you may want to invest in window shields that block 99.9% of UVA and UVB rays.

In areas where the inside of the car heats up quickly, you have to be very careful about hot buckles. When my kids were little, I would put a gel pack over the buckle when I would go into the store, and cover the seat with a beach towel that I kept in the car. This was inexpensive and worked great. They now have companies that offer this type of device: one is called COOLTECH, and another called Baby Bee Cool.

Sunburn soothers

No matter how hard you try and how often you lather your children up, they are bound to get sunburn at some point in their life. I was a maniacal mom with sunscreen and my kids still got the occasional burn. It was usually in a spot where I missed an area when I reapplied. Here are a few things you can do to soothe the pain.

Apply 100% aloe vera gel (keep in fridge) or, if you have a plant, open one up and use the pulp.

Soothe with a damp cool compress to the skin or cool with a caffeinated cold tea-soaked cloth placed on the skin. The tannic acid in the tea pulls the heat out of the skin (decaf does not work).

Use 1% hydrocortisone to decrease swelling (use as last resort as it is absorbed into the blood stream).

Try a pain reliever like acetaminophen.

Offer plenty of fluids.

Call the doctor if your child has extensive burns, is less than one year of age, has a temperature of >102 degrees, is lethargic, inconsolable, not eating, drinking, or urinating.

Do not use first-aid products that contain benzocaine, as it is a skin irritant.

Insect repellent

The American Academy of Pediatrics suggests avoiding bug bites with clothing. It is best to wear clothes to repel insects rather than to use insect repellent.

Do not dress your child in bright clothes or flowery prints that would attract insects and don't wear bright colors yourself.

Do not use scented soaps, perfumes, or hair sprays on or around your child.

Avoid areas where insects nest or congregate, such as stagnant pools of water, uncovered foods, and gardens where flowers are in bloom.

If you do need to use repellent, try to put it on clothes and shoes, instead of the child, if possible.

Avoid the skin around the eyes and mouth and possibly hands if your baby is constantly putting their hands in their mouth.

Read the safety label for age restrictions on all products to make sure it is safe for infants and children. Try to choose ones with the lowest concentrations when possible.

Active ingredients in most bug repellents are DEET, (N,N-diethyl-M-toluamide), citronella, soybean oil, permethrin, or picaridin.

DEET is considered the best all-purpose insect repellent, yet it can be toxic as it is absorbed into the skin and should be used only in low concentrations and stored safely out of reach of children. DEET is effective against mosquitoes, biting flies, gnats, chiggers, and ticks, yet it won't work against bees, wasps, or fire ants.

As per the AAP, until infants and children are at least two years of age, apply DEET sparingly. Weigh up the risk of exposure to potentially serious illness spread by insects and the possible risk of absorbing chemicals into the body. Remember, your skin is your largest organ.

If you do need to use it, never use it on a child less than two months of age. Some manufacturers say six months, so read the labels. I would also speak to your pediatrician before applying a bug repellent on a baby less than six months of age to weigh up the risks and benefits.

The AAP recommends repellants should have no more than 30% DEET. A maximum of 10% DEET repels for about two hours and 30% repels for about five hours.

Children should also be bathed as soon as possible with soap and water to wash any residual repellent off the skin before it absorbs.

Put on the repellent as infrequently as possible. Choose the lowest concentration to provide the required length of protection, and only a very light layer.

Do not use a combination sunscreen / insect repellent. Remember, you want to reapply sunscreen, and you want to limit the application of bug repellent.

Do not use multiple applications of repellents. Try to apply only once if possible.

DEET products can be applied to skin or clothing, yet it will damage plastics and spandex and will remain effective for hours.

Avoid skin near the mouth and eyes.

DEET should not sting the skin.

As an alternative to DEET, picaridin is available in the US in 5% and 10% concentrations.

There are natural alternatives to DEET. You might want to try to use a natural product first.

If you are worried about products containing DEET, you may want to try plant-derived products such as citronella, soybean oil, or essential oils.

Natrapel Plus has citronella as main the ingredient and no DEET.

Citronella candles and incense can also be effective in decreasing the number of mosquitoes in the area. We burn citronella around where we are sitting when we go camping.

Bite Blocker is a great natural repellent. It contains 2% soybean oil. It protects against 97% of mosquitoes even 3½ hours after application.

DoTERRA TerraShield has essential oils and coconut oil. We use this in our home all summer long as I am a big user of DoTERRA oils.

Products containing permethrin *should not* be applied directly to skin. This is the active ingredient used to treat lice and scabies. Permethrin is available in repellent spray for clothing and is an excellent repellent against ticks. This is great to use on shoes and/or a tent, or pants, when you are in an area that has deer ticks that can transmit Lyme disease.

For more information, you can contact:

The National Pesticide Telecommunication Network, open 24 hours a day, 7 days a week, for information about the active ingredients of insect repellents on 18008587378. For more information on insect repellants and safety and efficacy in children visit www.healthychildren.org and www.epa.gov

Don't spray the air around children with bug sprays. *Health warning: This is a respiratory irritant.

Sand flies cluster around heaps of seaweed and can be disease ridden. Insect repellents may help to keep them off, but it is best to just stay away from clumps on the beach.

To prevent rashes from parasites and algae in the ocean, rinse well between dips in the water and remove bathing suits as soon as possible.

If bumps appear and are itchy use calamine lotion or Aveeno anti-itch cream and, if severe, apply hydrocortisone sparingly in isolated spots.

Helpful beach tips

Bring along a spray bottle to spray off a pacifier and cool off. Baby powder also works well to help brush off sand. Just sprinkle the legs or arms that are covered with dried sand with the baby powder (*health warning: be careful to not let your little one inhale it,) and the sand wipes off like magic 😊

Stings: wasps, yellow jackets, and bees

If the stinger is embedded remove it with tweezers if possible. If no tweezers are available, you can scrape it with the edge of your fingernail or a credit card. Do not squeeze the stinger out, as this can release toxins into the skin.

Ice or a cold compress will decrease the pain and swelling. My mom's old remedy that worked well for me, as I was a magnet to bee stings, was a mixture of a meat tenderizer and warm water on a cotton ball applied to the tender area. This neutralizes the venom and decreases pain and swelling. The same thing works with baking soda and water on a cotton ball applied in the same manner. Both will also help pull the stinger out if it is embedded. After the stinger is removed, clean the area with soap and water.

Watch for symptoms of allergic reactions with all stings.

You may want to give an antihistamine like Zyrtec to decrease any itching and decrease an allergic reaction if you start to see swelling or any signs or symptoms of drooling, difficulty breathing or swallowing. If your child has an anaphylactic reaction, let your doctor know so they can give you a prescription for an EPIPEN.

In the warm summer months, it is not uncommon for babies to get heat rash or prickly heat. You often see these tiny red or flesh-colored bumps on the chest or in folds of their chubby little skin.

Treatment includes keeping the area cool and dry. After a bath apply baby cornstarch powder to the area. (*Health warning: Put this on your hand and pat it on the baby. Be careful not to let your baby inhale the powder.)

Travel / vacations

For travel outside the country, make sure all your child's immunizations are up to date. Then verify 4–6 weeks prior to travel that no additional immunizations are required or recommended.

Passport Health website www.passporthealthusa.com

Travel health and travel immunizations

Some ways to make traveling with children easier:

Start with check-in. If you are flying, take advantage of curbside check-in.

You may not want to preboard with your little one, especially if you have assigned seats. Instead, let your little one get out some excess energy; they will be sitting long enough. Wait until the last possible moment to get on the plane.

If you are traveling with another adult, however, let them preboard with the diaper bag and other baby paraphernalia and get ready for you to board with your little one at the last minute.

Bring a change of clothes for all family members in your carry-on. Bring a sweater for your child as well, or layer clothes, so if it gets too hot you can take something off. I have been on flights when the air conditioning on the plane is not functioning. It is also not uncommon for your child to vomit due to turbulence.

Bring one diaper for every hour of the flight.

Check your stroller and car seat at the gate rather than checking with baggage. You do not want these to possibly be lost. It is also convenient to have them when you get off the plane. If the plane is not full, they will allow you to bring your infant car seat on the plane even if you did not buy a ticket, as long as it is FAA approved (look for a sticker on your car seat).

For take-off and landing, offer a bottle, sippy cup, or pacifier. Babies should suck and swallow to equalize the pressure in their ears.

The Baby B'Air vest on Amazon is perfect for a lap child and an extra safety measure to help with turbulence.

When you arrive at your hotel or location make a quick safety sweep. You may want to bring along outlet plugs and a couple of other safety devices.

If possible, try to get a room with a fridge to keep snacks and milk, etc. If you tell the hotel you have a baby, they should provide a fridge for you at no charge even if one does not come as standard.

If traveling by car, you can help to avoid motion sickness by feeding the baby prior to the trip rather than when in motion. If possible, also have them sit in the middle of the backseat so they are not looking out the side windows. Crack the window slightly as fresh air can have a calming effect. Travel at night as motion sickness is associated with vision and your child might sleep the entire journey.

Going out to breakfast can be a hassle so you might want to buy fruit and cereal for your little one and yourself. Respect your child's routine. Try to stick to the same time zone if you are staying less than a week. Or you might split the difference if you are crossing a couple of time zones.

When going to a public place, may want a child harness / backpack if your child is walking. Put your cell phone number on your child's clothing. Dress your child in a bright color or something easy to spot.

This is my first-aid kit

Saline eye drops

Bandages (all types and sizes)

Antibiotic ointment

Saline or antiseptic wash, e.g., Bactine or hydrogen peroxide

Hydrocortisone cream

Antihistamine Zyrtec

Acetaminophen

Medicine dropper

Thermometer

Tweezers and small scissors

Sunscreen sample size

Cotton pads and swabs in a plastic baggie

Chemical ice pack

In the car / purse

Small flashlight

Lip balm

Extra water and snacks at all times

Keep a blanket and extra water in your car at all times.

This chapter could go on and on. I could not possibly tell you everything there is to know about traveling with an infant or every product on the market. This was just meant to give you a jump start and some ideas. Vacations can be great fun, or they can be more trouble than they are worth. If one parent generally provides the majority of the childcare, the other will have to pitch in during a vacation or it will only be a vacation for one. Take turns sharing the workload and that way everyone will have a great time.

CHAPTER 20

SWIM LESSONS: TRADITIONAL VS. SURVIVAL SWIMMING

"Telling a mom to not worry about her child is like telling water not to get wet."

- Author Unknown

Drowning / water hazards / risks

*In Arizona, drowning is the leading cause of death among children aged 1–2 years.

The American Academy of Pediatrics states that, each year, approximately 1,000 children under the age of 20 drown. Infants are most likely to drown in the bathtub, toddlers in swimming pools, and older children and adolescents in fresh water such as lakes, rivers, and ponds.

In Arizona, my state, most children drown in swimming pools because there are so many. However, other bodies of water can also be dangerous. Anything that holds enough water to submerge a baby's face is a danger:

Buckets and pails, especially 5-gallon buckets.

Ice chests with melted ice during or after a party.

Toilets. Little ones are very top heavy and drop things into toilets then bend over to retrieve them.

Hot tubs, spas, and whirlpools.

Irrigation ditches, postholes, wells, fishponds, and fountains.

Dog dishes (inside and out).

Pull pool covers tight as infants and toddlers have been found crawl out onto them and drown on puddles that form on the surface.

Again, anything that can hold a little bit of water is dangerous to an infant or toddler.

Other risks to infants and toddlers that involve being in water include hypothermia. Their little bodies can't regulate their body temperature like an older child or adult.

Water intoxication is also a risk. This is when babies drink too much water. This risk also includes what is called dry drownings.

Dry drowning

I want to talk about dry drowning as I have had a personal experience with a very good friend's little guy and dry drowning. I want to share the story so you will know what to watch for. When my girlfriend and her husband were in the backyard pulling toys out of the pool and cleaning up for the night, her little boy slipped off the edge and slipped under the water. He came right up, and they pulled him out and he seemed perfectly fine. He just coughed once, but otherwise appeared normal. They all got ready for bed and the event was forgotten.

The next day, as they were starting their morning watching cartoons, my girlfriend saw her son turn blue before her eyes. His eyes rolled back in his head and he stopped breathing. She called 911 and did rescue breathing. When he got to the ER, they found his lungs full of water. They asked if he slipped under the water in the tub or the pool and she remembered the event from the night before. She asked if such a quick event could cause this extreme outcome they were witnessing and was told this was called dry drowning. I tell you all this story so that if your little one has an event where they could have inhaled water, it is best to be safe and have your child seen to make sure their lungs are clear.

Water safety

The spread of communicable diseases can also be a risk. This can occur in public pools as well as freshwater areas. We have an area in Sedona, Arizona, that often closes due to E. coli.

Lakes and ocean water may be home to microorganisms that can cause a cut or scrape to become infected.

Keep your baby's head above water until they learn to hold their breath, as they may swallow too much water.

Water in the ear canal can lead to outer ear infections. This is different than an inner ear infection that often goes along with a cold. This is an infection of the ear canal. It can be fungal or bacterial and it will not go away on its own. One way to tell if your little one has an outer ear infection is that there is severe pain when you tug slightly on the ear lobe. (This can often be prevented by using swim ear drops if you find your child is prone to swimmer's ear.)

The American Academy of Pediatrics recommends waiting until at least two months of age before you take your infant in the water and many sources suggest waiting until six months as infants under 12 months cannot regulate their body temperature well. Limit pool time to between 10 minutes and 30 minutes and if they start to shiver, it is time to get out. If the water feels chilly to you it will be worse for your baby. The American Academy of Pediatrics says water temperature below 85 degrees is too cool and water above 100 degrees is too hot (no hot tubs under the age of three).

Whenever infants or toddlers are in or around water, an adult should be within arm's reach, providing touch supervision.

Always have your phone with you by the pool so you can call 911 if needed.

Remove all toys from the pool when not in use, so children are not tempted by them. Many children who drown fall in reaching for a toy that was left in the pool.

Recommendations for water conditions

Water should be crystal clear not green.

The water temperature should be 86 degrees or above and not lower than 85 degrees.

Chlorine levels should be 1.0–3.0 parts per million. Higher concentrations irritate skin and lower will not kill bacteria. (Several studies have also linked breathing issues for some children to chlorine.)

pH should be 7.4–7.8, higher or lower can cause eyes to sting.

Chlorine from a pool can deplete the skin of natural oils. You should rinse kids off after swimming, the sooner the better. Especially kiddos with eczema.

Saltwater pools have less chemicals, but they are still not chemical free.

Floatation devices

Floatation devices can give parents a false sense of security and parents may pay less attention to children in the water. They can also make kids who cannot swim overconfident and often a child who is accustomed to wearing water wings will forget he or she does not have them on and jump into the water.

When one of our best friend's boys was little, they had come over for a barbeque and swim party one evening. He had his water wings on, but they were not inflated as we were not planning on swimming until after dinner, but he wanted to wear them, so Mom let him. He walked straight into the deep end of the pool thinking he had his water wings on so he could float. Three adults went into the water after him fully dressed.

The American Academy of Pediatrics urges parents to think of flotation devices as toys rather than safety devices.

When my cousin was a baby, he was wearing one of the swimsuit rings and somehow, with all the big kids playing around him, he flipped over, and the ring actually held him under the water.

To say the least I am not a fan of floatation devices. Not only because of the reasons I mentioned above but they do not teach kids the proper body mechanics to swim. In order to swim or float, you need to be horizontal in the water not vertical, which is how most floatation devices hold kids up.

Swimming lessons and ISR

I am, however, an advocate for survival swimming classes for infants and toddlers. I will talk about these classes in a minute, but I want to first give you information from the American Academy of Pediatrics, so you also know their take on swimming lessons for infants and toddlers.

Here is an abstract from the American Academy of Pediatrics (AAP):

"Children develop at different rates, and not all are ready to begin swimming lessons at exactly the same age. When making your decision, keep your child's emotional maturity, physical and developmental abilities and limitations, and comfort level in the water in mind.

The AAP recommends swimming lessons as a layer of protection against drowning that can begin for many children starting at age one.

Parent–child toddler and preschool swimming classes are beneficial for many families:

- Recent studies suggest that water survival skills training and swimming lessons can help reduce drowning risk for children between ages 1 and 4. Classes that include both parents and their children also are a good way to introduce good water-safety habits and start building swim readiness skills. If your child seems ready, it is a good idea to start lessons now.

Swimming lessons for children ages four and up are a must for most families:

- By their fourth birthday, most children are ready for swimming lessons. At this age, they usually can learn basic water survival skills such as floating, treading water, and getting to an exit point. By age five or six, most children in swimming lessons can master the front crawl. If your child has not already started in a learn-to-swim program, now is the time!

Does the American Academy of Pediatrics recommend infant swimming classes?

- No, because there is currently no evidence that infant swimming programs for babies under one year old lower their drowning risk. Infants this age may show reflex "swimming" movements but cannot yet raise their heads out of the water well enough to breathe. It is OK to enroll in a parent–child water play class to help your infant get used to being in the pool though; this can be a fun activity to enjoy together.

Remember, swimming lessons do not make kids "drown proof."

- Always keep in mind that **swimming lessons are just one of several important layers of protection needed to help prevent drowning.** Another layer includes constant, focused supervision when your child is in or near a pool or any body of water. It also is essential to block access to pools during <u>non-swimming time</u>. The Consumer Product Safety Commission found that 69% of children under the age of five years were not expected to be in the water at the time of a drowning.

Now, I usually agree with the American Academy of Pediatrics but on this issue, I am not 100% on the same page. I enrolled my daughter in the parent–child swimming programs where we sang songs and blew bubbles in the water. Although she loved them, if she were to slip in the pool there would be no chance whatsoever of survival if an adult was not around to scoop her out of the water. We had / have a pool in our backyard and, in Arizona where I live, almost every person I know has a pool, including all my neighbors and friends. I did not know there was any other option for swimming lessons out there besides the traditional parent–child swimming lessons. One night, however, my husband and I were watching an episode of Dateline and they had a segment about infant and toddler survival swimming called ISR. At the time it stood for Infant Swimming Research. The name has since changed to Infant Swimming Resource. We could not believe what we were watching, and it was at that moment we both looked at each other and said we needed to find this.

Now this program may not be for everyone. I wanted to give you all an opportunity to consider it as an option out there as I had a challenging time finding an instructor or a program. That was 23 years ago my daughter was about one year old. Now it is much easier to find. I just wanted to offer you one alternative to the typical swimming lessons.

We took these classes as just one more safety precaution, and my husband and I think it was one of the very best decisions we have ever made.

This in no way should take the place of constant parental supervision and, even if your child successfully completes the course and demonstrates all his/her skills with the instructor Your child could still be at risk of drowning if he or she falls into the pool after ISR lessons if they fall into the pool unsupervised. It does not mean they are drown proofed. I feel it is one more safety step you can take, similar to the pool fence, the lock, etc.

With any aquatic program there are health risks with ingesting too much water, dry drowning, and hypothermia, to name a few. This program takes all those risks into account, however, and monitors each child very carefully.

Each ISR lesson is one-on-one at the instructor's home. Each lesson is individualized for each child's needs and abilities. Lessons, which can start as early as six months of age, are five times per week for approximately 10 minutes per lesson and, depending on the age of the child, it takes 4–6 weeks to complete the course.

To provide the safest lessons possible, your instructors should monitor a "BUDS" sheet, which stands for bowel, urine, diet, and sleep. They monitor this daily for safety prior to each lesson.

The ISR instructor training includes a minimum of 60 hours of supervised water training, plus education and testing in subjects such as psychology, physiology, and behavioral science. Plus, every ISR instructor must complete re-certification annually to maintain his or her affiliation with the program. Each instructor studies with a certified master instructor. ISR feels that the retention of the skills taught to the baby will obviously depend upon the quality and manner of the instruction.

Swimming must be taught to the baby as a sensory motor skill. The skills cannot be combined with games and songs. If swimming is presented as an intellectual skill, then yes, he or she will probably forget the games and songs and how to swim. ISR retention figures range from 94–100% after one year of no lessons. Since research shows that 86% of the infants and young children who drown every year in the United States drown while fully clothed, a safe progression towards floating fully clothed is also included in the curriculum. They also teach the parents how to play with their child in the pool to retain the skills they learn. www.infantswim.com

A friend in my bunco group signed her son up at the same time I signed Dylan up when they were both nine months old, even though she did not have a pool. Her parents did and her mom watched her son. That winter, during a family get-together, her son slipped outside and fell in the pool fully clothed, in the cold water. He remembered how to float six months later, and they heard him crying. They were able to get him out of the water and prevent drowning. I think this is an amazing program.

A more powerful story that my parenting moms insisted that I add to this book was told to me by a Master ISR instructor. This happened somewhere back east. A toddler fell in a lake. This lake had boat docks and this child had been missing for quite some time. They told the parents it had been almost two hours so this was probably going to be a recovery mission at this point if he was in the water. The mom insisted they keep looking. She said, "My baby had ISR instruction and he is floating somewhere, you need to keep looking and find him." Sure enough, over two hours later this little guy was found floating under a boat dock. Now this is the hard part to hear (as if the rest has not been tough enough): The reason they didn't find him sooner was that under the dock was a wasp's nest and every time he floated up to get air, he was getting stung. So, this sweet baby was only staying up long enough to catch his breath and going back under again. The story ends with a happy ending and, wow, what a testament to the program.

Again, I know this is not going to be the program for everyone. It is quite the commitment. Not everyone lives in a state like Arizona or has a pool in their backyard either. This may be too intense a program for everyone. I also know that it is not backed by the American Academy of Pediatrics. I rarely disagree with the American Academy of Pediatrics but in the case of ISR, I am a personal fan of this program.

The next three chapters I debated about including or eliminating from this book.

I include the topics in my parenting classes as a glimpse of what is to come in the next few months to years.

Although each chapter has a small amount of information that pertains to the first year, the majority of the information is for the older infant, toddler, and child.

I took a survey with the moms who had taken my class over the years and it was an overwhelming majority that felt I should include these next few chapters. They all felt that this is information that is helpful with parenting and, since I only plan on writing this one book, I have decided to leave the chapters in as bonus chapters.

I hope you enjoy them and that they give you a head start and a glimpse ahead for the next few months to years.

BONUS CHAPTERS

CHAPTER 21

NATURE VS. NURTURE

"Children smile 400 times a day on average ... adults 15 times. Children laugh 150 times a day ... adults 6 times per day. Children play between 4 and 6 hours a day ... adults only 20 minutes a day. What's happened?"

— Robert Holden

Nature is our genetics. It is the temperament we are born with.

Nurture is our supportive relationships and love relationships we encounter and develop throughout our lifetime.

I am not sure we will ever see a time when people stop questioning if boys and girls are actually born differently or if society is responsible for gender differences. Because I believe they are both responsible!

In her book *Bright from the Start* Jill Stamm says:

"The old thinking was that biology was to be your destiny. It was thought that IQs were born not made. Although some kids seem smarter from the get-go, we now know that a baby's intellectual capacity is not fixed at birth. A baby is born with an IQ range that can vary by as much as thirty points. An average IQ is 90–100, above 120 is considered a high IQ, and over 140 is considered a genius.

While genes and physical health set the stage for some of a child's future behavior, we now know that a child's IQ and the ability to function well also depend on the environmental experiences that they are exposed to on a consistent basis."

Dr. Jill Stamm says, "Think of healthy brain development as a dance between biology and early care. The two are so intertwined that scientists are now examining factors in the environment that can either hinder or facilitate the way that genes operate. We used to think genes functioned in a static way. If you had a gene for something, you had that trait. That is so with eye color or hair color but that is not so with all genes. Now we know some genes can be dormant and whether or not they turn on depends on experience."

In Dr. Stamm's book, she references a study to prove this very point. This study was done on rhesus monkeys and describes the power of life experiences that can actually overrule genes. It was shown that monkeys born with a particular variation of a gene would grow up to be extremely aggressive when they were poorly bonded with their mothers during infancy. However, other monkeys who also had the same gene will not continue with aggressive behaviors if removed from those moms who were not nurturing them and placed with a loving, nurturing mother.

The study went on to say that, since female monkeys often mimic the same kind of attachment relationships with their babies as they themselves experienced, it's possible the behavioral tendencies that were long believed to be transmitted through genes may be through social learning instead.

Dr. Stamm says, "The classic debate of nature vs. nurture and what shapes intelligence and personality is over. The two are intertwined.

A child grows up to be bright independent of his parents' intelligence levels and a child who is born bright can sustain or exceed that intelligence depending on life experiences."

Biological differences

Camilla Berlow and Julian Stanley from Johns Hopkins University studied gender differences in more than 100,000 children over 15 years and concluded without a doubt that some gender differences have a biological influence.

Girls

Girls, for example, are more sensitive to hot and cold, sounds, and touch.

Girls are also more interested in human faces.

Among the many differences, girls show greater communication skills.

Girls generally become verbal earlier than boys and are more relational.

Boys

Male fetuses tend to be more active (I personally can vouch for this one, having had one of each).

Boys are drawn to movement.

Boys generally are further ahead with large motor skills earlier than girls.

Various studies have found that, as early as infancy, boys prefer toys that are mechanical or moveable, while girls like those items that can be cuddled.

I saw an experiment done on an episode of *Good Morning America* years ago. They had a doctor on that studied newborns in the nursery just hours after they were born. I can't remember his name as it was so long ago. He had a mobile on one side and a woman on the other side. The boys looked toward the moving mobile whereas the girls looked toward the woman.

Dr. Jill Stamm explains this experiment in biological terms. She says it has to do with the difference in cells in the eyes. She did similar research where they placed a moving mobile on one side of an infant's bassinet and a pleasant human face on the other. The girls turned more consistently to the face and the boys to the moving mobile.

She and her team found differences in visual preferences as early as one day of age, before culture can exert influence. They felt physical differences in the formation of cells connected to the retina of the eye may be the reason for this preference.

Dr. Stamm explains that girls have more P cells that are linked to color-sensitive cones in the retina. These cells are found primarily in the center of the visual processing area of the eye that processes color and texture of mostly stationary objects; they help answer the question, "What is it?"

Interestingly boys have more M cells that are wired to rods in the retina and record black, white, and shades of gray. They are distributed throughout the retina and process primarily moving objects. M cells help answer the questions "Where is it?" and "Where is it going?"

Cell level gender differences in the eyes can also be seen impacting performance later in the preschool setting. This can be seen in children's artwork. Boys typically will choose six or fewer colors with a focus on the crayon colors of grey, black, silver, and blue. They love to draw verbs such as cars moving, rocket ships, and action things. Girls, on the other hand, will use ten or more crayons in vibrant colors and subtle shades. Girls tend to draw stationary objects and nouns such as flowers, trees, and houses.

In addition to drawing and coloring, boys show greater visual spatial abilities. This gives them an advantage with three-dimensional thinking with things like math, mazes, and puzzles.

This does not mean that one sex needs to be better in those skills, for example, girls may be better at solving a math problem if stated in verbal terms and boys may find it easier to solve if they use images.

Doctors from Johns Hopkins say, "The process of developing gender identity goes on internally before kids are verbal enough to talk about it, so it is difficult to know exactly how they come to understand that they are male or female."

Yet they have shown through PET scans and MRI that there are differences in images in brain function between adult males and females. For example, women possess a stronger connection between the two hemispheres of the brain and display more intense brain activity when they are recalling sad memories.

However, there is controversy over whether these differences in brain activity are inborn, or they are a result of early experiences, since these PET scans and MRIs are done later in life.

Many experts feel that men and women exhibit distinct neurological makeups simply because, as children, they were urged to play with different toys and develop different emotional characteristics.

"When your baby was born most of the major organs were fully formed but just on a miniature scale. This is not true for the brain. The brain begins its life outside of the womb. At birth the brain is only about a quarter of its eventual adult size. Before the second birthday, however, it will be up to three quarters of adult size. By the age of five it will be almost that of an adult in weight and volume (90%). That does not mean, however, that 90% of the information a person will know is learned in the first five years though. Every waking hour of every day from birth on, new neural connections are formed and modified." (Jill Stamm)

Scientists know that environment plays a crucial role in determining the structure of a child's brain. The stimulation a baby receives during the early years of life actually creates, strengthens, and reinforces neural pathways (physically organizes the brain as it develops).

The current belief about what makes us who we are is a combination of several factors.

The first factor is cognitive development: Infants learn to make sense of their world by sorting and categorizing, and looking for patterns in people and things. Even very young babies are able to distinguish between the way males and females move and speak. At first, babies are only aware of differences.

By three years old at the latest, a child looking at a picture should be able to tell if it is a man or a woman / boy or girl and know his or her own gender, says Anita Hurtig, PhD, professor of pediatric psychology at the University of Illinois. (I tested this with my son Dylan when he was just shy of three. I asked him about our labrador, Abbey. I asked him, "Dylan, is Abbey a boy or a girl?" He said, "She's a boy." I thought, "OK. He is not there yet". 😊) Dr. Hurtig says by the time your child is four, he or she typically understands that gender is permanent.

Society's impact

Most researchers feel culture has the greatest impact on how kids develop a gender identity. To determine what being a boy or girl means, a child learns the most by looking at how other boys and girls dress, act, and talk. Society and culture exert enormous influence on our kids and are very much a part of what makes a "boy a boy" or a "girl a girl." Society may influence as early as birth when the hospital attaches their name to a pink or blue tag. They often put little girls in pink hats with a bow and a boy in a blue one. We give girls pink balloons and boys blue ones.

It's impossible to entirely eliminate the subconscious stereotyping we impose on our children. Even the most well-meaning parents who are trying to stay gender neutral are affected by their own upbringing.

Parents often unknowingly insert gender cues by how they talk to their infant / child, for example: "How is my handsome boy?" or "How's my pretty girl?" I find myself doing it even though I teach this class year after year. When a new mom has her baby, and I see him or her for the first time, it would seem like an odd phrase for me to say, "She is a handsome girl" or "He is such a pretty boy." The words just do not seem to go together. This is our society. This is how we are raised to speak. It is our language, our culture.

Studies show parents spend more time talking to baby girls than they do to baby boys. (This one is hard for me as I had five years in between my kids, and I was all alone with each one of my kids, so I talked both their ears off all day long. Now it could be that Taylor would sit in my lap for hours to read books and Dylan was too busy to sit still very long. So, is that genetics?)

This means that girls are often socialized differently for interpersonal exchange. Remember, you must first receive language to speak it.

Studies also show that parents of little girls tend to hold their daughters more frequently. Now again, I go back to my two kids. My son literally would push off me to get down as he had too much to do. Nature or nurture?

Parents with boys tend to play more actively with boys and let them explore more than girls. Parents encourage and reward kids for identifying with the same sex parent. Fathers, in particular, describe their sons in terms such as sturdy, strong, and handsome. Dads describe their daughters as fragile, pretty, and dainty. Mothers tend to talk more about emotion with their daughters than they do their sons.

One study took 11 mothers and a 16-month-old infant.

Prior to the study, mothers were asked a series of questions about various things which included gender stereotyping. The mothers all agreed that parents should not treat male and female children differently.

Yet despite their best intentions, when they introduced an infant dressed in blue as "Adam", the mothers gave "him" things like trains to play with and when they introduced the same infant dressed in pink as "Beth," they gave "her" things like dolls to play with.

Media and TV also play a big role in gender stereotyping. We often get messages on TV about society's ever-changing definitions of "acceptable" gender behavior. Over time we are slowly adapting to these changes. When your child is older and watching TV, you may want to limit commercials. Watch more educational TV like PBS for preschoolers, as commercials tend to be very stereotypical.

Personality can also influence a child. An outgoing child, for example, may be more influenced by his or her peers' behavior because he or she is so tuned in to them with play, as opposed to a child who plays alone. The child who is not constantly engaged with others is less likely to be influenced by his or her peers as there is less interaction with them.

The situation and context can also influence a child's sex-role behaviors, i.e., a boy may act differently towards girls when with a group and chasing them around the playground versus when he is home alone with his beloved baby sister or, in my case, his beloved big sister.

We cannot keep children from all the messages of sexism they receive from society, no matter how hard we try. Messages can come from schools, churches, daycare, and peer groups. Yet, parents can play a critical role in helping children find healthy ways to cope with gender bias.

Dr. Brad Sachs, PhD and director of the Father Center in Maryland says, "Whether your child's interests are traditionally feminine or masculine, you need to find creative ways to help encourage and support them."

Dr. Patricia Bauer, PhD, at the Institute of Child Development at the University of Minnesota says, "We all have both masculine and feminine traits."

Parents need to help children find a way to balance the traditional and non-traditional aspects of their personality.

As women we look for a husband that will be a nurturing, caring, compassionate, loving, yet strong father. Little boys need to be taught those characteristics growing up. Men want strong, capable, self-assured, yet nurturing wives. Little girls need to also be taught these characteristics growing up.

Research indicates that those adults who are able to express both stereotypical female traits (nurturing and compassionate) and male traits of "independence, toughness, and achievement" are the most well-adjusted and self-assured adults. This is our goal and challenge as parents: Helping kids find a balance in a very gender-stereotypical society.

Do not limit your children by forcing them to adapt to traditional stereotypes ("boys need to be tough") or by depriving them of their right to act out traditional roles that they enjoy, like allowing a little girl to play dress up and put on fake makeup.

Surprisingly, the best way to encourage this balance in your children is *not* by treating them all the same. The best way to encourage this balance is to give a little more emphasis to those qualities in each child that need encouragement.

A child who is born overly sensitive may need inspiration to be tough and stand up for themselves. You might say, "Grace has been waiting patiently for a turn. It is her turn now," helping her to learn to stand up for herself. Or if a child takes a toy away from your little one and he is not bothered by it instead say, "Let's take turns. Liam was still playing with that. You can have a turn next." Then give the other child another toy and show your child it is OK to stand up for themselves. They will realize they can still make and have friends this way. This teaches them to be assertive.

Whereas another child may need extra lessons in empathy and caring about other people's feelings. If your child was more the aggressor, you step in and say, "Lilly was still playing with that toy. You can have a turn in a minute and you can play with this while you wait your turn." Take the toy away from your child and hand it back to the offended child and give your child another toy to play with in the meantime.

I am not saying you need to worry if your child embraces a strong gender type early on. This can help a child feel more secure with gender identity and, in turn, that security will help them to recognize that they do not have to be so rigid in their thinking.

However, it is a normal stage of development to experiment with sex roles. For example, boys wanting to wear nail polish or, in our house, princess shoes or clothes like his sister.

My husband cried when the ultrasound tech said it was a girl, but not because he was so happy about the miracle of life he was seeing on the monitor. He teared up because he was disappointed it was not a boy. He had already named our "son." He was so sure I was carrying a boy he had already purchased a miniature football. He wanted a boy, so he could do "guy" things with him. He wanted a little sports buddy. Yes, my husband was that guy. Now don't get me wrong, like most guys who say they want a son and have a daughter, he fell instantly in love with her, and she had him wrapped around her little finger within minutes and still does to this day. However, he did have this ideal image of what having a son would be predispositioned in his head and was over the moon when Dylan was born. Now, I tell you this back story so you understand why this next part is a big deal. One night we were getting ready to go to dinner. Dylan was about two at the time and was playing dress up with his sister. He had on a white glitter dress with feathers along the bottom, a pink feather boa, pink plastic princess shoes, butterfly barrettes in his hair, and a tiara on his head. When I said, "Let's get changed to go to dinner," my little man had a meltdown. He wanted to wear his princess outfit to dinner. My husband had no trouble with my son playing dress up with his sister, wearing nail polish, playing in her pretend kitchen, or with her dolls and stroller at home, but he lost his mind when Dylan said he wanted to wear his ensemble to a bar and grill for dinner. He said, "Absolutely not." I thought he looked adorable and had no issue with him going to dinner like he was, so I told my husband this was his battle.

Well, my son got his strong-willed nature from my husband and those two went round and round, "negotiating." My son compromised. He agreed to take off the long white dress, the pink feather boa, and the tiara, but he was sticking to his guns on the pink plastic princess shoes and butterfly hair barrettes. My husband, hungry and exhausted, finally said, "You know what, I don't care, let's just go."

I couldn't believe it. I was so proud of my husband because I knew that was difficult for him. I knew he was worried about what the other guys in a sports bar would think. As we walked through the patio of the restaurant, I was shocked at the response we got, and I think my husband was too. My husband was supported by the other dads there. Wow, what a great lesson that was for Dylan and my hubby. My husband got a high five and a "great job, Dad" from a couple of other dads as Dylan went clomping by in his high-heeled princess shoes. I really think that *single* experience changed my husband's perspective on how he felt about how other people perceived him and he supported our nonconformist. This allowed Dylan to stand up for himself later on.

And stand up for himself later on he did! My son, as I mentioned, was a competitive gymnast on a boys' team. He worked out with boys much older than him, most in their teens, in high school. Having an older sister, he loved spending time with her. One of the ways he would do that was by letting her paint his nails. He just loved the attention. When he was about seven, his sister had a slumber party. The girls were doing manicures and pedicures, and he wanted to be a part of things. So, he let them all do his nails. He had quite the rainbow on his hands and feet. This was before guys were routinely wearing nail polish as they are now. Well, Monday came around and I forgot to take his polish off. It dawned on me about midway through practice. When I picked him up, I said, "Hey buddy, how was practice." He said it was fine. I said, "I am so sorry I forgot to take your polish off, did you get teased?" He said, "Well, yes, at first the guys teased me but then I said, 'If you had a bunch of girls that wanted to paint your nails, I bet you would have let them.'" He said they all said, "Yes, we would have" and that was the end of it. I just smiled and was so proud that he stood up for himself and was not embarrassed in the least.

As I just mentioned above in my two stories, Mom and Dad don't necessarily have to be passive observers. Support your nonconformist. They may even need to be defended until they are old enough to stand up for themselves.

Conversely, if your child adheres to a particular gender stereotype, celebrate the strengths, yet point out ways to help them look beyond the stereotype. If you have a rough and tumble boy who wants to dress up like a superhero, let him, and talk about how superheroes help people too. If your daughter is all about wearing princess dresses and fake makeup, help your daughter to realize that it is not all-important to be beautiful on the outside but to be a beautiful person inside too.

Teach girls about anger. Allow a boy to express fear and talk about emotions. Cheer a boy who wants to cook or clean. Encourage a girl who wants to build and play with trucks.

You can help by setting and pointing out examples. The jobs in the home are family jobs. Mom and Dad both cook and clean. Mom and Dad both take out the trash and do yard work. There are no male or female jobs, but jobs that need to be done.

Some startling statistics on self-esteem:

By kindergarten, five-year-old little girls are six times as likely to use the word "love" than little boys are. There is a sharp drop in self-esteem between elementary school and high school. Most elementary school girls, when asked, felt good about themselves and happy. Unfortunately, by high school, only 29% of girls agreed with the statement, "I'm happy the way I am." Dr. Friedman feels it is because society is giving little girls the message that looks are more important than achievement.

Parenting our girls

You cannot change culture, but you can start in infancy to give your little girl a sense of strength and independence. Talk to her often and use words that describe characteristics you want to encourage in her: "That was so brave of you to climb the steps all by yourself",

"You are such a fast runner!", "You built that tower so tall." Offer her trucks and cars to play with. Give her blocks and balls. Allow her to climb and ride on toys that develop large muscle coordination. Give her toys like puzzles that teach her about spatial relationships. Help her to feel competent, self-assured, and self-sufficient. Let her do for herself what she is capable of doing on her own. Let her problem solve on her own first. Do not rush to solve her problems. Let her feel you have confidence in her abilities. Offer her choices when possible and urge her to take responsibility for the decisions she makes. Let her explore and get dirty. Encourage active games like tag and soccer. Put her in a little gym class.

Studies have shown that girls who participate in sports have higher self-esteem and a more positive body image. Yet even before they are old enough for organized sports, girls can develop coordination by kicking or throwing a ball, climbing on playground equipment, doing summersaults, running, and jumping.

When they are babies, you can encourage coordination by having them climb over pillows. Make an obstacle course with a collapsible tunnel. Encourage them to hop like a bunny in play. Anything that develops large muscles and motor skills will develop coordination and increase self-esteem.

Do not focus on the importance of physical appearance. That is not to say you cannot tell her she is beautiful but that is not all she is. Many girls are basing their self-esteem on looks, so talk more about what she can accomplish than how cute she looks.

Parenting our boys

Boys tend to be urged by parents and peers to be independent and achievement-oriented with not as much emphasis put on caring and empathy. As a society we do not talk enough to little boys about expressing feelings. We do not teach healthy ways to express anger with words rather than actions. As a result, violence is primarily a male problem. Men often have fewer close friends and weaker family ties than women do. Boys need help in feeling comfortable with nurturing and attachment.

Begin with plenty of physical attention. Little boys need just as much cuddling as little girls and just as much comfort when they cry. Little boys need to know it is OK to cry and that big boys cry too. Allow them to express sadness. You do not want them to suppress these emotions. Do not hide Dad's emotions from your son. Let your child see when you are upset and talk to him about your feelings. Spend time playing gentle games and continue to snuggle them as they grow. Talk to them often, encourage language development and conversation.

Provide them with all types of toys including dolls and dress-up clothes. Provide them with a kitchen so they can cook pretend meals for you. When your son plays with a doll let him know what a great dad he will be. Talk about feelings and how actions affect others. Offer constructive ways to work on conflict, especially working out conflict with words. Be careful of double standards, such as the old cliché "boys will be boys." If it would be unacceptable for a girl, it would be unacceptable for your boy as well. Let them help you with household chores and cooking.

Help our children to develop qualities that are valued in people of both sexes, such as confidence and compassion, and you can't go wrong.

Dads' role

Research has shown that fathers play an important role in encouraging children to break out of sex-role stereotyping. Someone other than a child's birth father can provide a beneficial male influence. Sons learn from their fathers what it is to be a man. Dads serve as role models for how men should act towards women. Boys learn how to treat women from their fathers and girls learn what to expect from men from their dads.

Boys whose fathers are actively involved in raising them are more likely to grow up with a healthy sense of gender identity, while those whose fathers were absent are more likely to be antisocial and possibly abusive and/or violent.

Dads do not have to be stay-at-home dads to have a positive influence on their kids. They just need to set aside time each day to spend time quality time with their kids. This could be in the form of hugging, reading, and playing. Studies show that working fathers spend one third less time than working mothers with their kids. Dads also play a vital role in encouraging independence and self-confidence in their daughters too. One study interviewed successful women and the one thing they all had in common was a father who believed in them. Girls whose father was the primary caregiver demonstrated a great sense of confidence and poise. Dads, however, can be less likely to encourage feminine values and find it easier to encourage independence in a daughter. By being involved in a child's life, a father demonstrates that a cherishing relationship is as masculine as it is feminine.

Dads also benefit from caring for their children. It brings about positive changes in fathers as well as the kids. Involved dads learn firsthand the value of nurturing and intimacy. Fathers who have been primary caregivers describe themselves as more patient, more accepting, and more sensitive to other people's needs.

I thought I would let Jane Nelsen's words of wisdom regarding nature versus nurture, from her book *Positive Discipline: The First Three Years*, close out this chapter:

"Popular magazines, books, and research journals are filled with new studies on human genes and their importance in how we live and who we become. Researchers believe that genes may have an even stronger influence on temperament and personality than we previously thought; many researchers believe that genes determine such qualities as optimism, depression, aggression, and even whether or not a person is a thrill seeker, which may be old news to parents who are forever plucking their daring toddlers from the tops of walls, jungle gyms, and trees. Parents may find themselves wondering just how much influence they have on their growing child. If genes are so powerful, does it really matter how we parent our children? The answer is that it matters a great deal. While a child inherits certain traits and tendencies through her genes, the story of how those traits develop has not been written yet. Your child may have arrived on the planet with her own unique temperament but how you and her other caregivers interact with her will shape the person she becomes. As educational psychologist Jane M. Healy puts it, 'Brains shape behavior and behavior shapes brains.' It is no longer a question of nature versus nurture. A child's genes and her environment engage in an intimate, complicated dance and both are part of who she will become. We parents, fragile and imperfect as we are, bear the responsibility for shaping our children's environment. We shape the very structure and wiring of their brains; we shape the people they become and the future they will have."

Sources for this chapter include:

Positive Discipline: The First Three Years by Jane Nelsen

Bright from the Start by Dr. Jill Stamm

Beyond Pink and Blue by Jenny Friedman, PHD

"Sugar and Spice" *Parenting*, September 2001

CHAPTER 22

SELF-ESTEEM

"Affirming words from moms and dads are like light switches. Speak a word of affirmation at the right moment in a child's life, and it's like lighting up a whole roomful of possibilities."

— *Gary Smalley*

What is self-esteem?

Self-esteem is the confidence and self-assurance each of us has in ourselves. It allows us to take risks and welcome new experiences.

Self-esteem comes from many places. There is not *one* thing that gives us self-esteem but a cumulation of events. A child's self-esteem must evolve over time. Self-esteem is not something we can just give to our children, although all parents wish we could.

Self-esteem comes from a person feeling capable, feeling valued, feeling loved, feeling a sense of worthiness, and belonging. The more positive a child's self-esteem, the more confident they will be and the more secure they will feel. Before a child starts school, the child's parents are the most important contributor to a child's self-esteem.

The more positive the parent's self-esteem is or appears to be, the more positive the child's will be. Children look at the parent as a role model.

Once a child starts school, teachers and friends also become an important part of the equation. Children with positive self-esteem will have an easier time making friends. They are not afraid to go up to a new group and introduce themselves, asking if they can join in.

Since we cannot give a child self-worth, how do we develop positive self-esteem? One of the best ways we can develop a child's self-worth is by giving them unconditional love.

Some other ways to encourage positive self-esteem include:

Encouraging independence

Independence starts out slowly and increases over time. Even a newborn demonstrates independence with gaze aversion. They look away when they start to feel over simulated. We teach independence when we teach self-soothing techniques where we help our infants learn to soothe themselves to sleep. When a baby cries and turns their head, refusing a particular food, they are demonstrating independence.

Make sure you are giving your baby quiet time alone. If they are playing quietly, start your own activity. Try to extend the time before you go to them to 10–15 minutes. Stall by talking to them rather than picking them up if they get fussy or frustrated and want your attention.

Hire a babysitter by at least six months. Being apart from you and then having you come back builds security, confidence, and independence. Relying on someone other than Mom and Dad helps your baby develop a sense of trust in other adults.

Toddlers seem to be declaring their need for independence all the time. The word "No" says it all. They use it for everything even when they do not mean it. "Do you want a cookie?" "No", then cry when you do not give them a cookie.

Toddlers want to try to do everything on their own. This includes feeding themselves, putting on their shoes, getting in their car seat, etc. Their need for independence dominates their day and can also be frustrating for them as well.

As parents we may need to cheer these first steps at independence as they enter into new challenges and situations. We encourage them and cheer when they try a new food. We praise them for getting through the first day of a new daycare / preschool or playgroup. When we react with enthusiasm when they do something on their own, they are more likely to repeat it. So, allow some extra time and allow them to try things on their own.

As we will discuss more in the discipline chapter, we want to encourage freedom within limits. Give them lots of choices when appropriate and encourage them to follow through with their decision. When kids learn they can tackle new challenges successfully on their own then they are less likely to rely on others next time. An independent child is more likely to experiment with different problem-solving techniques, which will serve them throughout their lives. Experts have found that children who are trained to be independent early on have a greater desire to achieve in school as well.

Karen Berberian, PhD, psychologist at St. Christopher's Hospital for Children in Philadelphia says, "Traits that characterize a self-sufficient child—a willingness to explore freely and the ability to feel good about accomplishments—are the ones that characterize a receptive learner."

"School phobia tendencies can be reduced or prevented by helping your child develop a sense of independence."

Building trust

When your child feels trust in the relationship this leads to positive self-esteem. The concept of trust starts to develop in infancy as well. Without trust in any relationship, it is impossible to feel safe, close, and comfortable. This is especially true for a helpless infant.

From your baby's perspective, reasonably prompt and consistent care is essential for developing trust. When their needs are met, such as feeding, changing, and snuggling, your baby develops a sense of safety and security. That leads to confidence and trust. Your baby feels valued and important.

You can maintain that feeling of trust as your child grows. One of the easiest ways to build trust is by having a routine to the day so your child can predict what is going to happen next. Consistent rules that have simple explanations that your child understands also add to a sense of trust, as well as setting reasonable limits. When children can predict what your responses will be, this helps build confidence in the relationship. So be consistent and follow through every time. Mean what you say and say what you mean.

Assertiveness

Teach your child to be assertive. An assertive child is one who will stand up for themselves. There is a difference between being assertive and aggressive. Assertiveness is letting people know your wants and needs. This is different from aggressiveness which is imposing those wants and needs on others. An aggressive child will try to manhandle a playmate out of a toy. An assertive child says they would like a turn next.

Granted, your child will not be able to say these words yet. Until they can stand up for themselves, you can demonstrate and say the words for them. Show them what is socially acceptable and give them the tools to do it themselves when they are old enough. Show them that standing up for themselves does not mean friends will not like them.

Many experts feel that assertiveness is partly inherited. Some children are shyer and more passive by nature. (You should not override natural tendencies by trying to force them into a role they are not comfortable in to boost their confidence, as this can have the opposite effect.) You can build on the small amount of assertiveness that every child has and help them to see how it can be useful. Teach shy kids how to speak up for themselves and show them and give them the tools to eventually do it themselves.

I taught this lesson with bubbles. I had one bottle of bubbles and taught taking turns, with me holding the bubble wand and making sure each child had a turn. Sharing / taking turns and assertiveness go hand in hand. If a child does not know what is expected of them then it is harder to be assertive. Help your child distinguish right from wrong rather than perceive the rules as arbitrary.

You are giving your child a gift. A pushy child will have a hard time making and keeping friends. Anything that promotes a healthy self-esteem promotes assertiveness. If a child feels good about who they are, they are more likely to assert themself.

Stuart Fischoff, PhD, professor of psychology at California State University says, "Being assertive helps in virtually every relationship, at school, at home, on the playground."

In the classroom, being assertive puts a child at an advantage because they are comfortable commanding the teacher's attention, raising their hand if they know the answer, and asking if they need extra help if they get lost. They will have an easier time making friends because they won't hesitate to ask, "Can I play too?"

Again, let them know it is OK to express their feelings. Feelings are never wrong, it's the actions that may or may not be socially acceptable and how they react to those feelings that may be inappropriate. Actions, not feelings, have consequences.

Dr. Fischoff also says, "All young children are self-absorbed, they think the world revolves around them." (In my house it does.) A child has to be taught to empathize.

Although it is age appropriate and normal behavior for a toddler to simply take a ball away from another child, you should correct them and ask them how she would feel if it were them. Just because it is age appropriate does not mean you should ignore it. Plant the seed early that others have feelings too.

Recognition and praise

Honest recognition and praise are a great way to build a child's self-confidence. Behavior that is noticed and appreciated is often repeated. Dr. Thomas D. Yarnell, PhD and clinical psychologist, says, "Honest praise is the quickest way to build a person's self-esteem." He suggests you try to find a way to encourage your child every day. Provide opportunities that are challenging but not so difficult that they cause frustration. Then cheer the accomplishment and tell them what an awesome job they did. It is also very important to acknowledge an attempt and offer encouragement even if they were not successful. Find something positive to say about the attempt so they try again. You may even give your child a task that you know they will be successful at to boost their self-esteem. This will give them a feeling of competence and confidence. Give your child age-appropriate responsibilities as early as possible. Do not do for children what they can do for themselves. If you do everything for them, they will doubt their own competence.

Jane Nelsen says it is important to "Balance our need to protect them with their need to take risks and tackle new challenges and explore their capabilities. Young children still need supervision and teaching about dangers, etc. However, encouragement does not mean making the world fit your child / toddler's every whim. Weigh your child's choices and environments to determine which experiences offer opportunities for growth and which are simply too dangerous. Allow your child to take reasonable risks and learn new skills."

Now praising your child for accomplishments can be a double-edged sword. You do not want your child to think they need to have your praise and approval for everything they do. This could backfire on you. Your child might think unless Mom and Dad praise me, I am not good enough. This could have the opposite effect of what we are going for. We do not want kids to feel they have to be perfect. Instead, encourage difficult tasks. Encouragement speaks to the effort, and praise speaks to the person. Encouragement is unconditional. Just get the message across that you have faith in your child and will love them no matter what.

Dr. Alison Arnold, life coach and author of *Scream and Run Naked* says it is important to praise children's character. Praise who they are, not what they do. This helps children learn that what they do does not define them. Praise their hard work. I am so proud of how hard you worked. This again goes more to character than achievement. Praise compassion towards others.

Use "You" statements that praise being: "Thank you, you are so helpful." Kids translate this into "I am helpful. I'm smart. I am talented." She says to praise giving and praise character. She states we live in a competitive culture and with comparisons comes pressure. Focus on what your child does well and the value they have within. Try not to be as achievement based as you are character based. You can't be the best if there is too much pressure. You have to feel good about who you are to feel good about what you do.

Respect

Show your child you respect them.

Showing your child that you respect them is another key component in reinforcing your child's self-worth.

There are several ways you can show respect for your children:

*You can offer them choices when appropriate then respect and abide by their choices.

*Another way to show respect towards children is to explain the reason behind the rules or explain why an adult made the decision they made.

*Avoid talking about children in front of children unless they are included in conversation. *If they are babies and you have had a day and a half and you need to vent to your spouse, wait until your baby is asleep to share.

*Help children learn that you accept them as a person even if you do not accept behavior: "I may not like this behavior, but I will always love YOU!"

*Criticize the behavior and not the child. "That was naughty behavior," not "you were naughty."

*If they feel from parents, "it's my way or the highway," they learn that speaking their mind gets them into trouble and they stop sharing with you.

*Let your children know you care about them no matter what. Mistakes can be fixed and don't take away from my love.

*Put a picture of your family where your baby can see it every day. This helps them to see they are part of a family. This shows them they are loved, cherished, they belong, and that they have support.

Physical activity

Physical activity / coordination and organized sports have a huge impact on positive self-confidence.

The *Good Beginnings* newsletter written by Dr. Ellen Abell, a child development specialist, says, "Self-esteem is a benefit of a child's confidence in their abilities to control their movements and muscles. Children who feel confident in their physical abilities will enjoy taking part in activities with other children. A child who throws a ball awkwardly or runs slower than other kids may avoid playing with other children. Mastering physical skills has a good effect on gaining independence, coping skills, forming friendships, and trying new things".

Prior to organized sports, just getting your child moving is important. Develop those large motor skills. Help them to feel confident in physical activity. In infancy encourage your little one to climb over things, under and around things. Have them first walk forward then backwards. Walk with their hands on their knees then with their hands on their backs. Put them in a park and recs class or little gym. As they grow, I personally find the value of being part of a team and being a "teammate" is a valuable thing for a child. Give them the discipline of attending practices. I think sports of any kind are an amazing gift we can give our kids. My daughter was a competitive dancer and, as you know, Dylan a competitive gymnast. Their coaches were other positive role models, building their self-esteem, and I am grateful for their influence over the years.

In my classes I give out this handout of a poem written by Diane Loomans entitled "If I had my child to raise over again." I thought I would also share it with all of you. It is so powerful.

If I had my child to raise all over again, I'd build self-esteem first, and the house later. I'd finger-paint more and point the finger less. I would do less correcting and more connecting. I'd take my eyes off my watch and watch with my eyes. I'd take more hikes and fly more kites. I'd stop playing serious, and seriously play. I would run through more fields and gaze at more stars. I'd do more hugging and less tugging.

- Diane Loomans, If I Had My Child to Raise Over Again

Here are some great self-esteem books and resources:

Hurray for You by Maryanne Richmond. For kids.

Stand Tall, Mary Lou Mellon by Patty Lovell. For kids.

Strong Mothers, Strong Sons by Meg Meeker MD. For Mom.

Strong Fathers, Strong Daughters by Meg Meeker MD. For Dad.

Free to be You and Me by Marlo Thomas (Music). For Kids.

Sources:

Dr. T. Berry Brazelton

Dr. Barton Schmitt

Positive Discipline, book series by Jane Nelson

Building your Child's Self-Esteem by Thomas D. Yarnell, PhD, clinical psychologist

CHAPTER 23

DISCIPLINE

"If we don't shape our kids, they will be shaped by outside forces that don't care what shape our kids are in."

— Dr. Louise Hart

The word "discipline" is derived from the Latin word *disciplina*, which means to teach. The aim of discipline is to define and reinforce limits. Goals of discipline are to protect our children from harm, teach them what is socially appropriate, and *eventually for them to learn self-discipline.*

Dr. T. Berry Brazelton, one of my favorite developmental pediatricians, has many wise quotes I have used throughout this book but here are three on discipline:

1. "What children learn first about limit-setting is the cornerstone of their moral development."
2. 2.) "Being able to set limits is a parent's second most important gift to a child after love."
3. "Reasonable limits keep us from raising spoiled children."

We appreciate our parents so much more after we have children. One thing my mom said about raising kids that I loved was, "You will always love your children but your goal as a parent is to raise children that others will love as well."

The disciplinary approach you use in the first three years of your child's life is critical. If you put in the time and energy now, you will reap enormous benefits later.

Even an infant can be taught limits and rules. An example of setting limits in infancy is putting your child down drowsy but awake; allowing your child to play independently; telling them at mealtime if they continue to feed their food to the dog from their highchair, you will take them down, and then following through. These are all discipline techniques.

Kids test limits to see what is and is not allowed. It is their job to test limits. This is developmentally appropriate. What we allow lets them see what is socially appropriate. By establishing firm limits, reinforcing good behavior, and building a trusting relationship, you can minimize the amount of discipline you will need when your child is older. Establishing limits will also influence how your child learns to distinguish right from wrong and also how well-adjusted and self-assured your child will ultimately be.

Michael Popkin, PhD, is the author of the *Active Parenting Today* discipline series. He says, "The problem most parents have is they don't have a consistent approach to parenting." He feels most people use a little of what their parents did, a little of the exact opposite of what their parents did, and a little of what they have picked up from friends, books, and magazines. He feels this can be OK as long as you avoid two discipline extremes: overly permissive and excessively authoritarian.

<u>He feels children of parents who are overly permissive</u> may have a tough time learning self-control and following limits and regulating their impulses. These kids may have a harder time adjusting to society's rules. This is usually most obvious when they start school.

<u>He conversely feels that children subjected to excessively authoritative / overly harsh and punitive disciplinary approaches (dictators</u>) can develop low self-esteem. These kids are at risk of becoming excessively timid and shy and self-conscious. Children raised by excessively authoritative parents can grow up rebellious and full of rage and act out aggressively. Studies have shown that young children who were raised with punitive punishment such as spanking are more likely to become bullies as they grow and use physical aggression through life.

He feels the key is to find a balance between the two extremes.

Democratic parenting

<u>Dr. Popkin calls this the "democratic" style of parenting or "active parenting,"</u> where the parent is the leader who encourages cooperation and stimulates learning. There is order and routine and every person is an important member of the family. Children are treated with dignity and respect even when their parents discipline them. Children are entitled to express their thoughts and feelings. Dr. Michael Popkin says, "Democracy does not mean that you will always get your way, it means you will always get your say. Freedom within limits"

Jane Nelson, the author of the *Positive Discipline* books, calls this style of parenting "positive discipline."

I believe to discipline effectively you have to be willing to adapt.

1. You not only have to first <u>know the specific techniques.</u>

2. You then have to be able to adapt them to your child's temperament and needs.
3. You have to take into account the particular situation.
4. Remember, what may work for one child may not always work for another.
5. There is not just one right way to discipline.

Taken and adapted from *Your Child's Health* by Dr. Barton Schmitt:

Age-by-age discipline techniques

Birth – 4 months: No discipline measures needed.

4 months – 8 months: Mild verbal disapproval is all that is needed.

8 months – 18 months: Structure the environment, distract, ignore, verbal and nonverbal disapproval. Physically moving or escorting and temporary timeout such as in a playpen.

18 months – 3 years: All the proceeding techniques plus a temporary timeout / thinking spot or as my friend and child psychologist, Barb Grady, calls it "a peaceful place."

Reorganizing your home

Example of structuring the home / their environment:

Around 6–9 months safety becomes the most critical discipline issue. You want to give them the freedom to explore while making certain things off limits. In one word "childproof." Examples include putting breakable items out of reach, setting up a gate, using safety latches, locking off certain rooms.

Toddlers are programmed neurologically to explore. If a child's explorations are met repeatedly with negative feedback, they may stop investigating the world around them, which is the way they learn. So, let us give them that freedom within *our* limits.

When Dylan was just shy of a year old, probably around 10 or 11 months, I came around the corner from the laundry room holding an armful of clothes. Instead of playing on the floor with his toys, I saw him literally swinging on the kitchen chandelier above our kitchen table. Yep, you read that correctly: He was swinging from the light fixture. I dropped the clothes and rushed as quickly as possible, without trying to frighten him, to pluck him off his makeshift jungle gym. I was completely freaked out, as you can imagine. I realized he had climbed up onto the chair and then up onto the table, stood up and then reached for the light fixture. So, I had to restructure his environment. When my husband came home, he looked around with a questioning look and asked me where all the kitchen chairs were. I told him the story and let him know our kitchen chairs now lived in the dining room behind the baby gate. They stayed there for several months, and the light was raised up several chain links. That is an example, albeit extreme, of structuring your environment.

Distraction, redirection, or diversion

To distract is to exchange one temptation for another one. This is a very helpful technique when out in public places. You can use a toy, food, books, or another activity. I always had a special "going-out bag" with toys and snacks that stayed in that bag and only came out at restaurants or the doctor's office, church, etc. Activities in my going-out bag were typically quiet activities like a felt board and an

Aquadoodle, search-and-find books, etc.: age-appropriate activities that changed as my kids did and their interests did.

Ignore the misbehavior

Dr. Schmitt suggests using this technique to eliminate behaviors that are harmless yet still unacceptable. Examples would be attention-getting behaviors such as tantrums, whining, pouting, and/or interrupting. The proper way to ignore your child is to move away from them. Turn your back and avoid eye contact. Stop all conversation or arguing or negotiating. You may even need to leave the room.

Parental verbal and nonverbal disapproval

<u>Verbal correction</u>: A change in the tone of your voice may be all that is needed to stop or change misbehavior.

<u>Non-verbal</u>: Would be a change of facial expression, it could be a concerned, sad, or a stern look. Sometimes all they need is a look from you to stop unwanted behavior. Children want to please you and often look to you for reassurance before they try something new.

Another non-verbal cue would be telling them, "One minute, please" when you are talking by holding up a finger. Now, little ones won't quite understand but when combined with, "Hold on one minute," they will eventually get it.

Other verbal mixed with non-verbal messaging is making sure you have made eye contact and using your stern or concerned face, and then adding your words such as "danger" or "no." The closer you are to the child, the more assured you are to have their attention and not raise your voice. Your comments can be made in a soft but disapproving tone.

Also, show your child the behavior you want repeated. For example, if they are pulling your hair, say "Ouch, that hurts." Use the word "gentle" and show them what you mean by using their hand to stroke your hair gently.

Make sure you have your child's attention before giving directions. Ask your child to stop and look at you. When they are old enough, ask them to repeat what you said to make sure they get it.

I have always said, "I need your eyes." Dylan was my stubborn one. I would say, "Mommy needs your eyes" and he would look everywhere but at me. I would wait there patiently until he looked at me. He was so darn cute that my most common mistake when I was so close, and he was rolling his eyes all over his head trying not to look at me, was smiling or giggling to myself.

Physically moving your child (manual guidance)

When your child needs to move but is refusing to go on their own, you might need to move your child from one place to another against their will. Examples of this are physically taking your little one to bed / crib, car, bath, car seat, or stroller.

Guide them by the hand or forearm and, if they refuse to be led, pick them up from behind. Give them a choice if they are old enough, "You can either walk to your bedroom with Mommy or I will have to carry you as it is nap time." When your child keeps playing and refuses to move you say, "I see you made your choice, you need

Mommy to help you." You then guide them or pick them up and take them to their room.

Temporary timeout

A temporary timeout can be an effective discipline technique for dealing with a misbehaving infant or toddler if it is not overused and if it is used in the correct way.

Timeout is a good technique to use to avoid injury. It is a safe place to have a tantrum and a good tool for disciplining aggression to gain control over their body. Timeouts can be used to help a child regain control of their body when redirection and other forms of discipline have not worked.

It is used to interrupt unacceptable behavior by removing the child from the original situation. It provides a cooling-off period for both parent and child.

Most providers feel that timeout should be replaced with logical consequences by age six.˙

A playpen or crib is a great place for timeouts. The purpose of timeout is *not* meant to be a punishment or meant to make a child feel isolated, but a way for them to gain self-control, so allowing them to be in a playpen with toys is OK. Remember the goal is self-control and calming down.

Chairs with a quiet book as the child gets older may be appropriate. You may call it their "thinking spot," "quiet place," "reading nook," etc.

Timeout should be short enough so the child has many chances to go back to the original situation and learn acceptable behavior.

Typically, this is one minute for every year of age. If your child wants to stay and play in the playpen that is OK, just give them the option to get out when time is up.

Understanding what is developmentally appropriate while teaching what is socially appropriate

Although most behaviors in infancy and toddlerhood are age-appropriate behaviors, you do not have to allow them. Stop inappropriate behavior immediately (even babies need to learn what is socially acceptable).

It is not uncommon for babies to poke, pinch, bite, or tug the hair of someone they love. They are busy exploring their world. This includes finding out what skin tastes like, how hair feels, and how a person reacts when pinched and poked. Since babies need repetition to learn a lesson, they are likely to do it over and over again. They do not realize that these things can hurt you or others. However, even an infant can be taught rules and limits. If the behavior would not be OK to do to another child, it should not be OK for you. To teach your child to respect others, you first have to teach your child to respect your rights.

If your little one pulls on your earring, or pokes you in the eye, remove their hand and say, "No, that hurts Mommy or Daddy," show them how to touch gently or you may just simply put them down. When you are holding a child that bites or pinches you, putting the child down is a form of timeout. It may take several times for them to correlate that every time they pinch Mom or pull her hair, they are put down. They will eventually learn this is not a behavior that is appropriate. If your child is biting you, you can put your hand over their mouth and say again firmly, "No, that hurts mommy. Mouths are for eating and kissing, not biting!" If your baby is biting you, set a good example by not giving them love bites or blowing on their bellies as they may get confused.

Alternatives to "no"

Between six months to one year, your baby discovers mobility. A newly mobile baby finds more and more off-limits objects within his or her reach and things to get into. You are going to find yourself saying "no" more than you would like.

I realize "no" can be the quickest and easiest way to get your child's attention and, at times, it is a reflex, but many experts say to save "no" for situations of danger, because if you overuse the word, they may learn to tune you out and it will lose its power. Keep in mind your child responds better to tone rather than the word until about 12 months. Some sooner, when they can grasp the meaning of the word.

A few alternatives to "no" to try:

I used the word "danger" for dangerous situations. Other words you might try are "hot", "ouch", "gentle", "danger." The earlier you start trying out other words, the more they will become second nature.

I will share a cute story with all of you about a mom I had in class several years back. After this lecture she went home to share the lecture with her husband and said they were using the word "no" too much and that they needed to come up with some other words. The following day she said he was so proud and wanted to show her how he found a new word that was working. I am chuckling as I type this. He said that, when his little guy went to grab the lamp, he yelled out "decoration." He was so excited it worked. I hated to tell her it was probably the way he yelled the word out rather than the word "decoration" itself, but I was excited he was taking my advice to heart. 😊

When you are tempted to blurt out "no," try to redirect your little one to another activity. Pause and consider what your child is doing and why. They may be reaching for the breakable glass because it is shiny. Offer them a child-safe mirror instead.

Remember to use your non-verbal cues and stern or concerned looks. Babies often glance at parents for reassurance when trying something new. You would be surprised at how often your little one actually knows they are probably not supposed to be touching that and will look at you to see if you will stop them. Try to stop behavior by giving them a stern or worried look without any words at all.

Rather than simply saying "no," show them the correct way to do something. For example, if your child is pulling on the dog's fur, rather than simply saying "no," show him how to stroke or pet and feel the dog gently.

Try to use "I" messages

Our goal is to prevent a defense reaction. This will be more helpful as they get older, but it is never too early to start. It takes practice to change the way you phrase things. So, start in infancy, and by toddlerhood it will be second nature for you. Starting off with "you" is accusatory and can trigger a defense reaction. (This works with spouses too 😉) Examples of starting with "I" are: "I get upset when…" "It makes me sad when…" "I am sorry you are so mad / so sad but we don't hit," rather than using "you" and starting with "You were naughty" or "You shouldn't have done that." Instead say "that was naughty behavior." This lets your child know it was the behavior you didn't approve of, not your kiddo. Now, you may say, "You must be really angry" or "That was naughty behavior, we never hit someone, it hurts," putting emphasis on the behavior not the child.

Make sure the message of love gets through

Children respond to discipline from people they feel loved by and want to please. Hug and kiss and smile at them often. The greatest gift we can give our kids is making sure they feel valued and loved every single day, even if they make mistakes. When they feel loved and important, they feel that they belong. This encourages positive self-esteem. Give them honest praise every day. Honest, earned praise. More on this to come...

They form opinions of themselves through their perception of how you feel about them. This gives them a strong foundation to develop to their full potential.

Correcting with love

Talk to your child the way you would want to be talked to. Avoid yelling or using a disrespectful tone of voice. If you lose your cool, don't be afraid to say you're sorry. Show them that even adults make mistakes and need to say "I am sorry" if they hurt someone's feelings. Give your children increased attention when they are not demanding it. Many experts feel that it takes several positive contacts to counter one negative one. My colleague calls these positive interactions "time-ins."

Explain the reason behind the rule: Children learn better when parents add age-appropriate explanations to why they are asking their child to behave in a certain way. The younger the child is, the more concrete the rule should be. Remember, babies aged 11–14 months of age understand more than 50 words. An 18-month-old can learn approximately nine words per day. So, they understand more than they can articulate: "Ouch, pinching hurts" / "No, danger" / "Mouths are for eating and kissing, not biting" / "Do not pinch your brother you will hurt him."

Children begin to understand the rationale behind the rules. Children who do not get clear reasons often come up with their own. Be careful how you phrase things. A child's interpretation may be different from yours. They may think, for example, you don't think they have the ability to do something and that is why you are telling them not to do it. Or they may feel they are personally bad, rather than that you are protecting them from something dangerous.

Again, make sure the message of love gets through, that you love them, you just do not like the behavior: "I love you, but I don't like it when you hit people. It hurts them. They feel sad. It makes their mommy feel sad to see them cry or hurt." Make sure they understand that they are not bad but that hitting is bad. Bring attention to the unacceptable behavior.

A cute story about a friend of mine demonstrates how a child may not always interpret things the way you do. When my friend was a little boy, he had surgery for a hernia and the surgeon told him he would not be able to climb a tree, run, ride a bike, etc. for a couple of weeks. When his mother came home from work, his bike was in the driveway and she found him up a tree. He was so happy to see his mother and, when she asked him what he was doing, he proudly stated the doctor said I would not be able to run, ride a bike, or climb trees, but he was wrong, I did all those things today. ☺

Be kind and firm

For most parents, it is very easy to be kind and difficult to be firm.

Firmness, however, means using appropriate parenting principles with confidence.

Kindness means maintaining dignity and respect for yourself and your child while using parenting principles. Play a mental game with yourself. Ask yourself, if someone recorded your discipline techniques and played it on national TV, how would you feel? If you feel OK, then chances are you are being both kind and firm.

Offer choices

By giving older babies and toddlers plenty of choices, they feel more in control (choices give the child a sense of independence). Offering choices helps decrease power struggles. You control the choices, and you set the limits. Whenever appropriate, give your child a choice between at least two _acceptable_ options. Acceptable means you are willing to accept either option the child chooses. Only offer choices you feel good about. Offer choices about things that really don't matter. Yet remember *not everything* is a choice. For example, it is not optional to sit in the car seat. There may be an option on how they get into the car seat, for example, "Are you going to climb in yourself or does Mommy or Daddy need to help you?"

Another example is if you say, "You can either sit down in your stroller or we are going home." IF they don't sit down, you need to follow through and return home. If you really don't want to go home, don't offer it as a choice! If you are struggling with control, make some practice runs when you really do not care if you go home. This will allow you to gain credibility.

Young children need limited choices. Two choices are enough. As they get older you may need to broaden your choices.

Offering choices can be a great way to get older infants and young toddlers to do things they don't want to do. For example, it is not a choice to brush your teeth or not, but a choice could be, "Do you want to brush your teeth with your Winnie the Pooh toothbrush or your Piglet toothbrush?"

Natural consequences

Natural consequences happen <u>on their own.</u> Children naturally learn some things if parents can resist the urge to rescue, lecture, or punish them. They learn for themselves and won't blame you for the consequence. You might point out the natural consequence after something happens. A child who deliberately spills their juice or milk will not have juice to drink. A child who feeds all their food to the dog is out of food. If they throw a toy in a tantrum and it breaks or, like in our house, over the baby gate, they won't have that toy to play with. If an accident happens after you have warned your child, point it out, "I am sorry that the dog knocked you down and you got hurt. That is why Mommy says not to lie on the dog." Or "If you squeeze the juice box you will get juice on you and you will be wet and sticky," etc. As children get older you can allow natural consequences to play out more than when they are little.

Logical consequences

Use a logical consequence when a natural consequence would not be appropriate.

You can use a logical consequence to prevent a dangerous situation from happening if you were to let a natural consequence play out. Or if a natural consequence would be unacceptable due to long-range results, like those from not brushing your teeth.

For example: "If you do not brush your teeth they will rot and fall out."

You cannot let a toddler learn through natural consequences that the oven is hot by touching it or what will happen if they run into the street. With logical consequences the parent or adult must get involved.

A logical consequence must follow the 3 *Rs:* it must be related, respectful, and reasonable. A logical consequence does not always have to be verbal either. If the child treats the dog aggressively, you can quietly remove the dog. You can say, "Mommy has told you not to pull on the dog's tail, it hurts Molly. Now Molly has to go outside." A child throwing sand who knows the rules is taken home. A child who runs into the street is taken inside.

Some rules for logical consequences include the following:

"If it is not obvious, it is not logical." For example, if your child scribbles on the wall, the reasonable, respectful, related consequence would be to give the child a cloth and have them help you clean it up. If they toss their food on the floor, it would be reasonable, respectful, and related to take them out of their highchair and have them help you pick up the food off the floor.

You need to continue to give children opportunities to learn responsibility through consequence. They will eventually get it.

Follow through

This and consistency are two of the most important rules of discipline.

Follow through can reduce frustration and conflict. Your child will learn that you mean what you say and that you say what you mean. You will always follow through with an appropriate consequence.

You need to be prepared to follow through with the consequence. If you tell your child who is throwing a fit in the grocery store, "You have to stop, or we will have to go out to the car until you can gain control of your body" you have to be willing to leave your cart for a time and go out to the car.

Make sure your words and actions match up.

Consistency

Consistency is a crucial component to discipline.

If you tell your child "only one cookie" and they are screaming and having a fit in front of someone and you give in, maybe to avoid a scene, you make them happy in the short term, but you have just lost credibility. The behavior is sure to be repeated.

Children are smart and they know how to push Mom and Dad's buttons. They will remember this incident and next time they want a cookie they will throw a fit again because it worked before. Children do what works! They have long memories.

It is important for both parents to be consistent. When Taylor was about a year and a half old, I was trying to do taxes, and I asked my husband to run some errands at Target and take our daughter with him. On the way out the door I reminded him to take the grocery cart seat. He acknowledged me and left. He came back a very frazzled dad and said, "I do not know how you do this all the time alone." I asked him what he meant, and he said she was a terror. He said she was running under the rounds of clothes and pulling things off hangers. He said it was horrible and very embarrassing and scary as she even hid once. I asked him if he forgot the cart seat. He said, "No I took it, but she didn't want to sit in it. I said, "Well, that was your first mistake. She should not have had a choice."

Now, fast forward a few days and I had to go to Walmart. I remember it like it was yesterday and my little pumpkin, who never gave me a hassle before, decided she didn't want to ride in her seat. She remembered her trip to Target with Daddy. She quickly realized Mom was not going to let her run around Walmart. I told her my job is to keep her safe and healthy and to do that she needed to ride in this cart. Now, in her defense, I am sure this was confusing. Well, she carried on and cried and I stuck to my guns. I held her little body in the cart with my arm over her legs as she kicked and screamed, and wow did I get looks. I just smiled at everyone walking by. When my little darling finally relaxed after what felt like an hour (probably 10 minutes), I said, "I am so glad you are feeling better. Are you ready to go shopping now?" Now to be honest that was the last thing I wanted to do. I was sweating up a storm and mortified, hoping not to have to see anyone in the store that passed me in the parking lot, but I knew I had to follow through. That was the last time she tested me. It was understandable that she would test the limits. That is what toddlers do, and Daddy changed the rules. Mom, however, reinforced those rules and she quickly realized Mom is going to follow through and she means business. Dad learned a lesson too 😉

Precede the consequence with only one reminder or warning

After the rule is clearly stated and <u>understood</u>, the warning is unnecessary. (With younger children you may have to give them a couple reminders to make sure they understand.) Avoid repeated threats of consequences if your child does not stop what he or she is doing. I am not an advocate of counting. Most children will wait until the final number to react. "You can climb in your car seat or Mommy can help you." If the child does not move say, "OK, I see you have made your choice, you would like Mommy to help you." You then pick the child up and buckle them in (while they are doing the alligator death roll).

Routines

As you all know by now, I feel routines are of extreme importance. Children need routines. Routines offer consistency and predictability. Setting routines helps your child know what to expect. Once the routine is in place, the routine is the boss and the parents do not have to continually give orders, e.g., bedtime routine, morning routine, bath routine, even brushing teeth.

Routines give children a sense of security and help them to transition from one activity to the next with less objection because it happens this way every single time, every single day.

Mistakes

Help your children understand that mistakes are opportunities to learn. We all make mistakes, even parents 😊 Don't hesitate to let your children know when you make a mistake. People are often very forgiving when you admit your mistake. Say you are sorry and try to solve the problem you created. Children are no different. "I am sorry Mommy yelled. I was running late, and it was not your fault ... I will do better next time."

Act more and talk less

Children tend to tune out parents if they talk too much. The younger the child is, the more concrete the explanation should be, as I mentioned previously. It is perfectly OK to lift a child up to bed rather than lecturing, ordering, or threatening. You have to sometimes get their attention before they hear you. Get on their level and make eye contact: "Mommy needs your eyes" or "Daddy needs your eyes."

Yelling can be an effective tool if you do not do it often. If you yell, "Stop, danger!" as your child is running for the road, and you do not yell often, you are more likely to have an immediate response. If you yell consistently, children tend to tune you out until you reach a certain decibel.

Control

The only behavior we can control is our own. Our goal as parents is to teach our children self-control. Let your child figure it out on his/her own. Do not be too fast to fix a problem for your child. Let your child try to figure it out him or herself first. Frustration can be a powerful learning tool. Children realize they can do this on their own and develop a sense of accomplishment. They are more likely the next time to try to problem-solve on their own. Allowing your child to try will increase their independence and promotes healthy / positive self-esteem. If you rush to help them too fast, they may think that even Mom or Dad thinks they can't do it.

Promises

Do not make them unless you intend to keep them. Promises come back to follow-through and consistency.

Try to figure out what is behind the behavior

A child may be reaching for the computer keyboard because they see Mom and Dad on it daily. Buy them toys that are like your adult items. A pretend computer, play vacuum, play doll, play kitchen, etc. This type of play is called symbolic play.

Feelings

Feelings are different from thoughts. Help your children learn that your feelings are different from your actions. What you feel is *never* inappropriate, it is what you do that sometimes is. Feelings describe something going on inside. They are not good or bad, right or wrong, proper or improper, logical or illogical, they are just feelings. Feelings can usually be described in one word: happy, hurt, angry, hungry, sad, irritated, embarrassed, etc. Tell children how you feel and help them understand and put a word to how they feel: "I know you are angry that we have to leave the park, but you can't hit Mommy, it hurts me and makes me sad." Read books about feelings starting in early infancy.

Tantrums are often a way of expressing frustrations when children cannot say what they feel. We may have been dragging them all over town and they are overtired. Give them the tools to deal with frustration, such as teaching them sign language, so they can express what they are feeling before they are verbal.

Special time together

It is important to spend one-on-one time together each day, every day. Play something fun, do something spontaneous. Especially if you feel as though your day has been spent on corrections and redirections.

Use a sense of humor

Put your child's behavior into perspective. Recognizing their behavior as age appropriate helps you to see an otherwise annoying behavior as cute. Looking back, it is much easier for me to chuckle at some of my kids' behavior. It is much more difficult to find humor when you are in the throes of a tantrum.

Take small steps

Say to yourself, "I am not perfect, and I am going to make mistakes."

Parenting does not always come easy. It is certainly not easy all the time and every child is different. Your children are not going to be psychologically scarred for life because you choose the wrong discipline tool or approach for a particular behavior. Chalk it up to a lesson learned and you will know better what to try next time. Spouses need to parent together and talk about discipline before you need it. You need to create a united front as they grow. As the children get older, involve them as well. Dave and I had a consequence chart on the side of the fridge when the kids were older so we could be on the same page whenever possible.

Discipline for clear intent

Interrupt your child before someone is hurt or damage is done. For example, if you see a child raise a toy to hit a playmate, intervene before the playmate is injured.

Apply the consequence immediately

Delayed consequences are less effective because young children forget why they are being disciplined. Correction should occur immediately, if possible, and by the adult who witnessed the behavior: A child needs to say they are sorry or clean up a mess, etc. As kids get older it is important for both parents to be involved in large issues. One parent should not always be the disciplinarian.

Make a one-sentence comment about the rule during correction

Avoid making a long speech. Keep it very brief. "You are in the thinking chair because you hit your brother." "You are in a timeout because you threw sand after Mommy asked you not to." Yet keep in mind that it is important to explain the reason behind the rule when you give the warning: "Jack, don't throw sand, it can hurt someone's eyes." "If you throw it again you will have to sit in timeout." The younger they are the shorter the explanation: "Ouch, biting hurts."

Make timeout brief

Again remember, timeout should be one minute for each year of age. Children should be able to have the opportunity to repeat the action with the correct behavior shortly afterwards if possible.

Ignore your child's arguments during correction

Under three years of age, children mainly understand action rather than words.

Follow the consequence with love and trust

Welcome the child back. Do not comment on the previous misbehavior or require an apology for it. Now, Super Nanny says you should require an apology, and I actually think it is important that they are accountable to others' feelings, but make it short and do not dwell on it.

Direct the correction against the misbehavior, not the child

"It is never OK to hurt someone," rather than, "You are a bad girl."

Positive reinforcement for desired behavior

Dr. Barton Schmitt feels that "Behavior is predominantly shaped by consequences. Behavior that results in a pleasant reward or praise is more likely to be repeated." Positive reinforcement can be verbal or non-verbal with hugs and snuggles (time-ins). Watch for behavior you like and then praise your child. You can say things like, "I like the way you..." or "I appreciate..." or "I am proud of the way you..." Move close to the child, look at him or her, smile, and be physically affectionate. This does take time and energy. Yet a parent's affection and attention are your child's favorite reward.

Praise the behavior, not the person. Sharing toys, petting the dog gently, stroking your hair, giving kisses rather than biting, etc. Praise them for trying a difficult or undesired task, "That was so brave of you to..." Try to catch your child's good behavior and comment on it three times for every one time that you discipline or criticize.

Positive reinforcements are especially helpful when they are having a rough day. Just like us when we are having a trying day, someone can go out of their way to say something nice, and it can turn your day around. A hug from a loved one can make everything OK.

You can use material reinforcers which act as incentives. Examples are an extra book to read at bedtime if we can get through the bedtime routine quickly or a reward of a cookie *after* shopping. These are used as incentives for increasing the frequency of more responsible behavior.

Positive reinforcement

A reward is something kids can work towards and feel proud about. The younger the child, the sooner the reward should follow the behavior. Be careful not to overuse rewards or they may grow to expect one every time they cooperate. For example, if you play quietly while Mom takes this call, when I am off the phone, we will do a puzzle together.

Bribes are different from rewards. A bribe is a pay-off in advance and, because they are given before a child cooperates, a bribe is often doomed to backfire. An example of a bribe is, "I will read you one more story if you promise to go to sleep afterwards." Or giving the cookie at the beginning of the shopping trip and saying, "I will get you a cookie if you promise to sit quietly in the cart while we shop."

The power of positive reinforcement is great. For most kids, your undivided attention is the greatest reward of all.

Timeouts: the pros and cons

Pros to timeouts

Timeouts can be used to help a child gain control when redirection has not worked. Timeouts can be used to avoid injury. It can be a safe place to have a tantrum. It can create a safe place where your child can calm down. Creating a safe place is different than the traditional timeout where a child is forced to sit facing a wall or isolated. It should not be a punishment. Timeout is meant to remove your child from a dangerous or overwhelming situation and allow the child to gain self-control and calm down. As my friend Barb Grady says, "Discipline begins when both parent and child are calm." A timeout is effective in a family that has lots of positive attention and positive reinforcement.

Jane Nelson from Positive Discipline says, "Timeout can become an empowering experience for children instead of punitive and humiliating. Timeout is encouraging when it gives the child a chance to take a short break and then try again as soon as they are ready to change their behavior. Kids do better when they feel better. You do not motivate them by making them feel worse through punitive timeout."

Timeout is used to interrupt unacceptable behavior by removing the child from an area of trouble to a place that gives them peace. It provides a cooling-off period for both parent and child. For a child less than two years old, timeout is mainly a change in environment or a distraction. Dr. Barton Schmitt feels that there is nothing better than timeout for most of the irrational behavior of toddlers. He states that it is much more effective than shouting, threatening, or spanking. If it used appropriately, it could change <u>any</u> childhood behavior. He says timeout is your trump card. The American Academy of Pediatrics suggests using timeout as your last resort when other techniques have not worked.

Misbehavior that responds to timeout may be aggressive, harmful, or disruptive behavior that cannot be ignored. Timeouts are most effective when not overused, again pick one or two things, for example, biting and pushing. Timeouts are unnecessary for most temper tantrums and can be replaced with logical consequences by age six.

When you are holding a child that bites or pinches you, putting the child down is a form of timeout. A playpen or crib is a convenient place for timeouts. Playpens are good for infants and toddlers under 18 months because the child might be frightened if not in the same room as you. Or a child's chair with a few books in it as kids get a bit older. Taylor had a big, red, stuffed Elmo chair and Dylan sat on the stairs with a basket of books next to him.

Timeout should be short enough that the child has many chances to go back to the original situation and learn acceptable behavior: One minute for every year of age. A timer with colors and sound is great for young kids.

Give your child the opportunity to make things right, e.g., if your child made a mess during a tantrum, allow your child to help you clean up the mess they made or redirect them to another activity and give positive reinforcement when they do it. Notice something positive as soon as possible. If the behavior is repeated, you should start the whole process over again. Do not think of a timeout as a punishment, rather a way of helping your child stop what they are doing, calm down, and change the behavior.

Enforce immediately. If your child calms down before the end of the set time, let them up and congratulate them for regaining their composure: "I am glad you are feeling better now." Children under two are just learning how to handle frustrations and may not have the ability to remember why they are in timeout.

Cons to timeouts

Dr. Robert Mckenzie, author of *Setting Limits: How to Raise Responsible, Independent Children by Providing Clear Boundaries*, says, "timeouts can be a misused and abused form of discipline." He states, "too often it is applied with anger, which rather than teach, breeds resentment." "Parents may rely on it too much and expect too much from it."

Many experts believe that, until age two, little ones cannot understand a timeout. For children under two, the value of timeout comes in the first few seconds when they are insulted that you stopped their activity. Opponents argue that timeout sends a message that whenever you are upset or angry, you should be isolated. They also worry that you run the risk of turning a safe haven, e.g., a crib, into a place with negative associations.

One expert says she put her 21-month-old in a new timeout chair, trying to be calm and cool, and she said that it all dissolved and turned into an episode of the Keystone Cops. The child thought it was fun and learned nothing. She says not to get roped into a power struggle: it is better to be brief and successful than to get into a big battle.

Before the child is able to control impulses, it's best to try to distract, redirect, and ignore minor misdeeds and closely supervise to prevent.

(I don't disagree with trying these things first. I believe, like Dr. Barton Schmidt, to use your timeout as your trump card.)

Disagreements between parents

Co-parenting does not mean that parents have to think and act exactly alike with their children. There should be mutual respect in the relationship. Children have no trouble learning Dad does things one way and Mom does things another. This is not confusing to kids. However, you cannot let kids manipulate one parent against the other. Agree to disagree on some issues and appreciate each other's differences.

However, on big issues such as overall discipline techniques, e.g., as whether or not to spank, try to come up with a game plan. Both parents should be on the same page. Read books, attend parenting classes, and discuss each other's views and feelings on parenting and discipline styles. When possible, discuss issues before they come up to. If you disagree on how a situation was handled by your spouse, discuss this when your child is not around. Only step in if your child is in danger or the other parent is losing control.

The American Academy of Pediatrics says that telling your child how to behave is an important part of discipline but showing them how to behave is even more significant. Children learn a lot about temper and self-control from watching their parents and other adults interact. If they see adults relating in a positive way toward one another, they will learn that this is how others should be treated.

Spanking

"In the US approximately 33% of parents use spanking as a form of discipline. This has decreased from approximately 50% in 1993", says Serena Gordon, *HealthDay News,* July 27, 2020.

Reasons not to spank

Most child development experts are firmly opposed to spanking as a means of discipline. In 1998 the American Academy of Pediatrics took an official stance against spanking, stating that it has negative consequences and is no more effective than other approaches.

The research overwhelmingly shows that positive discipline techniques are the most effective, according to Irwin Hyman, author of *The Case Against Spanking: How to Discipline your Child Without Hitting*, says, "Spanking lowers self-esteem and teaches kids that the use of force is a way to solve problems. Spanking has been linked in studies to increased aggression in preschool and school-age children."

Dr. Barton Schmitt states, "We can raise children to be agreeable, disciplined, responsible, productive adults without ever spanking them. He says parents who turn to spanking as a last resort to break a child's will, may find they have underestimated the child's determination."

Spanking carries the risk of injury.

Physical punishment usually makes aggressive behavior worse.

It teaches a child to hit when he or she is angry.

Other forms of discipline are more constructive and leave a child with some guilt and the early formation of a conscience.

American Academy view on Spanking from the AAP

*The American Academy of pediatrics strongly opposes striking a child.

*It may work for the moment, but it is no more effective in changing behavior than a time-out.

*Spanking increases aggression and anger instead of teaching responsibility

*Parents may intend to stay calm yet often do not and regret it later.

*Because most parents do not want to spank, they are less likely to be consistent.

*Spanking makes other consequences less effective such as those used at school. And gradually spanking loses its impact.

*Children who are spanked are more likely to be depressed, use alcohol, have more anger, hit their own children approve of and hit their spouses and engage in crime and violence as adults.

*Spanking teaches a child that causing others pain is justified to control them even with those you love.

*If the spanking is spontaneous parents should later explain calmly why they did it, the specific behavior that provoked it and how angry they felt. They might apologize to their child for their loss of control because that usually helps the youngster understand and accept the spanking.

*They feel although spanking may relieve a parent's frustration for the moment and extinguish undesirable behavior for a brief time it is the least effective way to discipline.

*It is harmful emotionally to both parent and child. Not only can it result in harm but also it teaches children that violence is an acceptable way to discipline or express anger.

*While stopping the behavior temporarily it does not teach alternative behavior.

*It also interferes with the development of trust, a sense of security, and effective communication. (As spanking becomes the communication method.)

*It also may cause emotional pain and resentment.

If you do decide to spank however there are guidelines for safe physical punishment-

*Hit only with an open hand. Hitting your child with any instrument interferes with your ability to measure the amount of force you are applying. Paddles and belts often leave bruises often not intended,

*Hit only on the buttocks, hands, and legs. Hitting a child on the face is demeaning as well as dangerous.

*Give only one swat that is enough to change behavior. Hitting the child more than once is more to relieve your anger than to teach the child anything additional.

*Do not spank children less than one year of age. Spanking is inappropriate before your child has learned to walk. You should also cease spanking when a child reaches 5-6, this is when negotiation and discussion should be used.

* If you feel you must spank to make a young child behave, reserve it for situations where you want to have an immediate impact on

the child and show that the action is not only forbidden but also dangerous. An example would be spanking when a child runs into the street or turns on the stove.

*Do not use physical punishment more than once a day. The more the child is spanked the less effect it will have.

*Do not use physical punishment for aggressive misbehavior such as biting, hitting etc. Physical punishment under such circumstances teaches a child that it is all right for a bigger person to strike a smaller person. Aggressive children need to be taught restraint and self-control. They respond best to "time-outs" and an opportunity to think about the pain they caused another.

*Never shake a child because it can cause internal bleeding in the brain and blood clots in the brain.

*Do not allow babysitters or teachers to spank your child.

*Never spank a child when you are out of control, scared or have anything to drink.

I will share my personal struggle in my marriage over the spanking debate. Before we had kids, I took several discipline classes in order to give advice on discipline. My husband and I had quite a few discussions where we realized we had very different feelings about discipline. Most were minor, but the big one was he believed in spanking, and I did not. He agreed to try it my way "first" and try the positive discipline approach and use the thinking chair. Taylor was a very easy child in hindsight after having Dylan. My husband and I can both agree on this after the fact but at the age of 3 she went through a pretty typical stage of defiance. She was having some tantrums where during the tantrum she would roll on the floor and would kick the wall. This was so out of character for her that my husband said what we are doing with "time out" is not working. I think I want to try spanking. I was so shocked by this I wasn't sure what to do. It was against everything I believed but we had tried it my way first. So, in my infinite wisdom I said, "Well her 3 year well visit is coming up you can talk to the pediatrician. You can explain what is going on. If she agrees with spanking, then I will give it a try." In my head I thought, I am so smart she will never agree with this and then I will not be the one to say no. The following week when we were at the well visit our wonderful, trusted pediatrician asked, "How is disciplining going." My husband says funny you should ask this and goes into his story. What she said shocked me. I was speechless. She said, "Well I believe in trying positive discipline techniques first but if used correctly and in a loving manner a spanking can be effective. She said only spank with an open hand only swat the buttocks and give a warning prior." I do not think I said a word all the way home, I was in shock. Weeks went by and all was well. No toddler meltdowns. It was about a month later when we were in California at My husband's aunt's house (Grandma to the kids.) Her house is pristine white and perfect. She was overtired from being at Disney and had a full-blown meltdown. I moved her into the guest room to calm down and relax (her makeshift thinking spot or time out spot) when she started to kick the walls with her shoes on. Like I mentioned before, the new behavior she had recently started. I went to go to her, and my husband stopped me saying, "I've got this." My heart skipped a beat as I knew what was coming. I sat outside the closed door, and I heard him tell our daughter if you keep kicking Grandma's walls Daddy is going to have to spank you. Now Taylor had no idea what a spanking was so she kept kicking the walls as toddlers will test. The next thing I heard was my daughter screaming and then quiet. Then nothing for about 30 minutes. When my husband came out his eyes were red from crying and my daughter was asleep on the bed. He looked and me and said we are going back to time out. I asked what had happened and he said I cannot do that again she asked me, "Daddy why did you hit me." ☹

In hindsight I am glad we allowed him to figure out on his own that this was not the discipline technique for us. This was just a temporary stage and it soon passed with positive discipline techniques.

A self-control trick.

Anger is a right brain response.

If you do a left-brain response right away as soon as the feeling of anger starts it will slowly go away.

The quickest left-brain response is counting. Count to 10-100 whatever it takes.

There is scientific evidence that this works to calm you down. Give it a try.

"Too often we forget that discipline really means to teach, not to punish. A disciple is a student, not a recipient of behavioral consequences." Daniel J Siegel "Disciples choose to follow out of love and trust, not coercion and fear. Parental discipline must also be based in a relationship with so much love and trust that our children choose to learn from us, not from fear of punishment, but because our example is worth following." Dulce Chale

Some discipline resources See also Bibliography:

Positive Discipline series-Jane Nelsen

Active Parenting books-By Michael Popkin

Your Child's Health by Dr. Barton Schmitt

FINAL WORDS FROM THE AUTHOR

This first year is so special, and I feel honored that you chose this book to share some of these first experiences with me. I hope it met your expectations and you were able to gain valuable information and insight. I truly love teaching and although I wish I could have been in front of each of you in a classroom setting, I feel like this is the next best thing. I hope it allows parents all over, who would otherwise not be able to attend my classes, gain the value of a parenting class. I would love your feedback. If you liked the book, please leave a review on Amazon. Keep up the hard work, it is worth it. The time and energy you put in now will pay off when you have young adults that are ready to face any challenge this big world throws at them.

> *"You will never look back on life and think,*
> *'I spent too much time with my kids."*
>
> *— Unknown*

> *"It's not what you do for your children but what you have taught them to do for themselves that will make them successful human beings."*
>
> *— Ann Landers*

SPECIAL THANK YOU

I would like to thank the clinical experts who helped make this book happen and aided in assuring I had the most up to date advice as possible. The field of pediatrics is constantly changing. By the time this book gets to print there may already be changes. So, make sure you keep up to date on Healthy Children.org- https://www.healthychildren.org. This is the American Academy Pediatrics website which will always keep you up to date on the latest information in the field of pediatrics.

A special thank you goes out to Dr Jeffrey Siegel M.D., a board-certified pediatrician at North Scottsdale Pediatrics/ Arbor Medical Partners who spent countless hours away from his own family editing each chapter. This book would not be possible without your expertise and feedback. Thank you is not enough!

Dr. Ron Fischler M.D., a board-certified pediatrician, thank you for taking the time to review in detail the chapter on sleep and giving me an enormous amount of support and advice, on not only sleep but on the book in general and being my overall pediatric mentor and teacher over the years.

You have both been instrumental in my career and love of pediatrics. You have encouraged my love for teaching and triage over my 30 year career. You have both been friends and mentors and I am so grateful to have started my nursing career with you both.

Dr. David J. Reeder M.D., a board-certified physician in asthma, allergy and immunology, thank you for your advice on all thing's allergy and immunology and reviewing that material. You are one of the most selfless people I know. You give your time to your patients so willingly and you are always looking for ways to help others. Your patients are so lucky to have such a caring physician and I am personally blessed to have you as a physician and friend. Thank you for your time and advice.

Last but not least thank you Melissa Thomson, a certified infant massage therapist and fragile infant specialist, for reviewing the content on infant massage.

Finally, to my family, friends and past students, who encouraged and supported me to put my lectures and stories to print, without all of you, this book would not be complete!

INDEX

3-dimensional thinking
    386
5-gallon buckets
    369
5-point harness
    226
32-page booklet, free
    224
45-degree angle
    172, 225
70-degree day
    228
505-BABY
    223
1877lifebankusa
    47

A

AABR (Automated Auditory Brainstem Response);AABR (Automated Auditory Brainstem Response 32
AAP- American Academy of Pediatrics
    27
AAP-American Academy of Pediatrics
    196
AAP (American Academy of Pediatrics);AAP (American Academy of Pediatrics
    24, 27, 48, 86, 105, 134, 146, 162, 167, 189, 225, 332, 354, 360, 372, 379, 440, 525
AAP Committee
    105, 216
AAP- Estimated
    260
AAP Guide
    164
AAP policy statement
    49
AAP/Ross Laboratories
    276
AAP- Toys
    328
Abbey
    2, 388
abdomen
    80, 114, 117, 222
Abell, Ellen
    409
absolutely not
    393
Academy
    48
    g-screening/American
    33
Accidental poisoning
    197
accident history
    340
accidents
    55, 57, 60, 197, 206, 213, 227, 426
    auto
    226
Accreditation Criteria
    343
accuracy
    168, 287
Acetaminophen
    99, 114, 220, 237, 247, 267, 354, 360, 367
aching joints
    101
acid
    71
    tannic
    100, 360
Acne
    69
ACTH
    334
actions match
    428
Activated Charcoal

205
active ingredients
  262, 357, 361, 363
 main
  357
Active parent
  414
Active Parenting
  413, 446, 525
Active Parenting Publishers Inc
  525
activities
 age-appropriate
  340, 417
 daily
  189
 everyday
  184
 increased
  120
 little
  158
 long involved
  316
 new
  178, 279
 outdoor
  218
 physical
  119, 336, 409
 quiet
  416
activity gym
  173, 317
activity mat
  279, 323
activity playmats
  64
activity stations
  64
Adam
  389
Adaptability-How

282
Adolescence
  526
adolescents
  369
adult auto
  261
adult head size
  165
adulthood
  39, 288
adults
  41, 44, 71, 73, 141, 147, 233, 292, 295, 332, 337, 382, 440
 disciplined responsible productive
  441
 self-assured
  391
adult size
  200, 387
adult spider
  222
Advantages of breastfeeding-;Advantages of breastfeeding
  86
adventure, new
  281
advice
  2, 8, 17, 123, 133, 148, 196, 203, 244, 306, 422, 444, 448
 adopted
  2
 changed triage
  259
 expert
  2
 giving parents
  3
 medical
  1, 255
affection
  180
 parent's;parents

435
affiliation
377
affirmation
401
Affirming words
401
African American Babies
39
African Americans
34, 44
afterbirth
15
age
37, 140, 147, 159, 165, 172, 184, 224, 235, 247, 263, 280, 291, 297, 302, 312, 330, 343, 374
  appropriate
152
  child's;childs
295
  crises
287
  earlier
187
  early
290
  good
279
  older
88
age-appropriate explanations
423
age babies
151, 281
age children
348, 435
age colors start
168
age discipline techniques
415
age group
227, 321, 330, 348
age guidelines
330
age love
330
age love rhythm
330
age range
58
age restrictions
361
aggression
399, 442
  disciplining
419
  increased
441
  physical
414
Aggressive children
444
aggressive diaper changer
124
aggressiveness
405
aging
43
  premature
357
Agriculture
220
air
56, 70, 100, 102, 108, 217, 231, 245, 286, 315, 363, 378
  cold
233
  cold freezer
233
  cool
228
  fresh
122, 128, 206, 367
  stale
136
airborne

245, 248
air bubbles
53
air conditioning
221, 366
air ducts
218
air exposure
66, 73, 241
air filters
218
air fresheners
201
air-permeable mesh surface
139
air pollution
218
airway
54, 135, 198
  best
136
  wide-open
136
alarms
216
alcohol
67, 98, 171, 202
alcoholic beverages
202
alcohol poisoning
202
alert state
271
  wide-awake
271, 276
alignment
167, 264
allergens
126, 218, 250, 305
Allergens/Molds
218
allergic basis
106
allergic reactions
251, 254, 259, 299, 364
  severe
197, 251, 308
allergies
71, 87, 218, 261, 298, 306, 314, 358, 449
  dairy
302
  egg
305
  environmental
307
  lifelong
307
  nickel
253
  severe
305
  symptoms of
299, 303
allergists
72, 259, 308
  pediatric
71, 251, 308
allergy situations
259
Allison Arnold Life
408
aloe vera gel
360
Altaf Ul Qadri
52
Altman
525
Amaryllis
203
amazon
267, 356, 366, 447
American Academy
324, 442
American Academy of Audiology
33
American academy of pediatrics
28, 48, 86, 134, 189, 316, 317,

320, 332, 333, 354, 372, 379,
440, 525
American Academy of Pediatrics
formula
105
American Academy of Pediatrics
Guide
526
American Academy of Pediatrics
website
8
American Academy Pediatrics
448
americanbaby.com
349
American coffee
12
American College
10, 13
American Journal
129
Americans
44
American Sign Language
192
a monique moment
118
amount
102, 106, 112, 131, 256, 307, 311,
325, 332, 443, 448
  high
    11
  ideal
    266
  increased
    16
  large
    239
  lesser
    103
  minimal
    312
  pea-sized

266
reasonable
284
sized
265
small
13, 66, 75, 114, 216, 239, 266,
303, 380, 405
unique
333
anaphylaxis
254, 307
anesthesiologist
124
anger
277, 293, 350, 395, 397, 439, 442,
446
anger fear
295
animal bite
254
animal kingdom
16, 311
animated American Sign Language
dictionary
193
Anita Hurtig PhD
387
ankles
69, 71
annual maintenance fee
50
Anterior fontanel
37
antibacterial
262
antibacterial cleansers work
262
antibacterial products flooding
262
antibiotic drug
262
antibiotic eye

34
antibiotic ointment
    40, 255, 257, 367
  topical
    250
antibiotics
    18, 102, 219, 241, 245, 310, 354
  oral
    250
  oral prophylactic
    253
antibodies
    5, 81, 86, 104, 308
  producing excessive
    126
anticipation
    293
antihistamine
    250, 305, 365
antihistamine, children's;antihistamine, childrens
    299
Antihistamines block
    308
Antihistamine Zyrtec
    367
Anti-inflammatories
    354
Anti-inflammatory cream
    252
anxieties
    229, 291, 316
anyways, rare
    27
a peaceful place
    415
APGAR score
    23
apnea
    4, 136
apologize
    2, 442
apology
    435
apples
    14, 198, 302
  example Gala
    302
apple sauce
    240
applesauce
    300
  fiber includes-;fiber includes
    301
  rice
    239
Appliance latches
    208
appliances
    216, 342
  fuel burning
    217
  household
    208
application
    362
applications, multiple
    362
applied minutes
    72
appointments
    79, 251, 354
approaches, consistent
    413
Approach- Withdrawal-How
    282
approximate time
    203
apricots
    243, 301, 312
aqua doodle
    325, 417
Aquaphor
    65, 70, 242
ARA
    105
Arbor Medical Partners

448
arch
  26, 185
area
  anal
    70
  bad
    252
  burned
    257
  crowded
    122
  freshwater
    371
  irrigation
    221
  kitchen
    344
  main
    70
  perineal
    115
  remote
    204
  sleeping
    216
  small
    72, 242, 355
  sore
    267
  tender
    101, 364
  vaginal
    75
area bleeds
  256
areola
  93, 100
Arizona
  3, 29, 46, 72, 84, 87, 228, 257,
    359, 369, 376, 379
Arizona Black
  222
Arizona Newborn screening program
    29
Arizona Newborn screening program screens
  29
Arizona parenting
  351
Arizona passenger restraint law
  224
Arizona Scorpions
  219
Arizona State University
  3, 193
arms
  26, 77, 168, 171, 180, 278, 287,
    292, 321, 364, 372
arms fly
  26
arms, upper
  248
arm swings
  284
arrival, new
  126
article
  best
    16
  first
    304
articulation
  192
Asia
  29
Asia infants
  139
Asian patients
  44
Asians
  44
ASL interpreter
  193
Asparagus
  14
aspirin

457

206, 247
assertiveness
   405
assessments
   25
  baby's;babys
   38
  neonatal maturity
   25
asthma
   71, 126, 215, 261, 307, 337, 358, 449
Asthma/Allergist/Immunologist
   306
asthma attacks
   127
asthma, exacerbate
   218
attachment
   280, 288, 292, 350, 397
  emotional
   288
  strong
   178, 269, 292
attachment relationships
   383
attention
   167, 175, 186, 189, 272, 281, 283, 293, 394, 417, 424, 431, 435
  child's;childs
   418, 421
  decreased
   215
  medical
   77, 237
  physical
   397
  positive
   437
  teacher's;teachers
   406
  undivided
   333, 436
Audiology

33
auditory brainstem
   32
Australia
   29, 134, 139
authoritarian
   413
Authoritative Guide
   525
Author Unknown
   230, 369
Automated Auditory Brainstem Response (AABR);Automated Auditory Brainstem Response (AABR
   32
automatic stop mechanisms
   213
Aveeno
   247, 364
Avent
   22
Average hours of sleep-;Average hours of sleep
   140
average IQ
   382
average milestones
   169
average norms
   185
average size
   11
average time
   298
average weights
   166
aversion
   299
  gaze
   402
avobenzone
   357
avocados

14, 301, 304
awake
    103, 144, 150, 153, 172, 256, 271, 278, 318, 413
  half
    293
  jerk
    111
  wide
    271
awakenings
  brief
    141
  frequent
    143
  partial
    151
AZ
  219, 369
Azalea
  202

B

ba
  178, 186
babble
  173, 176, 186, 189
babble sounds
  183
babble/talk
  284
babbling
  174, 176, 186, 281, 315
  normal
    55
babies and toddlers
  226, 261, 348
Babies' chin;Babies chin
  93
babies cry
  41
  new
    146
babies drink
  370
babies grunt
  68
babies habituate
  145
babies hide
  282
babies love
  319, 329
Babies-R-Us
  55
babies slept
  273
babies slipping
  58
babies sneeze
  41
babies start
  156, 159
babies use
  193
babies use rolling
  179
babies wake
  141
Babo
  358
baby
  12, 16, 21, 29, 40, 52, 103, 120, 125, 133, 156, 225, 234, 261, 266, 297, 311, 353, 420
  active
    324
  blind
    293
  breast-fed
    67, 81, 86
  breastfed
    87, 94, 105, 143, 244
  colicky
    336
  convulsions

41
cousin's;cousins
   251, 289
crying
   275
easy-going
   278
female
   36
first
   2, 104, 387
full-term
   11, 69
fur
   126
healthy
   170
help
   80, 329
hypersensitive
   278
little
   120
mind
   272
month
   280
new
   121, 128
newborn
   92, 292, 317
older
   56, 158
premature
   84
saved
   229
screen
   29
second
   211, 289
sensitive
   278
spoil

188
sucking
   54
sweet
   378
teething
   267
term
   269
unborn
   215
wake
   90, 92, 142
young
   71, 140, 387
baby babbles
   189
Baby B'Air;Baby BAir
   366
baby bath
   67
baby bathtub
   58, 70
baby bathtub/foam bathmat
   65
baby bee
   359
baby blues
   127
baby books
   297
baby boys
   35, 389
baby breathe
   64
Baby Bug Magazine
   331
baby burn
   355
baby button, smallest
   59
baby chances
   325
baby colors

330
baby cries
    146, 152, 272, 277, 291, 319, 402
baby experience
    317
baby faces
    318
  board books
    330
baby food
    300
  preparing
    300
baby fussing
    38
baby gates
    58, 207, 416, 426
Baby gates-Baby gates
    58
baby-gazing
    77
baby girls
    35, 186, 358, 389
baby graze
    143
baby guzzles
    90
Baby Hotline
    223
baby inhale
    365
baby latch
    93
baby leans
    62
baby lotion
    69
baby naps
    121
baby outdoors
    122
baby paraphernalia
    366
baby pauses

109
baby powder
    201, 364
baby pull
    329
baby rolls
    140, 278, 318
baby rubbing
    71
baby's ability;babys ability
    32, 287
baby-safe feeder
    235
Baby Safe Feeder
    64, 267, 302
Baby's age;Babys age
    195
baby's arrival;babys arrival
    125
baby's birth;babys birth
    40, 50
baby scribble
    325
baby's cries;babys cries
    188
baby's ears move;babys ears move
    97
Baby's Emotions;Babys Emotions
    330
baby's equipment;babys equipment
    77
baby's habits;babys habits
    342
baby shampoo
    73
Baby's hands;Babys hands
    30, 173, 322
baby's head;babys head
    26, 32, 76, 180, 371
baby's heel;babys heel
    30
baby sign language
    191
baby sister

390
babysitter
 122, 290, 342, 347, 402, 444
baby sleep
 146, 526
baby smiles
 277, 319
baby's mouth;babys mouth
 96, 101, 109
baby socks- nothing
 22
baby sparks
 342
baby's preferences;babys preferences
 301
baby's ques;babys ques
 314
baby's skin;babys skin
 31
baby's sounds;babys sounds
 77
baby's stimulation threshold;babys
  stimulation threshold
 336
baby stations
 57
Baby's teeth;Babys teeth
 263
baby stools
 80
baby studies
 276
baby sunglasses
 354
baby's way;babys way
 267
baby swings
 59
baby syndrome
 82
baby teeth
 264, 267
  child's;childs

 264
healthy
 268
baby themself
 324
baby time
 138
baby tooth
 265
baby toothbrush
 264
baby touch
 319
baby upright
 82, 176, 322
baby ventures
 181
baby vomits
 238
baby wakes
 151, 158
Baby Walkers
 57
baby watch
 329
baby wear
 139
Bachelor
 3
backfire
 407, 436
backs
 37, 76, 135, 336, 410
backseat
 229, 367
backwards
 89, 410
backyard
 370, 379
bacteria
 11, 24, 107, 126, 234, 261, 306,
  310, 372
coliform

12
harmless
262
surface
310
bacterial conjunctivitis
244
bacteria plenty
262
Bactine
367
Bactroban
250
Badger
358
bag
 102, 241, 325, 416
 canvas tote
 326
 going out
 416
 multi-compartment
 46
 small
 102
baking soda
 70, 242, 254, 258, 364
balance
 57, 130, 306, 350, 351, 391, 407, 414
 fine
 157
Ballantine Books
 526
balloons
 199
 pink
 388
balls
 180, 187, 199, 286, 326, 328, 396, 406, 410
 cotton
 254, 364
 large

326
 red
 330
 Balls and small toys
 199
bananas
 171, 240, 300, 317
 chilled
 235
 frozen
 267
banana toothbrush
 267
 little
 264
Bandages
 367
bank
 45
 for-profit cord blood
 49
 least expensive
 46
 private cord blood
 50
 private family
 43
 public
 50
 public cord blood
 48
banking
 42, 47, 50
Bantam Books
 525
Bantam Books1998
 526
bar
 58, 60, 393
 expanding pressure
 58
barbeque grills
 222
Bard, Elizabeth

463

339
bark
   219
bark, decorative
   219
Bark scorpions
   219
barrel cactus
   258
barrier
   71, 242
barrier diaper rash cream
   69
Barr, Ronald
   272, 274
Barton
   525
Barton Schmitt M
   33
Barton Schmitt MD
   40
Barton Schmitt states
   441
Barton Schmitt Triage
   259
Barton Schmitt- Your Child's Health;Barton Schmitt- Your Childs Health
   164
basin
   63, 218
  clean removable
   63
basket
   213, 326, 438
bassinet
   61, 77, 82, 111, 126, 146
  infant's;infants
   385
bath
   58, 72, 115, 123, 248, 252, 275, 320, 365, 418
  calming
   290
  cool
   73, 258
  daily
   72
  luke-warm
   237
  oatmeal
   247
  shallow
   323
  sponge
   67
  warm
   119, 163, 242, 276
bathing
   67, 73, 188, 355, 364
Bath rings and bath seats-;Bath rings and bath seats
   58
bathroom
   57, 111, 115, 207, 218, 344
  darkened
   276
  steamy
   231, 233
bathroom scales
   211
bath routine
   430
bath seats
   58
bath time
   72, 252
bath toys
   325, 328
  multiple
   326
bathtub
   208, 246, 258, 326, 369
  clean
   116
bats

64, 173, 254, 322
batteries
    153, 202, 209, 211, 215, 293
  coin lithium
    210
battle
    393, 439
Beach Tips
    364
beads
    199
  little
    67
beans
    161, 243, 308, 312
  green
    301
  kidney
    312
Becoming Baby Wise
    164, 526
bed
    59, 111, 114, 136, 144, 150, 155,
    160, 178, 221, 231
bed clothes
    146
bed/crib
    418
bedding
    56
  baby's;babys
    210
bedroom
    151, 418
bed sheets
    221
bedtime
    82, 137, 147, 149, 155, 161, 256,
    277, 290, 320, 336, 436
bedtime, regular
    157
bedtime routine
    72, 157, 159, 291, 320, 430, 436
  basic

277
calm relaxing
    162
calm/soothing
    148
bedtime story
    157
bedtime wake
    256
beef
    12, 312
beeps
    78, 236
bees
    361, 364
Bee sting
    254, 364
behavior
    192, 194, 281, 286, 406, 409, 417,
    420, 423, 428, 431, 433, 442
  acceptable
    419, 438
  acceptable gender
    390
  age-appropriate
    420
  aggressive
    383, 441
  antisocial
    288
  baby's;babys
    272, 315
  changing
    442
  childhood
    437
  child's;childs
    433
  child's sex role;childs sex role
    390
  correct
    434
  disruptive

438
exploratory
280
good
413, 436
irrational
437
naughty
409, 423
new
180, 445
normal
406
peer's;peers
390
responsible
436
restricting
343
unacceptable
419, 424, 437
Behavioral Development
525
behavioral science
377
Behavior Problems
525
belief
151, 387
old
193
bellies
191, 421
little
4
belly button
113
belts
226, 228, 443
strong
62
Benadryl
251
benefits

1, 15, 84, 88, 313, 320, 334, 337, 355, 357, 409, 413
clear
205
medical
27
possible
16
Berlow, Camilla
384
berries
203
holly
214
Berry Brazelton Touchpoints
164
Berry M.D
525
Beth
389
bewitching hour
272, 275, 279
BF babies
94
Bibliogoraphy
446
Bibliography
525
bike
424
bilirubin
79
extra
80
yellow
79
bilirubin level
79
high
79
Biologic Differences
384
biologic terms

466

385
Biologist Julie Mennella Ph
13
biology
382
Biology Pre-med
3
birth
4, 20, 23, 30, 42, 117, 119, 167, 170, 225, 269, 311, 316, 382, 387
  child's;childs
197
  giving
120, 131, 350
Birth-4mo
415
birth anyways
75
birth babies
292
birth canal
24, 33, 36, 40
birth control
88
birthday
185, 235, 375, 387
birth length
167
birthmark, flat
39
birthmarks
40
birth process
35
birth trauma
34
birth weight
30, 67, 92, 95, 142, 166
birthweight, double
166
birth weight doubles
96
birth weight, low

26, 358
bit backwards
75
bit bow
38
Bite Blocker
363
bite breaks
219
bites
219, 222, 253, 256, 420, 438
  black widow
223
  initial
222
  stork
39
bite site
223
bit swollen
34
bit watery
299
black residue
218
black widow, male
222
Black Widow Spider
222
black widows, young
222
Black widow webs
222
bladder
36, 114, 117
blanket
21, 59, 61, 71, 74, 126, 137, 160, 280, 329, 347, 368
  bili
80
  soft
21
  warm

467

139
bleach
    218, 262
bleach cleanser
    262
bleeding
    24, 28, 66, 74, 99, 113, 117, 257
bleeding diaper rash
    70
bleeding nipples
    93
bleeds, longer
    24
blinds call
    212
blink
    41, 171, 206
blisters
    247, 249, 257
  cloudy
    247, 250
  open
    257
  small thick-walled water
    249
  thin-walled water
    247
blocked mucus glands
    35
blocks
    58, 122, 164, 328, 359, 396, 526
  large
    326
blood
    30, 34, 36, 42, 46, 67, 75, 79, 95, 100, 237, 240, 256
  baby's;babys
    30, 35, 81, 312
  banked
    45
  clotting
    24
  donating

47
  suspect
    95
blood cancer
    44
blood cells
    215
  dead red
    240
  red
    79, 81
blood clots
    444
blood disease
    44
blood disorders
    43, 49
blood group incompatibility
    81
blood poisoning
    223
blood pressure
    307
blood stream
    360
blood sugar
    204
  newborn's;newborns
    25
blood test
    80, 131
blood thinners
    204
blood types
    25, 81
bloody
    115
blotches
    39
  red
    38
Blue Lizard
    358
blues

168, 318
bluish
    68, 231
bluish-gray
    39
BM pattern babies, infrequent
    94
board
    366, 416
board-certified pediatrician
    448
boat docks
    378
body
    39, 79, 88, 93, 98, 100, 104, 248, 271, 310, 315, 336, 338, 354, 419
  large black shiny
    222
  little
    238, 336, 370, 429
  upper
    138, 173
  woman's;womans
    131
body hair
    37
body language
    174, 296
body mechanics
    57, 373
  appropriate
    57
body temp
    108
body temperature
    73, 157, 370, 372
body wash
    21
body weight
    131, 216
bombing stirs
    112
bond

125, 187, 320
  parent child
    329
bone fractures
    88
bone marrow
    42
bone marrow transplants
    43
bones
    76
  soft pliable
    76
bone strength
    88
bonus chapters
    380
boo
    159, 181, 283, 291, 316, 326
book Baby's feelings;book Babys feelings
    294
Book Hurray
    411
book Positive Discipline
    399
books
    6, 133, 162, 318, 320, 323, 329, 333, 378, 412, 416, 438, 440, 447
book sign
    193
book Touchpoints
    272, 280, 348
booster
    226, 246
booster seats
    226
  children use
    226
  harness-type
    226
  shoulder strap

226
border patrol
    85
borders
    70, 85, 101, 242
boredom
    279, 316
born deaf
    33
boss
    125, 352, 430
bottle bag
    63
bottle feeding
    40, 84
bottle nipples
    101
bottles
    25, 52, 88, 95, 104, 107, 143, 150,
    178, 265, 289, 293, 298, 303
  favorite
    52
  milk-based
    240
  new Avent
    52
  peri
    70, 74, 115, 241
  peri wash
    115
  regular
    53
  spray
    310, 364
  sterilize
    107
  wide-mouth
    53
bottle types
    52
bounce
    62, 183, 286, 324, 331, 338, 356
bouncy seat

64, 279, 317, 323
bowel habits
    282
bowel movements
    41, 68, 119, 241
  soft
    94
bowels
    111, 119, 377
bowl
    257
  warm
    99
boxes
    200, 328
  jabber
    184
  little
    200
  small shoe
    326
  supply
    344
boys
    27, 43, 65, 74, 166, 186, 212, 382,
    384, 388, 396
  boy a
    388
  circumcised
    28
  handsome
    388
  infancy
    385
  little
    258, 370, 373, 391, 395, 424
  old cliché
    397
  tumble
    395
boys cry
    397
BP medication

470

204
brace
    59
Brad Sachs PhD
    390
bradycardia
    4
brain
    15, 24, 32, 80, 83, 105, 329, 336, 386, 399, 444
  baby's;babys
    288, 316
  child's;childs
    332, 387
  developing
    216
  growing
    76
  healthy
    288
brain activity
    386
  intense
    386
brain aneurysm
    289
brain development
    272
  baby's;babys
    336
  better
    335
  early
    332
  healthy
    383
brain function
    386
Brains shape behavior and behavior
    399
brakes, working
    62
branches, low

213
brands
    53, 67, 99, 139, 207, 226, 241
  changing diaper
    69
  great
    65, 303
  popular
    358
  probiotic
    241
Brat Diet
    240
Brat diet bananas
    239
brave
    395, 435
Brazelton
    272, 277, 279, 288, 525
Brazelton, Berry
    2, 25, 195, 270, 276, 348, 411
Brazelton Neonatal Behavioral
    25
Brazelton's method;Brazeltons method
    275
breakdown
    94
  approximate pound-by-pound
    10
breast
    53, 87, 90, 96, 98, 110, 143, 148, 150, 297
  opposite
    91
  pump
    103
  strength
    239
Breast and Bottle Feeding
    84
breast cancer
    88, 358
breastfed children

87
Breastfed stools
94
breast feeding
41, 84, 88, 95, 110, 297, 312
breast-feeding
104
breastfeeding
3, 4, 13, 25, 84, 96, 98, 100, 104,
108, 137, 297
breastfeeding burns
88
breast feeding delays
88
Breast-Feeding Jaundice
81
breastfeeding medication
85
breastfeeding moms
11
breastfeeding mothers
106
breastfeeding nurse
151
breast infection
101
breast milk
13, 16, 85, 95, 102, 149, 151, 153,
156, 238, 297, 303, 311
breastmilk
14, 85, 98, 106, 156, 239, 297
 increasing
313
breast milk intake
299
breast milk jaundice
81
breast pads
171, 317
 mother's;mothers
171
breast pumps
53, 102
breasts soften
96
breasts softening
93
breast tissue
11
breathable mattresses
139
 new
139
breathe
4, 139, 171, 216, 233, 375
breathing
23, 41, 136, 231, 270
 diff
254
 difficulty
77, 237, 250, 307, 365
 irregular
141
 rescue
371
breathing co fumes
217
Brian
2
bribe
436
bridge
5, 39
Bristol England
104
Britax Regent
226
broccoli
14, 97, 243, 301
broken blood vessel, little
34
bronchiolitis
87
brother
53, 84, 424, 434
Browns
40, 52, 63
Brown's brand;Browns brand

82
bruises
40, 443
brush
184, 221, 310, 426
  rooting reflex
  93
brushing
266, 427
bubbles
376, 405
bubble wand
405
Buckets
356, 369
buckle
223, 228, 359, 430
buckles, hot
359
Buckman Robert M.D
526
buddy
394
  little sports
  392
budget
310, 351
BUDS
377
bug bites
68
  avoiding
  360
building blocks
42, 105
bulging
77, 237
bumper jumper- Hangs
64
bumpers
56, 138
bumps
38, 68, 364
  flesh-colored

365
  little white
  39
  pink
  72
  raised
  242
  small
  69
bunny
191, 396
Burke, Leo
133
burn candles
218
burn citronella
363
burning
210
  stops
  257
burns
108, 205, 208, 210, 228, 257, 354, 359
  acute blistering
  353
  blistered
  257
  degree
  257
  potential
  203
burp
77, 82, 91, 109, 227
burp cloths
64
Burping
109
burst
118
butter
305
  peanut

198, 305, 312
buttocks
    39, 70, 249, 443, 445
button batteries
    199, 210
  small
    202
buttons
    161, 199, 211
  dad's;dads
    428
bye
    183, 192, 285

C

cabinets
    207, 327
  locked
    208
  medicine
    207
cables
    210
  charging
    210
Cactus/Foreign body
    258
Cactus spines
    258
Caesar dressings
    12, 306
caffeine
    12, 98
caffeine intake
    12
cake
    289, 327
Caladium
    202
Calamine
    247
calculators
    211
California
    48, 445
California State University
    406
call maintenance
    118
call Newborn
    7
Call poison control
    203, 220
call satellite spots
    242
calories
    81, 88, 155, 156, 311
  daily
    311
Canada
    84, 136
cancers
    27, 42, 47
  cervical
    28
  common childhood
    44
  common form of
    353
  ovarian
    87
candies, hard
    22, 198, 305
candles
    218
  burned
    218
  flameless
    211
canines
    263
cans, open
    208
cantaloupe
    301
capabilities

407
capacity
    307
    intellectual
        382
Caput
    36
carbohydrates
    106, 311
    primary
        106
Carbon monoxide
    216
carbon monoxide detectors
    215
carbon monoxide poisoning
    216
Cardboard books
    328
cardiac arrest
    197
cardiologist
    4
care
    78, 84, 120, 125, 128, 292, 294, 350, 351, 355, 409
    consistent
        404
    early
        383
    good
        268
    limited neonatal
        335
    little extra
        23
    medical
        262
    special vaginal
        115
    taking
        121
career

3, 448
    long
        3
care giver, regular
    286
caregivers
    343, 399
    changing
        288
    child's;childs
        296
    primary
        398
    secondary
        138
Care of bottles-;Care of bottles
    107
care provider
    345
care seat
    224
caring
    83, 125, 337, 351, 392, 396, 398, 525
Caring Kids
    295
caring, nurturing
    391
caring physician
    449
Carolyn Rovee-Collier PhD
    193
carrier
    61
    front infant
        146
    style front
        61
carriers/Front carriers
    61
carrot juice
    13
    pregnant women

13
carrots
   240, 300, 305
  cooked
   243
  raw
   198
cars
   216, 224, 228, 328, 386, 396
  passenger
   224
cart
   213, 428, 436
cart flips
   213
cases poison control
   203
cataracts
   354, 357
cat dander
   261
categorizing
   387
cat jumping
   127
cats
   126, 209
Caucasian babies
   34
Caucasian patients
   45
Caucasians
   39, 44
causality
   280, 283
cause cancer
   354
cause cavities
   151
cause cord blood
   50
cause damage
   80, 236
cause dehydration
   354
cause disease
   261
cause eyes
   372
cause GI
   214
cause infection
   114
Cause of allergies-;Cause of allergies
   308
cause pneumonia
   205
cause restlessness
   161
cause scrapes
   40
cause sedation
   98
cause skin irritation
   258
cause skin thinning
   72, 252
cause suffocation
   198
cause symptoms
   131
cause tipping
   62
Caustic chemicals
   205
cavities
   265, 268
cc
   306
CCHD (Critical congenital heart disease);CCHD (Critical congenital heart disease
   31
ceilings
   213, 219
celebrate
   6, 68, 110
  gender stereotype

394
Celebration Stem Cell Center
  46
Cell level gender differences
  386
Cell phone Charging cables
  210
cells
  47, 50, 385
  banked
    45
  denser
    186
  immune
    261
  white
    42
cells help answer
  385
Central America
  29
cephalohematoma
  37
cereals
  13, 119, 181, 239, 297, 367
  enriched
    312
  iron-rich
    299
  rice
    299
certification
  347
  complete re-;complete re
    377
Certified infant massage therapist
  449
Cesarean
  116
cesarean birth
  114
Cetaphil
  72
CETIRIZINE DOSING

260
chain links
  416
chair
  9, 60, 163, 322, 416, 419, 439
  child's;childs
    438
  folding
    60
chair backward
  214
Chalk
  433
change
  7, 34, 71, 74, 76, 97, 111, 115,
    125, 131, 159, 243, 250, 417,
    437
  fast
    131
  positive
    398
  routine
    229
change air filters
  218
change behavior
  443
change culture
  395
change diapers
  144
change misbehavior
  417
change sleep habits
  153
Chapter, important
  133
characteristics
  emotional
    387
  neuromuscular
    25
Charcoal

477

206
charcoal grills
    216
charge
    47, 366
  taking
    123
charred skin, white
    257
cheeks
    39, 71, 96, 101, 249, 322
  baby's;babys
    26, 96
  little chubby baby chipmunk
    200
cheese
    12, 204, 243
  cottage
    68, 302
  imported
    12
chemical changes
    131
Chemical ice pack
    368
chemicals
    56, 67, 308, 358, 373
  absorbing
    361
  toxic
    56
Cherry tree
    202
Cheryl M.A
    525
chest
    24, 79, 139, 171, 231, 335, 365
chest, mother's;chest, mothers
    292
chest palpitations
    130
chew
    198, 235, 256, 264, 331
chickenpox

247
chicken pox vaccine
    246
child
    126, 150, 162, 183, 197, 226, 243,
    250, 264, 293, 303, 311, 329,
    345, 351, 360, 365, 390, 399,
    415
  10-pound
    227
  active
    60
  aggressive
    405
  assertive
    405
  easy
    444
  final
    4
  first
    20, 155
  growing
    399
  independent
    403
  offended
    392
  older
    162, 370
  outgoing
    390
  parent
    376
  pushy
    406
  self-sufficient
    404
  young
    198, 305, 443, 525
childbirth
    84, 124, 131
child breaks

265
child breathe
233
child calms
439
childcare
3, 368
childcare centers
349
childcare provider
229
childcare setting
348
child cries
150, 293
child development
343, 390
child development specialist
409
child discomfort
236
child gain control
437
child harness/backpack
367
child health
104, 135
childhood
83, 86, 126, 133, 230, 245, 288, 315
childhood asthma
14
childhood diseases
198
childhood rite
230
child ingests
204, 206
child locks
207
child magazine
82
child- manual guidance

418
child panics
156
childproof
207, 415
child proofing
317
Childproofing
207
childproofing ways
207
child relax
337
children
57, 196, 215, 224, 230, 245, 294, 302, 329, 340, 347, 353, 359, 372, 397, 407, 412, 423, 428, 439
  allergic
    308
  encouraging
    398
  female
    389
  helping
    390
  independent
    439
  non-allergic
    307
  older
    308, 369
  painful
    249
  small
    234
  spank
    443
  spoiled
    412
  young
    191, 206, 215, 220, 233, 258, 307, 312, 330, 332, 378, 406, 414,

426, 434
younger
  332, 430
children ages
  307, 369, 375
children drown
  369
children hurt
  212
children love
  210
Children of moms
  155
children opportunities
  428
children pass
  249
children's art work;childrens art work
  386
children's artwork;childrens artwork
  344
Children's Chewables;Childrens Chewables
  259
children self-control
  431
Children's Hospital;Childrens Hospital
  83
children smile
  382
children sound
  345
children sprout
  263
Children's Sleep Evaluation Center in Pittsburgh;Childrens Sleep Evaluation Center in Pittsburgh
  155
children teach
  129
children wiggle

60
child restraint laws
  224
child restraints
  224
child ride
  213
child safety
  212
Child safety seats
  224
  installed
  226
child's appearance;childs appearance
  237
child's arguments;childs arguments
  435
child scribbles
  427
child's crib;childs crib
  137
  older
  161
child's day;childs day
  344
child's doctor;childs doctor
  230, 356
Child's Emotional and Behavioral Development;Childs Emotional and Behavioral Development
  525
child's explorations;childs explorations
  416
child's feet;childs feet
  62
child's head;childs head
  225
Child's Health;Childs Health
  33, 80, 134, 261, 306, 446, 525
child's interpretation;childs interpretation
  424
child's IQ;childs IQ

330, 383
child size
   200
child's jawbone;childs jawbone
   135
child's mouth;childs mouth
   203
child's outcome;childs outcome
   350
child spits
   136
child's self-confidence;childs self-confidence
   406
Child's Self Esteem;Childs Self Esteem
   411
Child's Sleep;Childs Sleep
   164, 526
Child's Sleep Problems;Childs Sleep Problems
   526
child's symptoms change;childs symptoms change
   256
child studies
   287
child's understanding;childs understanding
   329
child surviving
   226
child throwing
   428
child/toddler
   407
chill
   103
chin
   26, 39, 41, 71, 172
China
   106
chlorine

372
choices
   16, 49, 62, 72, 84, 348, 396, 403, 408, 418, 425, 429
   child's;childs
      407
   limited
      426
   personal
      27
choking
   200, 298
   fraternity party
      200
   mild
      109
choking hazard
   209, 236, 267, 298, 302, 317, 322
   common
      199
Choking/respiratory arrest
   197
choline
   14
chores
   120, 123
   household
      121, 397
Christmas Cactus
   214
Chronic sun exposure
   353
Chron's disease;Chrons disease
   87
chubby
   61, 365
chubby bunny
   198
chubby gum massager
   267
chuckle
   174, 433
chunky board books

481

331
churches
  390, 416
Churchill, Jill
  19
cigarette smoking
  137
circuit breaker
  342
circulation
  79
circumcise
  18, 27, 65
circumcision
  27, 36
circumference
  165
citronella
  361, 362
citronella candles
  363
citrus
  249, 300, 305
clap
  315, 331
classes
  2, 6, 9, 15, 118, 136, 206, 211, 293, 332, 374, 380, 410, 421, 447
  childcare
    346
  grade
    193
  infant swim
    375
  in-person
    84
  little gym
    396
  preschool swim
    374
  recs
    410
  swimming

374
classroom
  295, 406
  daughter's;daughters
    200
  old kindergarten
    194
classroom setting
  447
classroom success
  295
class year
  388
cleanliness
  344
climber
  209, 219
clinical outcomes
  48
clinical psychologist
  407
clips
  62, 199
  harness
    225
clock
  150, 196
  biological
    157
  little internal
    149
Clogged milk duct
  99
clogged nothing
  76
closed space
  156
closet 210
cloth 427
  caffeinated cold tea-soaked
    360
  soft baby wash
    76
  warm moist

99
wet
75
cloth diapers
64, 69
clothes
23, 122, 137, 210, 211, 355, 361,
366, 392, 397, 416, 429
baby's;babys
56
bright
360
layer
366
new
253
outfits-;outfits
22
pre-pregnancy
111
clothing
54, 66, 161, 206, 221, 359
children's;childrens
211
child's;childs
367
tight-fitting
82
Clothing/How
73
clots
114
small
114
clouds rainbows
323
clusters
39, 363
cochlea
31
codes
121, 342
lock key

342
cognitive advantages
191
cognitive process causality
329
cognitive science
187
Cohen
526
Coins
199
cola
12, 24
Colace
119
Cold cabbage
99
cold call
257
cold compresses
257, 364
cold drinks
249
cold meds
232
cold Popsicle
256
colds
230, 234, 346
minor
231
Colds/flus
87
cold water
102, 216, 257, 378
coli
305, 371
colic
52, 107, 274
colic, inconsolable fussy period
274
colic symptoms
53
collapsible tunnel

396
collection kit
   49
college
   4, 129, 200, 221, 282
color change
   40
colored bulbs, bright
   213
colors
   23, 34, 37, 61, 79, 94, 219, 222,
   230, 239, 301, 321, 327, 385,
   438
  blue
    233
  bold
    169
  bright
    360, 367
  bright primary
    168
  crayon
    386
  crayons vibrant
    386
  darker
    240
  eye process
    385
  grey
    231
  pink
    244
  purple
    70
  yellow
    79
  yellowish
    79
colossal change
   125
colostrum
   93
  thick yellowish

98
Columbus
   167
combat turnover
   345
comfort
   90, 145, 151, 156, 159, 188, 281,
   284, 288, 290, 293, 319, 324,
   397
comforting
   125, 159, 281
comfort level
   374
comfort measures
   233, 274
Comfort objects
   55, 160
commercials
   390
common cause
   38
common household poisons
   201
Common Illnesses
   525
common place
   257
common sleep problems parents
   163
common variable
   5
communication
   185, 191, 271, 315, 336
  average rate of
    186
  baby's brain-body;babys brain-body
    336
  effective
    443
communication disorders
   315
communication method
   443
communication milestones

189
communication newborns
146
communication skills
384
community birth ingest
16
companies
3, 17, 46, 207, 359
  alarm
342
  great
112
  reputable
17
compartment
209
compassion
293, 397
competence
337, 407
competitive dancer
410
complicated designs
168
complicated events
162
component
428
  main
155
compounding pharmacies
70, 242
comprehension
184, 191
  child's;childs
184
compress, cool
360
compulsively
112
computer
32, 328, 349, 432
computer keyboard

432
Concentrated
107
concentrations
56, 259, 362
  low
361
  lowest
361
concentrations irritate skin
372
concept
283, 327, 404
conditions
28, 42, 72, 82, 131, 238, 247
  allergic atopic
307
  atopic allergic
307
  common skin
71
  genetic
5
  medical
4, 109, 136, 274, 313
  odd-looking skin
38
cone-shaped head
36
cones, sensitive
385
confidence
83, 123, 272, 295, 337, 396, 397, 401, 407, 425
  child's;childs
409
confirmation
18
conflict
397, 428
confusion
217, 247
congratulate

439
Conjunctivitis
    244
cons
    27, 355, 437, 439
consciousness
    217, 247, 255
  stages of
    270, 273
consequence chart
    433
consequences
    227, 406, 426, 434, 442
  appropriate
    428
  behavioral
    446
  logical
    419, 427, 438
  natural
    426
  negative
    441
consistency
    94, 153, 299, 428, 430
Consistent rules
    404
consonants
    186, 189
consonant sounds
    187, 190
consonant vowel combination
    178
constipating
    243, 299
constipation
    14, 119, 243, 335
constriction
    233
constructive ways
    397
consumer product safety commission
    146, 212, 375
consumption

11
human
    16
contact
    11, 76, 78, 102, 156, 206, 231, 234, 248, 253, 308, 356, 363
  close
    155
  direct skin-to-skin
    88
  middle-of-the-night
    151
  peer
    295
  physical
    284
  positive
    269, 423
  rapid respiratory rate
    231
  short
    152
  social
    351
  warm personal
    272
contact case
    21
contact dermatitis
    252, 258
containers
    102, 242, 325
  unbreakable
    328
contaminate
    215
contamination
    12
contentment
    292
context
    188, 390
contractions

113
painful afterbirth
113
uterine
99
contrasting colors
320
bold
330
strong
318
contributor
261
important
401
control
118, 127, 222, 226, 298, 304, 425, 431, 442, 444
better
168
child regain
419
disease
129
help regain
117
losing
128, 440
normal bladder
117
pest
222
poison
203, 222, 342
control group
335
control impulses
439
controlled setting
308
controversy
386
convalescence
16
conversation
86, 191, 285, 397, 409, 417
convulsions
41, 306
cooing
172, 272
baby's;babys
188
cook
16, 120, 122, 310, 395, 397
safety tip-;safety tip
305
cookie
403, 428, 436
cookie dough
306
cool TM
359
cooperation
414
actions stimulate
315
Cooperative Extensions
220
coordination
57, 173, 396, 409
developing hand eye
175, 321
increased hand eye
176
large muscle
396
muscular
336
practice hand eye
321
coos
187, 276
Copycat grief
293
cord
24, 46, 66
spinal

487

15
umbilical
 42, 66
cord blood
 25, 42
 baby's umbilical;babys umbilical
 25
 bank Dylan's;bank Dylans
 45
 child's;childs
 47, 50
 donating
 42, 49
 infant's;infants
 42
 son's;sons
 46
 storage of
 47
 umbilical
 48
cord blood banking
 42, 45, 48
 private
 49
 public
 48
cord blood collection
 25
cord blood donations
 50
Cord blood harvesting and storage
 45
cord blood kit
 22
cord blood registry
 46
cord blood transplants
 48
cord care
 66
cord clamp
 24
cord foundation

48
cords
 blind
 56, 161
 dangerous
 209
cord stump
 24
 umbilical
 66
core strength
 318
corner drug
 251
corner posts
 56
corners
 93, 96, 210, 222, 240, 283, 322,
 329, 416
 rounded
 331
cornerstone
 412
corn sweeteners
 106
correction
 433
Cosmetics-Nail polish
 201
Cotton pads
 368
cotton, thin
 74
couch
 179, 322, 324
cough
 77, 230, 232
 croupy
 232
 fake
 280
 over-the-counter
 232
cough sounds

232
Coumadin
    204
counter Lotromin
    70
countertops
    62, 262
country
    2, 106, 226, 261, 365
country faces
    261
couple
    2, 22, 25, 54, 71, 120, 131, 155, 241, 293, 366, 393, 424
couple, first
    69, 113
couple reminders
    430
couple times
    352
cousin
    251, 289, 373
Covid tests
    18
coworkers Brian
    1
cows
    106, 310
cow's milk;cows milk
    105, 312
cow's milk formulas;cows milk formulas
    105
coxsackie
    249
CPR
    197, 340, 345
CPR classes
    136, 197
  infant-toddler
    197
CPR, pediatric
    346
crackers
    240, 305
thin
    198
cradle
    61, 147
Cradle Cap
    73
cradle fidgeting
    145, 271
cramped quarters
    38
crawl
    182, 210, 221, 255, 292, 344, 370
crawling
    57, 176, 179, 182, 215, 221, 255, 325
  started
    209
crawl upstairs
    182
crayons, broken
    199
crazy
    9, 45, 94, 200, 217
crazy childproofing
    207
cream
    69, 91, 100, 116, 242, 250
  antibiotic
    250, 253
  antifungal
    70, 242
  anti itch
    364
  antiitch
    247
  free
    252
  topical anesthetic
    29
creative ways
    182, 390
credibility, lost

428
credit card
    221, 254, 364
Creeps
    182
crib
    55, 59, 76, 82, 138, 145, 151, 156, 160, 194, 199, 209, 320, 323, 438
  baby's;babys
    149
  down
    55
  portable
    59
  standard
    139
crib accessories
    56
crib mattress
    56
  organic
    56
crib mobiles
    56
crib regulations
    55
crib sheets
    111
crib side
    55
crib tent
    127, 209, 221
crib wedge
    82
Criticizing
    409
croup
    232
croup symptoms, mild
    233
crowd
    214
crowded place

214
crowded spaces
    214
cry
    77, 154, 171, 174, 273, 280, 284, 286, 289, 292, 300, 320, 397
  basic
    277
  distinct
    277
  painful
    234
crying
    41, 130, 134, 145, 149, 151, 156, 158, 171, 174, 271
crying it out
    289
crying newborn
    111
crying period
    288
crying state
    271
Cryobanks International
    47
Cryocell
    46
Cryocell.com
    43
crystals
    67, 372
  urate
    67
C-section
    4, 113, 116
cuddle
    145, 180, 189, 257, 286, 291, 326
cuddle time
  extra
    155
  great
    288
cuddling

490

146, 155, 274, 397
cues
 121, 296
 baby's;babys
 153
 nonverbal
 337
cues/demands
 278
cultural studies
 337
Culturelle
 241
cultures
 290, 351, 385, 388
 competitive
 408
 rapid strep
 18
cup
 12, 15, 103, 184, 187, 242, 303,
  310, 327
 sippy
 151, 234, 266, 297, 303, 331, 366
 stackable measuring
 327
 suction
 58
 trainer
 179
 two-handled
 179
cup vinegar
 310
cup water
 310
curl
 26, 292, 331
curling irons
 208, 257
curves
 38, 319
cushions
 116, 208
donut
 120
customer service
 200
Cuts
 255
CVID
 5
 immune deficiency
 5
cycle
 115, 273
 normal sleep
 144
Cyrocell.com
 43
Cystic Fibrosis
 30
cysts, little
 35

D

dada
 182, 187, 190
dadda
 184
daddy
 187, 191, 214, 420, 425, 429
daddy, kicking Grandma's walls;daddy, kicking Grandmas walls
 445
daddy why did you hit me
 446
dad praise
 407
dads
 3, 123, 125, 144, 148, 188, 193,
  280, 283, 286, 393, 398, 430,
  432
 early 1990's;early 1990s
 124
 frazzled

429
　stay-at-home
　　352
　weekdays
　　124
dads benefit
　337
Dad's role;Dads role
　123
Dahl, Robert
　155
daily allowance
　266
dairy
　71, 97, 240, 243
damage
　24, 205, 434
　cause brain
　　236
　cell
　　358
　root
　　265
damage plastics
　362
damp
　144, 252, 360
danger
　57, 146, 207, 214, 262, 369, 407,
　　417, 421, 440
danger/Mouths
　424
Dangle
　318
Daniel J Siegel
　446
dark
　114, 221
dark greenish
　94
dark iris
　34
dark place, cool

219
darling, little
　429
Darrow, David
　235
Dartmouth Medical School review
　54
date
　9, 22, 102, 122, 128, 255, 295,
　　345, 365, 448
　due
　　9
　expiration
　　358
date advice
　448
Dateline
　376
daughter
　45, 53, 85, 154, 200, 206, 376,
　　389, 392, 395, 398, 445
daughter screaming
　445
Dave
　351, 433
David
　525
David L Katz
　129
David Reeder M
　306
day
　38, 68, 75, 83, 90, 103, 120, 142,
　　149, 157, 161, 191, 252, 270,
　　277, 299, 333, 382, 407, 421
day care
　350
daycare
　232, 249, 261, 347, 390
daycare costs
　351
daycare-preschool
　343
daycare/preschool, new

492

403
daycare, private in-home
  340
Daycare Provider
  339
daycare setting
  232, 348
day.Children
  382
day Fussy time
  272
daylight
  79, 291
daylight aids
  80
day mom
  123, 127
daytime feedings, frequent
  143
day work
  90
d-blood-banks
  48
Dean's list;Deans list
  4
deaths
  24, 60, 112, 135, 198, 211, 217,
    224, 227, 369
  crash-related
    226
  reducing
    224
  reducing toddler
    224
Debasish Mridha
  263
decaf
  100, 360
Decayed baby teeth
  265
Decedron
  233
decision
  17, 27, 42, 45, 130, 341, 349, 374,
    396, 403, 408
  mother's;mothers
    350
decoration
  421
DEET
  361
DEET picaridin
  362
DEET repels
  362
Defects
  31
Defrosted milk
  103
degrees
  78, 103, 112, 174, 208, 231, 237,
    249, 257, 345, 360, 372
  baccalaureate
    343
  science
    3
  degree wash area
    257
dehydration
  92, 142, 238, 240, 249
Delaware
  295
delay
  149, 192
delay, baby walkers
  57
Delayed consequences
  434
delay feeding
  149
delay speech
  192
delight
  314
delivery
  15, 20, 27, 30, 34, 37, 49, 99, 112,
    123, 127, 130
  baby's;babys

49
regular
  117
vaginal
  119
delivery process
  37
Democracy
  414
Democratic Parenting
  414
Democratic style
  414
Dental
  263
dental habits, good
  267
Dental lecture
  298
dentists
  265
  pediatric
    265
dentist's preference;dentists preference
  22
Denver Developmental Screening
  317
Department
  9
depression
  129, 200, 399
  perinatal
    130
  peripartum
    131
  postpartum
    16, 129, 131, 337
  woman's;womans
    131
Dept
  220
dermatologist
  357
  pediatric
    72
Desired Behavior
  435
detector
  218
  broken
    217
detergent
  252
detergent, new
  69, 253
detergent packets
  201
determinant, main
  269
Developing language
  328
development
  165, 169, 280, 283, 287, 312, 315, 321, 332, 335, 345
  abnormal testes
    358
  child's;childs
    274
  cognitive
    387
  emotional
    269, 280, 296
  healthy
    185, 287, 525
  human
    135
  large muscle
    396
  mature neurological
    335
  moral
    412
  physical
    280
  social

293
developmental abilities
    374
developmental achievement
    279
developmental challenges
    162
developmental pediatrician
    274
  world-renowned
    25
Developmental psychologist Tiffany Field
    335
developmental stage
    272, 275
  normal
    272
devices
    58, 60, 137, 200, 359
  child passenger restraint
    224
  floatation
    373
  flotation
    373
  recording
    22
DHA
    14, 105
diabetes
    261, 337
  insulin-dependent
    87
Diagnosis of RSV
    234
diaper bag
    63, 199, 366
diaper call
    74
diaper change
    69, 74, 242
diaper rash
    69, 101, 144, 241
  bad
    70
  regular
    241
diaper rash cream
    64
diaper rash treatment
    70, 242
diapers
    21, 36, 63, 74, 82, 95, 121, 125, 144, 242, 346, 366
  disposable
    67
  messy
    75
  regular
    241
  stooled
    96
diarrhea
    87, 107, 235, 238, 306
diary
    252, 307
Dieffenbachia
    202
diet
    14, 18, 30, 71, 89, 97, 243, 312, 377
  child's;childs
    252
  healthy balanced
    97
  mother's;mothers
    14, 98
diet change
    72
Dietz, Patricia
    129
differences
    49, 144, 169, 242, 282, 357, 367, 385, 405, 440
differences girls

384
differences, physical
385
difficulty digesting
106
difficulty swallowing
220, 307
Diffuser-Candles
21
digestible proteins whey
86
digestion
86
digestive system
107, 278, 335
  immature
  40, 68, 82
digestive tract
68, 240
dignity
414
  maintaining
  425
Diller, Phyllis
128
dining room
416
  formal
  207
dinner
373, 393
Diphenhydramine
259, 299
dips
101, 364
direction
26, 138, 173, 177
  front-to-back
  115
  normal
  38
director
390
  clinical

83
Disadvantages of breastfeeding
89
Disagreements
440
discharge
30, 35, 75, 114, 230, 244, 253
  green
  66
  vaginal
  114
  white
  35, 75
discharge timing
30
disciple
446
disciplinarian
434
disciplinary approach
413
discipline
3, 340, 346, 410, 414, 419, 423,
  428, 433, 436, 439, 446
discipline classes
444
discipline extremes
413
Discipline for clear intent-;Discipline
  for clear intent
434
discipline lecture
59
discipline measures
415
discipline, positive
411, 414, 437, 446, 525
discipline resources
446
discipline styles
440
discipline techniques
346, 413, 425, 440, 446
  effective

419
positive
441, 445
discipline tool
433
discoloration
67, 72, 252, 265
discomfort
114
 relieve hemorrhoid
120
disease ridden
363
diseases
30, 39, 43, 47, 48, 86, 248
 communicable
371
 critical congenital heart
31
 developing heart
312
 fatal
48
 fifth's;fifths
248
 host
43
 immune
261
 life-threatening
42
 transmit Lyme's;transmit Lymes
363
 transmitted
27
dishes
370
 heavy
214
dishwasher
53, 102, 108, 208
dishwasher detergent/pods
201
disinfectant

262
disks
198, 306
dislikes
292, 300, 342
dislocation
38
 hip
38
Disney
214, 445
disorders
30, 47
 amino acid
30
 endocrine
30
 fatty acid oxidation
30
 immune
42
 lysosomal storage
30
 metabolic
30, 49
 neuromuscular
30
 organic acid
30
disorientation
217
display
386
 early
293
displeasures
182, 189, 284
disposition
352
disruption
144
 hormone
358
distance

497

    84, 167, 173
distance vision
    169
distract
    296, 415, 439
Distractibility
    282
distraction
    274, 437
divert
    416
doctors
    8, 17, 29, 66, 68, 79, 114, 119, 128, 137, 231, 240, 245, 298, 308
dogs
    126, 219
  hot
    198, 305
  prairie
    254
Dogs/Animals
    126
dolls
    328, 389, 393, 397, 432
  life-sized
    126
  rag
    180
Domonic Barone
    351
donation
    42, 45, 47, 50
Donation Gilbert Az
    47
donation, organ
    47
donor
    43
donor family
    49
donor, matching
    44
donor samples

    48
DON'T;DONT
    73
doors
    206, 221
  appliance
    208
  heavy
    209
doorstops, hinged
    209
doorway
    58, 323
dose
    24, 85, 251
doses, small
    217
Doterra oils
    363
Doterra Terrashield
    363
downstairs
    208
  fallen
    58
  upstairs
    123
drainage
    244
  green
    234
drawers
    207
  use oven
    208
drawstrings
    211
dream feed
    150
dreams, lovely
    111
dress
    73, 122, 354, 360, 367, 391, 395
  long white

393
white glitter
  393
dressing
  184, 188
drills
  215, 346
drink Caffeine
  13
drinking
  244, 298, 327, 360
drink milk
  97
drink plenty
  117
Drink plenty of fluids
  119
drooling
  179, 233, 251, 298, 365
drooling, excessive
  220, 307
drooling rash
  70
droplets
  232, 246
  infected
  245
drown
  21, 369, 372, 378
drownings
  58, 197, 369, 374, 378
  dry
  370, 377
drowning water hazards/risks
  369
drown proof
  375
drowsy
  145, 152, 157, 271
  down
  145, 278, 413
Dr's;Drs
  161
Dr's office;Drs office

78
dry cleaning bags
  210
dryers
  209, 216
dry flaky
  73
drying rack
  108
dry mouth
  238
duct leaks
  76
duct massage
  76
ducts
  75, 99, 102, 218, 245
  clogged
  76, 102
  plugged
  101
Duffy
  525
Dulce Chale
  446
dump
  98, 210, 325
duration
  140, 273
dust
  218
dust mites
  218
duties
  341, 351
dyes
  67, 252
Dylan
  4, 45, 72, 86, 154, 192, 331, 351,
  354, 388, 393, 410, 416, 438,
  444
Dylan's condition;Dylans condition
  45
Dylan sign language

193

E

earbud
31
  small
  31
earbuds-Hospitals
21
ear canal
371
ear drum
234
ear infections
87, 215, 234, 244, 371
  bilateral
  289
  inner
  371
ear lobe
371
Early artic explorers
313
Early Childhood Programs
343
Early diagnosis
247
early experiences
386
  positive
  329
early introduction
305
early prenatal
49
Early signs of infection
66
early spring
248
earphones
31
  small

32
ears
  34, 190, 234, 244, 366, 389, 420
  baby's;babys
  31
  elephant
  202
  inner
  32, 53
  newborn's;newborns
  33
  swim
  371
  swimmer's;swimmers
  371
ears wiggle
97
earth
51, 311
ear thermometers
78, 236
ear thermometer type
63
eater, adventurous
304
eating
  13, 60, 90, 130, 143, 146, 156, 276, 299, 303, 360, 421, 424
  comfortable
  299
  intoxication form
  313
  normally
  153
  recognizable
  172
eating foods
106
eating sugar
310
echo
32
  reduced

32
E. coli
    12
eczema
    71, 252, 261, 307, 373
eczema patches
    71
eczema, severe
    71, 305
edge
    34, 55, 62, 254, 364, 370
  straight top
    58
edges sword, double
    407
education
    48, 340, 346, 377
  early childhood
    343
  little child-related formal
    343
educational psychologist Jane M
      Healy
    399
educational purposes
    1
educational TV
    390
education courses
    345
education journey
    3
effectiveness
    138
effects
  alcohol's;alcohols
    98
  ill
    289
  negative
    332
eggs
    14, 300, 305
egg sacks

222
egg sacs
    222
Electric shock
    197
electrodes
    32
  sticker
    32
electrolyte requirements
    260
electrolytes
    240
electronics
    332
Elemental
    107
elevate
    116, 119, 231
Elizabeth
    526
Elmer's glue;Elmers glue
    258
Elmo chair
    438
emergencies
    18, 125, 211, 215, 342, 345, 525
emergency endoscopy
    211
emergency numbers
    342
emergency room doctors
    217
emergency surgery
    211
emotional leap
    287
emotional roller coaster
    350
emotions
    189, 277, 283, 288, 292, 389, 395,
        397
  basic

295
expressing multiple
284
hide Dad's;hide Dads
397
mixed
349
strong
284, 294
empathy
288, 293, 392, 397
Empty boxes and containers
329
emptying
  frequent
    117
  good
    91
encapsulation
  16
  placental
    17
encouragement
  351, 391, 407
endocrine disrupter
  358
endocrinologist
  84
energy
  130, 298, 413, 435, 447
Engorgement
  98
Enhanced formulas
  106
Entrapment
  58
environment
  252, 308, 383, 387, 399, 407, 415, 437
  children's;childrens
    399
  marine
    11
  noncompetitive
    348
  outdoor
    348
  safe
    344
Environmental threats
  215
enzyme deficiencies
  30
enzymes
  81, 86, 262
epidemiologist
  12, 129
EPI pen
  365
Epi Pen Jr
  308
episiotomy
  115
episiotomy stitches
  116
episodes
  83, 87, 238, 376, 385, 439
epithelial pearls
  35
Erections
  36
Eric Church
  111
errands
  341, 429
Erwin
  525
Erythema toxicium
  68
Erythema Toxicum
  38
escape ladders
  215, 342
escape route
  342
esophagus
  205, 210
Essential Reference

525
Establishing limits
413
estrogen
35
  extra
  35
  female hormones
  131
ethnic/minority populations
50
Eucerin
72, 252
Europe
29, 134
evaporating
262
Evenflo
57
Evenflow
227
everyday
82, 198
everyday patenting Problems
525
evolutionary terms
289
example girls
386
Examples of foods
97
excess
313
excess energy
365
excessive dryness
71
excessive lethargy
231, 237
exchange
416
  interpersonal
  389
excitement thresholds

336
exclamation
190
Exersaucer
57, 279, 323
exhaust fans
221
exhaustion
101, 351
experience
1, 8, 15, 98, 119, 121, 125, 179, 235, 249, 383, 407, 437
  environmental
  383
  first
  447
  personal
  133, 302, 370
  sensory
  330
  single
  394
  unique
  111
experiment
194, 287, 385, 392, 403
expert crawler
183
experts
88, 98, 106, 186, 191, 287, 293, 403, 421, 423, 439
  child development
  441
  clinical
  448
  multiple
  8
experts call
145
exploration
176, 279
Expose
70
exposure

503

215, 218, 249, 251, 261, 361
early
    261
expressionless
    194
expressions
  facial
    174, 192, 292, 295, 320, 417
    people's;peoples
    283
exterminator
    221
extinguishers
    215, 342
Extra tummy time
    158
extremities
    248
eye color
    383
  newborn's;newborns
    34
eye contact
    237, 272, 278, 284, 291, 319, 417, 431
  close
    319
eye discharge
    180
eye hook
    213
eye infections
    24
eyelids
    34, 39, 244, 355
eye muscles
    167, 318
eye orbit
    76
eye orbit/socket
    245
eyes
    33, 76, 167, 173, 180, 206, 244, 271, 319, 354, 361, 385, 410, 418, 431
  baby's;babys
    73, 75
  button
    161
  close
    62
  green
    354, 359
  naked
    258
  saline
    367
  eyes cross
    175
  eyes roll
    371
Ezzo
    526
Ezzo, Gary
    164

F

FAA
    366
FAAP
    49, 525
fabrics
    319
  coarse
    171
  soft
    322
faces
    39, 54, 77, 138, 162, 276, 319, 322, 330
  human
    319, 384
  new
    175
facial features
    284, 319
Fahrenheit

231
fair skinned child
    359
fairy godmother
    197
fake
    391, 395
familiarity
    320
families
    44, 46, 49, 106, 120, 122, 130, 327, 349, 374, 378, 409, 414
  extended
    351
  young
    45
family bed
    146
family editing
    448
family history
    42, 47
  strong
    126
family members
    47, 72, 95, 127, 290, 354, 366
family member's home;family members home
    215
family photos
    323
family planning
    115
family recipes
    13
  traditional
    13
family schedule
    277
family's feet;familys feet
    118
family shares
    50
family's use;familys use

49
fan
    62, 74, 373
  ceiling
    74, 137
  personal
    379
Fanconi's Anemia;Fanconis Anemia
    43
Farber, Harold
    126
farm animals
    261
fasten
    59, 62
fasten harness clips
    225
fat
    10, 86, 106, 185, 312
Father Center
    390
fatherhood
    125
  new
    125
fathers
    125, 187, 389, 398
  baby's;babys
    263
  child's birth;childs birth
    398
  strong
    391
  working
    398
Father's time;Fathers time
    124
fatigue
    131, 217
fat intake
    312
fat pad
    185
fatty acids

505

12, 14, 105
  digestible
    86
fat yogurt
  302
favorite developmental pediatricians
  270, 412
favorites
  53, 63, 168, 358
  child's;childs
    331
favorite time
  331
fearlessness
  336
fears
  136, 155, 162, 228, 336, 395, 446
  greatest
    134
feedback
  344, 447
  negative
    416
  personal
    16
feeding
  71, 82, 85, 90, 98, 103, 108, 123, 125, 143, 149, 271, 403
  consecutive
    79
  finger
    181
  last
    91, 147, 150
  small
    143
feeding maxing
  109
feeding multiples
  91
feeding periods/cycles
  273
feeding problems

52, 299
feeding solids
  281
feeding twins
  85, 103
feeling justice
  111
feelings
  120, 127, 130, 292, 296, 317, 397, 401, 404, 429, 432, 439, 440
feelings of competence
  337, 407
feelings of competence and confi-
    dence
  337, 407
Feelings of loss of body and self
  132
feeling stress
  132
feet tall
  84
feet touch
  322
female black widow
  222
Female Genitalia
  35
females
  28, 386
females move
  387
female spider, mature
  222
feminine
  390, 398
feminine traits
  390
feminine values
  398
fenugreek supplements
  84
Ferber
  526
Fertilizers

202
Fetal monitors
40
fever
68, 76, 101, 116, 230, 234, 241,
248, 267, 346, 354, 356
fever reducer
246
fiber
14, 243
Fifth disease
248
filter
63
  removable
  63
Final words
447
finger brush
264
finger foods
302, 322
  junior
  303
finger injury
213
fingernail
254, 364
finger-paint
410
fingers
26, 54, 113, 173, 181, 191, 203,
209, 212, 249, 267, 287, 325,
410, 417
  index
  181
  little
  392
  pinky
  93
finger stick
313
Firmness however

425
first Aid kit
342, 367
first breast
90
first cycle
145
first dental
265
first immunizations
122
first law
226
first molars
263
first month
94, 108, 117, 121, 165, 172
first spoken word
188
first start
104, 183
first tooth
179, 263
first trimester
13
first vaccination
24
first year molars
264
Fischler, Ron
133
fish
11, 305, 307
Fisher Price Sights
163
fish intake
106
Fishoff
406
fists
181, 298
  closed
  173
  tight

170
fit
    7, 55, 61, 153, 210, 221, 226, 331, 428
  good
    19
  perfect
    17
  right
    347
  shoulder belt
    226
fix it
    273
flaps, little
    35
flare
    72, 307
flashlight
    144, 222
Flat heads/back
    76
Flat pink birthmarks
    39
flavors
    13, 98, 301, 312
  vinegary
    310
flight attendants
    128, 351
flights
    366
flipping
    158
float
    328, 373, 378
floating
    375, 378
Flood
    206
floor
    151, 168, 207, 221, 282, 318, 326, 329, 333, 416, 427, 444
floor playing
    324
floppy
    171, 180
Florajen
    241
Florida
    46
flow
    114, 136, 278
  vaginal
    115
Flower/garden
    202
flowers
    203, 317, 361, 386
flu
    217, 247
fluid pools
    234
fluid requirements
    306
fluids
    35, 39, 53, 77, 97, 103, 119, 234, 237, 249, 258, 306, 360
  amniotic
    11
  clear
    35, 255
  excess body
    95
  infected
    234
  lighter
    202, 205
  oral
    260
fluid use
    310
fluoride
    265, 297
fluoride, the1950's;fluoride, the1950s
    266
fluoride toothpaste

266
fluoride varnish
298
  applying
266
focus
    167, 321, 346, 350, 386, 396, 408
folate
    14
folate include- Strawberries
    301
fold, little
    60
folds
    72, 365
Fontanels
    37
food allergies
    306
  associated
    307
food effects milk
    97
food elimination
    308
food group
    308
food hazards
    305
food log
    300
food preferences
    14, 98
food proteins
    308
foods
    11, 97, 180, 198, 243, 298, 317, 413, 416, 426
  bland
    239
  canned
    266
  common allergic
    308
  constipating
    239, 243, 299
  correct
    308
  ethnic
    13
  first
    298
  gassy
    97
  high-fiber
    240
  ideal
    86
  ingredient
    302
  jarred
    302
  new
    243, 251, 299, 403
  non-constipating
    243, 299
  organic
    309
  perfect
    304
  pureed
    304
  regular nonorganic
    309
  rich
    312
  safe
    325
  salty
    249
  soft
    304
  stage
    300
  suspected
    97, 308
  uncovered

    361
foot
  26, 124, 249
 baby's;babys
    194
force
  205, 227, 280, 289, 405, 412, 441,
    443
forehead
    39
forehead scanning type
    78
foreskin
  28, 36, 75
foreskin infections
    28
foreskin retraction
  28, 75
forgiving
  3, 431
forgot
  394, 429
forks
  210, 303
form
 abused
    439
 drinking
    202
 dry yellow scab
    74
 jarred pureed
    304
 language milestones
    190
 liquid
    205
 rare
    5
 raw
    304
formaldehyde
    252
formation
    385
 early
    441
 massage speeds myelin
    336
form sources
    276
formula
  53, 85, 88, 105, 150, 153, 156,
    238, 244, 289, 297, 303
 giving
  25, 299
 microwave
    109
 milk-based
    71
 mix
    297
 mixed
    109
 non-dairy
    71
 oz of
  108, 149, 156, 298
 preferred
    106
 supplemental
  25, 93
 taking
    299
formula amount
    108
Formula-fed newborns
    108
formula feeding
  80, 105
formula feeding basics
    107
formula intake
    298
formula intolerance
    107
formula manufacturers

    109
formulas, new
    105
formula temperature
    108
four-legged creatures
    187
fragments, retained
    265
fragrance
    67, 252
frame
    64, 324
  metal
    61
  working family
    351
Frankel's advice;Frankels advice
    125
Frankel, Valerie
    124
freckles
    354, 359
freedom
    269, 403, 414
freeze
    102, 122
freezer
    103, 233
  small extra
    122
frenulum
    256
frequency
    252, 436
Fresh Food Feeder
    64
fresh milk
    103
freshwater
    369
friction
    37
  normal

    37
fridge
    103, 108, 208, 310, 360, 366, 434
fridge magnets
    208
Friedman
    395
friend Barb Grady
    437
friendliness
    336
friend's baby, best;friends baby, best
    52
friends, good
    2, 204, 370
friendships
    294, 410
front
    26, 62, 97, 177, 227, 284, 318,
    321, 332, 409, 428, 447
  lower
    264
  united
    433
front crawl
    375
front office
    349
front seat
    229
frozen bagel
    267
frozen breast milk
    103
frozen milk
    103
frozen pieces
    16
fruit juice
    243, 300
fruits
    13, 119, 243, 267, 300, 310, 367
  frozen

235, 267
non-constipating
  239
fry, small
  85
FSA
  11
fuel-burning source
  216
fun
  134, 177, 299, 313, 337, 433, 439
fun activity
  375
function
  235, 311, 383
fun, great
  368
fun noises
  178
fun occurrence
  98
furniture
  183, 212, 325
  heavy
    209
  outdoor
    222
fuss
  92, 145, 153, 178, 279, 288, 292, 317
fussiness
  271, 274, 319
  increased
    234
fussing
  145, 149, 273
fussy
  53, 97, 120, 138, 146, 271, 277, 319, 326, 402
fussy period
  272, 279, 334
  active
    273
  predictable
    273
fussy stop
  316
fussy times
  273, 320

G

gain control
  419, 428
gain credibility
  426
gain self-control
  419, 437
Gala
  302
game Pat-a-cake
  315
game plan
  440
games
  156, 159, 181, 183, 194, 198, 209, 280, 283, 291, 315, 320, 327, 333, 377
  active
    396
  favorite
    285
  gentle
    397
  mental
    425
  portable video
    211
  separation
    155
  social
    326
  vocal
    281
games work
  316
gap

55, 96
garage
    56, 211, 217, 222, 342
Gary M.A
    526
gas
    23, 52, 82, 119, 178, 202, 206, 351
gas appliances
    217
gas company
    217
gas dryer
    218
Gas-fired heating systems
    216
gas fireplace
    209
gas, passing
    40
gassier
    40
gassy
    52, 97
Gastro-intestinal bug
    238
gate
    58, 366, 415
gaze avert
    278
Geburtshilfe Frauenheilkd
    15
gelatin capsules
    16
gender
    27, 387
gender bias
    390
gender cues
    388
gender differences
    382, 384
   studied
    384
gender identity
    388, 392, 398
   developing
    386
gender stereotyping
    389
General Motors
    224
genes
    383, 399
   child's;childs
    399
   human
    399
genetic basis
    311
genetic defect
    50
genetic predisposition
    126
genetics
    263, 382, 389
Genital care
    74
genital hygiene
    28
gentle caressing
    336
gentle guidance
    321
gentle words
    150
George J MD FAAP
    526
Gerber
    14, 300
Gerber Liquilytes
    238
Gerber Products Company
    14
Gerber Soothe
    241
German Medical Journal

16
germs
    261
germy/dirty
    20
gestures
    184, 190, 284, 292
get-go
    100, 382
gibberish
    190
GI bug
    240
GI flora, good
    240
gift
    197, 406
  amazing
    51, 410
  greatest
    423
  important
    412
  precious life-saving
    49
gifts, best
    133
giggle
    85, 178, 281
girlfriend
    370
girls
    75, 166, 186, 382, 384, 387, 392, 394
  bad
    435
  elementary school
    395
  girl a
    388
  handsome
    388
girls dress

388
Give Life
    47
giving birth use
    115
giving little girls
    395
giving older babies
    425
glad
    429, 439, 446
glasses
    21, 103, 168, 203, 259
  breakable
    422
Glenn
    125
Glenn, Stephen
    525
goal
    90, 141, 278, 391, 412, 419, 422, 431
  ultimate
    158
Good Beginnings
    409
goodbye
    290, 347
Good change
    310
Good childcare
    348
Goodman, Mary
    316
Good Morning America
    385
goose egg
    255
Gotham Books
    525
grab
    59, 100, 168, 212, 257, 295, 303, 421
grab ahold

100
grab items
213
Grace
391
Graco
64
Graco TM jumper
324
grade
331
  low
  236
grades, highest
295
grain bread
119
grains
309
Grandma
445
grandmother
200
grandparents
123
grandparent's meds;grandparents meds
203
Granted
405
grapefruit
310
  large
  113
grapes
198, 305
  prunes peaches
  243
grasping
283, 322
Gravity
99
gray

34, 40, 385
gray-blue eyes
34
gray eyes
34
grazing
143, 146
Great Self Esteem Books
411
Greek yogurt
14
Green Leafy Veggies- Including
14
greens
301
  leafy
  15
  spinach/dark
  301
greeting card
211
Gr Greer
125
grocery
310, 428
grocery cart
64, 82, 213, 262
grocery cart seat
429
Groggily
112
Groner, Judith
167
Gross motor movements
192
ground
16, 325, 343
  breeding
  218
group
13, 343, 390, 403
  bunco
  378
  environmental working

358
muscle
　57
new
　402
peer
　390
placenta ingestion
　16
group carrot juice
　13
group setting
　17
group sizes, small
　343
groups size
　343
growth
　165, 218, 312, 315, 332, 334, 407
growth and development
　165, 312, 315, 332
growth, rapid brain
　37
growth spurts
　92, 166
　large
　　166
　mini
　　166
grunt
　41, 77
gs/circumcision-by-country
　29
guests
　121
guide
　164, 296, 301, 418
gums
　35, 101, 198, 256
　baby's;babys
　　101
　sore
　　267
guns
　393, 429
gurgling
　172
gurgling sounds
　41
gut
　241
gut feeling
　19
gut flora, good
　241
gut instinct
　346
gut, parental
　8
gym, little
　410
gymnast
　209
　competitive
　　5, 394, 410
Gynecologists
　10
Gynecologists' position;Gynecologists position
　13
Gynecology
　9, 129

H

Haakkaa
　99
habit
　149, 153
　bad sleep
　　59
habits, bad
　146, 148, 152
hair
　37, 168, 184, 247, 393, 418, 420, 435
　blonde

359
dark
  37
long
  21
permanent
  37
red
  359
soft fine
  37
washing
  276
wet
  232
hair barrettes
  393
hairbrush
  184
  soft baby
  73
hair clips
  199
hair color
  383
hair products
  202
hair sprays
  361
hair tie
  21
Ham
  330
hand control
  321
hand foot
  249
hand movements
  285
hands work
  173
hand towel
  67
hand toys
  173
hangs
  325
mesh
  59
Happiest Baby
  526
hard surface, flat
  322
harnesses buckles
  228
harness slots, lower
  225
Hart, Louise
  412
harvests
  302
Harvey, David
  357
Harvey M.D
  526
hassle
  50, 367, 429
hats
  73, 137, 354
  pink
  388
  wide brimmed
  356
hay fever
  307
head
  24, 26, 36, 55, 136, 170, 209, 211,
    318, 321, 371, 375, 393
headaches
  130, 217
  severe
  102
head bobs
  172
head circumference
  165
head flops

517

170
head injuries
    255
head start
    380
head steady-Hold
    318
head teacher
    345
head trauma
    213, 255
healing
    100
  improper
    28
health
    4, 18, 154, 312, 365
  environmental
    216
  good
    25, 155, 298
  good gut
    241
health benefits
    311
health challenges
    5
health experts
    135
health issues
    4, 153
Health Lecture
    230
health policies
    345
health risks
    108, 377
health warning
    363
Healthy Children.org
    448
healthy sleep habits
    143, 148, 152
  encouraging

    133, 142
  good
    164
Healthy Sleep Habits Happy Child
    526
Hearing loss
    33
Hearing screening
    31
Hearing Screens
    31
heart
    4, 9, 37, 42, 66, 118, 165, 289,
      334, 422, 445
heart attack
    304
heart medication
    204
heart palpitations
    217
heart problem
    31
heart rate
    23
  baby's;babys
    270
heat
    54, 227, 248, 257, 357, 365
  applying
    114
  extreme
    227
  safety tip-;safety tip
    306
Heath, Kevin
    333
heating vents
    74
heat rash
    72, 365
heel prick
    30
height

518

24, 63, 167, 224, 255
manufacturer's;manufacturers
63
Heimlich Maneuver
199
help
14, 30, 40, 50, 91, 99, 112, 119, 126, 140, 145, 158, 275, 282, 321, 351, 374, 394, 425, 430
help brush
364
help children
346, 391, 409
helper
120
mother's;mothers
352
helpfultechnique
416
Helping kids
391
helpless
273, 275
helpless feeling
262
helpless individuals
352
help parents
149
help prop
138
help pull
100, 254, 364
help release
335
help soothe skin
258
help tone
126
hemispheres
386
Hemlock
202
hemoglobinopathies
30
hemorrhage
24
subconjunctival
34
hemorrhoids
119
HEPA-style air purifier
218
Hepatitis
24
herpes simplex
39
hiccups
68, 109
Hiccups- Hiccups
40
hide
155, 169, 183, 222, 282, 291, 327, 342
highchair children
60
highchairs
60, 214, 279, 282, 325, 413, 427
child's;childs
214
portable
60, 200
high fever
235
High humidity
218
high IQ
382
Hill
525
hind milk
91
hip fractures
88
hips
38, 137
infant's;infants

38
hip, tight
38
Hispanic patients
44
Hispanics
39, 44
historical study
16
history
354
  strong
  106
hitting
424, 441, 443
hives
250
  viral
  252
Holden, Robert
382
Holiday dangers
213
holiday ornaments
211
holidays
213, 341
holiday tablecloths
214
Hollandaise sauce
12
home
21, 80, 120, 155, 197, 199, 215,
251, 288, 310, 339, 347, 393,
424
  coming
  126
  instructor's;instructors
  377
home comfort measures
233
home dads
398
home monitors

138
home parents
351
home state
359
homework
17
Honduras
29
Honest recognition and praise
406
honesty newborns
65
honey
85, 304
Hong Kong
106
hood cords
211
hook
62, 122
Hopkins, John
386
horizontal Eustachian
235
hormonal changes
129
hormones
30, 130, 157, 334
  feel-good
  334
  given
  310
  given growth
  310
  maternal
  69, 75, 127
  producing
  88
hospital
17, 24, 31, 41, 75, 114, 116, 120,
123, 204, 289, 335
hospital bag

23
hospital floors
20
hospital gown
20
hospitalizations
21, 224
hospital noise
21
hospital personnel
25
Hospital Routine
20
hospital setting
21
hospital staff
23
hospitals use
32
hotel
366
hour intervals
112
hour nap wake
256
hours
29, 77, 89, 97, 102, 117, 120, 131, 140, 151, 161, 220, 237, 245, 254, 258, 273, 350, 362, 377
  extra
141
  half
82
  working
352
hours call
114
hours convulsions
77
hours eating
134
house
74, 77, 113, 121, 128, 184, 188, 202, 206, 215, 221, 406, 410
2-story
215
husband's aunt's;husbands aunts
445
messy
128, 352
two- story
342
housekeeper
128
bad
352
how is disciplining going
445
hrs
91, 150, 216, 238, 244
Hug and kiss and smile
423
hugging
398, 411
hugs
327, 435
extra
291
Human adults
112
human beings, successful
447
human bite protocol
254
human milk
86, 105
Human milk and infant formula
86
humans
15, 222, 254, 311
humidifier
63, 218
cool mist
218, 231, 233
humiliating
437
humor

118, 433
  little
    118
hunger
    92, 277
hungry
    141, 146, 156, 172, 271, 303, 393, 432
Hurtig
    388
hurts
    42, 67, 104, 117, 212, 293, 350, 418, 420, 423, 426, 432
  biting
    434
  pinching
    424
hurts mommy
    420
  no that
    420
husband
    84, 120, 207, 211, 214, 217, 370, 376, 391, 416, 421, 429, 444
husband Glen
    124
husband lol
    145
hydrocortisone
    116, 252, 360
hydrocortisone cream
    367
hydrocortisone, severe
    364
hydrogen peroxide
    367
hyperactive
    220
Hyperemesis
    4, 9, 45
Hyperemesis Gravidarum
    3
Hypersensitivity
    219
hyperventilation
    130
hypothermia
    370, 377

I

ibuprofen
    114, 236, 247, 257, 267, 354
ice
    108, 116, 220, 255, 364
  crushed
    100
  melted
    369
Ice chests
    210, 369
ice cube
    256
ice packs
    99, 115
ICU
    204
i do not know the cause
    246
IgCN
    1
ij.org/bonemarrowstatistics
    45
illegal steroids
    85
Illinois
    388
illness
    3, 5, 77, 131, 137, 154, 235, 245, 249, 252, 261
  first
    235, 267
  mild
    248
  new
    63, 159
  respiratory

104
terrible childhood
249
viral
217, 234, 238, 248
illness call
79
images
284, 386
correct
184
ideal
392
positive body
396
imaginary monsters
162
imbalance
261
chemical
130
imbed real words
190
imitate
174, 176, 188, 194, 320
imitate gestures
184
imitate sounds
173, 178
imitating
180, 184
imitating people
286
immune deficiencies
49
immune deficiency
primary
5
rare
45
immune globulin injection
254
immune system
42, 126, 240, 334
developing
261
immature
307
immune system disorders
30
immunity
43
mom's;moms
267
immunizations
122, 137, 365
child's;childs
365
Immunoglobulin
4
Immunoglobulin infusions
5
immunologist
45
pediatric
241
immunology
449
impacting performance
386
imperfections
33
Impetigo
250
improvement
107, 337
incentives
436
inches
33, 38, 55, 58, 78, 165, 167, 199, 221, 226, 228, 236, 250
inches, one/half
219
inches tall
166
inch projections

35
incision
117
abdominal
116
incisors
264
lower
263
upper
263
increased attention
423
paying
190
increased risk
359
twofold
12
incubation period
244, 249
normal
248
independence
269, 296, 391, 395, 398, 402, 410, 432
encouraging
398, 402
sense of
404, 425
wanting
292
Indeterminate state
271
Index
450
India and Asia infants
139
indicator, best
238
i need your eyes Dylan
418
infant acne

39
infant botulism
304
infant carriers
61
infant/child
388
infant communication
337
infant feeder
298
infant formulas
86, 89, 105, 266
infant glycerin suppository
244
infant massage
334, 449
infant nutrition
157, 297
infant rear
225
infants
24, 54, 58, 71, 78, 105, 136, 144, 148, 156, 186, 191, 297, 316, 343, 368, 372, 375, 387
breast-fed
313
formula-fed
87
healthy
135
helpless
404
human
86
male
28
misbehaving
419
older
148, 380, 426
premature
335
teaching

192
teething
267
ways
317
world
290
younger
284
infants age
61
infants and toddlers
214, 287, 317, 370, 374, 438
infant seat
63
  rear-facing
225
infant self-feeding
304
infant sign language
184
infant's milk;infants milk
309
infants outgrow
63
infants sleep
136
infants start
143
infant suffocation
147
infants wake
141
Infant Swimming Resource
376
infant swim programs
375
infection
  18, 24, 40, 66, 86, 116, 215, 219,
  230, 234, 253, 258, 268, 371
  bacterial
236
  cause gum

265
decreased
335
frequent viral upper respiratory
235
impetigo
250
lung
205
mild respiratory
233
outer-ear
371
respiratory tract
233
signs of
115, 119
sinus
230
staph
250
strep
241
urinary tract
27, 87, 117
vaginal
101
viral
247
watch for signs and symptoms of
223, 255, 258
infertility
358
influence
  biological
384
  little
311
  male
398
  positive
398
info-for-parents-disorder-info

29
information
    1, 7, 15, 216, 223, 229, 273, 276, 363, 374, 380, 387, 447
  baby's;babys
    342
  clinical
    16
  factual
    48
Infrequent bowel movements
  95
ingesting
  15, 311, 377
ingestions
  16, 203
ingredient, main
  363
ingredients, important
  288
inhale
  73, 364
Inhaled poisons
  206
injuries
  40, 60, 83, 208, 212, 224, 253, 419, 437, 441
  external
    83
  fatal
    227
  pens-Many playpen
    59
  sustain
    61
  unintentional
    224
injuries result
  60
injury prevention
  226
inner ear organ
  31
Insect repellent

360, 363
  best all-purpose
    361
insects
  222, 360
insects nest
  361
insects, repel
  360
inspection locator
  223
inspection sites
  223
install latches
  207
institute
  45, 104, 390
  national
    135
institutions
  288
  accrediting
    50
instruction
  377
instructions, special
  75
instructor
  376
instructor, certified master
  377
instructor studies
  377
instructor training
  377
insurance
  42, 339, 346
insurance agent
  339
insurance policy
  45
intake
  156, 304
  baby's;babys

300
daily fluid
299
inadequate
81
intellectuals
278
intelligence
185, 383
intensity
274, 282
intentions, best
389
interest
  baby's;babys
    57
  child's;childs
    316, 390
  decreased
    131
  heightened
    279
interrupt
419, 434, 437
interruptions, brief
80
inter-uterine growth restriction
4
intervention, effective
32
interview
8, 17, 339
interview process
339
intestines
240
  baby's;babys
    81
intolerance
106
intuition
8
  mother's;mothers

45, 341
investment, great
158
Involved dads
398
ipecac
204
IQ
191, 330, 382
IQ, lower
215
IQ range
382
iris
34
iron
14, 106, 204, 297, 312
iron, extra
299, 312
iron level
312
  baby's;babys
    297
iron pills
205
Irrigation ditches
370
irritability
98, 131, 217, 220, 234
irritants
28, 41, 215
irritate
71, 75, 241
Irwin Hyman author
441
is a bit misleading
141
isles
118, 213
isolation
351
  social
    132
ISR

374, 376, 379
Israel
    29
ISR instruction
    378
itching
    255, 365
itchy
    71, 246, 248, 250, 253
itchy use Calamine lotion TM
    364
items
    59, 65, 122, 156, 161, 211, 213, 228, 325, 347, 385
  adult
    432
  cold
    235
  dropped
    177
  favorite
    267
  high priority
    352
  large
    319
  putting breakable
    415
  safe
    327
i told you that you had to go
    118
Itsy-Bitsy Spider
    329
iu
    105, 313
IV infusion
    4
Ivy
    202
Izard, Carol
    295

J

jabbering sounds
    188
Jack
    434
Jane
    525
Jane ED
    525
Jane Greer Ph
    125
Jane Nelsen Positive Discipline
    400
Jane Nelsen's words;Jane Nelsens words
    399
Japan
    29
jaundice
    30, 79, 80
  mild
    79
  normal physiologic
    81
  normal physiological
    81
jaw glides
    96
jaw, lower
    171
Jeffrey Siegel M
    448
jelly
    116, 236
Jenny Friedman PHD
    400
jerky
    11, 170, 175, 271, 273
jewelry
    199
  flashing
    211
Jill Stamm Bright
    400
Jill Stam's book Bright From;Jill Stams

book Bright From
    186
Jill Stam's book Bright From The Start;Jill Stams book Bright From The Start
    316
Jimson Weed
    203
jitteriness
    41
jobs
    6, 128, 144, 164, 211, 271, 294, 340, 350, 395, 407, 413, 429
  female
    395
Johns Hopkins University
    384
John's Hopkins university;Johns Hopkins university
    187
Johnson
    312
Johnson- Pediatric Nursing
    312
Johnston, Richard
    261
jostling
    83
  little extra
    82
  regular
    83
Jot
    170
Journal
    10
journey
    1, 367
joy
    189, 295
judgment
  best
    311
  impaired

    217
juice
    204, 235, 239, 265, 299, 426
  avoiding
    240
  avoid- Unpasteurized
    12
  pasteurized
    306
  prune
    312
juice box
    426
Julie Menella PhD
    98
Jullian Stanley
    384
jump
    186, 272, 324, 373
jumper, free-standing
    324
jumping
    325, 396
jump start
    368
jungle gyms
    399
Justice Bone
    45

K

Kaiser Permanente Medical Program
    28
kangaroo care babies
    335
Karen Berberian PhD
    404
Karen Kay Imagava
    83
Karp
    526
Karp, Harvey

529

164
Kartini Diapari-Oengider
　353
Kegel
　117
Kelly King Alexander
　187
Kentucky
　9
key component
　408
key fobs
　211
keystone cops
　439
kick
　　173, 214, 284, 292, 444
　meds
　　251
　splash
　　323
kicking
　　396, 445
kiddos
　　21, 154, 179, 355, 373, 423
　sensitive
　　70
kids
　　2, 18, 191, 196, 205, 211, 245,
　　249, 261, 294, 327, 332, 343,
　　373, 386, 398, 407, 414, 433,
　　444
　amazing
　　1
　older
　　71, 344
　raising
　　2, 6, 412
　teach
　　373
　young
　　438
kids ages

226
kids-Alfalfa sprouts
　305
kids allergic
　308
kids foods
　306
kids playing
　373
kids test limits
　413
kindergarten
　395
kindness
　352, 425
king mackerel
　11
kink
　84, 136
kisses
　327, 423
　giving
　　435
　giving air
　　192
kissing
　421, 424
kitchen
　207, 215, 327, 393, 397, 432
kitchen bar area
　62
kitchen cabinets
　327
kitchen chairs
　60, 416
kitchen chandelier
　416
kitchen duct
　218
kitchen knives
　210
kitchen sink
　73, 310
kitchen table

530

416
knees
  61, 71, 179, 182, 410
  head shoulders
  190
knowledge
  1, 6, 192, 211, 229
KY
  78, 236

L

Lab Abbey
  388
labeled lox
  11
labels
  102, 122, 356, 361
labia
  75
labor
  49, 123, 350
Laboratories, Ross
  195, 317
labs in-house, basic
  18
lactation consultant
  41, 91
lactobacillus GG
  241
lactose
  16, 86, 106, 240, 311
lag
  186
  jet
  149, 157
lakes
  11, 369, 378
Lakes and ocean water
  371
Lamott, Anne
  334
Landers, Ann

447
language
  32, 186, 192, 284, 323, 388
  foreign
  321, 324
  second
  193
  spoken
  32
language development
  269, 330, 397
  slow
  332
language games
  190
language skills
  330
lanolin
  100, 252
Lanugo
  37
lap
  177, 226, 324, 331, 389
lap belts
  226
lap child
  366
lap, parent's;lap, parents
  187
Large building blocks
  328
large chalk
  325
large chunks
  302
large crayon
  325
Large dogs cause
  219
Large dolls
  328
large doses
  98
large issues

531

434
large muscles groups
  176
Laser treatment
  40
lashes matting
  76
latch
  99, 101
Latin word disciplina
  412
laughs
  85, 112, 118, 174, 178, 187, 284
 belly
  281
 times.Children
  382
laundry
  113, 120, 241, 341
 hospital's;hospitals
  23
 liquid
  201
laundry detergent
  122
laundry detergent/pods
  201
laundry room
  217, 416
Lavender
  21
law states children
  226
laxative
  119
laxative effect
  300
laxative, natural
  95
layer
  374
layers, important
  375
leak

  99
 small
  218
learning
  185, 187, 192, 271, 279, 282, 292,
  315, 327, 332, 346
 best
  348
 first
  185
 rapid
  283
 social
  383
learning dad
  440
learning language
  32
learning play
  315
learning program
  348
learning tool
  431
lectures
  2, 7, 163, 211, 229, 421, 426, 449
 childproofing
  317
 emotional
  316
leg relax
  338
legs
  38, 41, 58, 72, 79, 119, 171, 287,
  292, 335, 336
 baby's;babys
  58
 little
  61
 lower
  38
 nonskid
  59
 one-inch

222
Legumes
    15
length
    198, 219, 234, 275, 316, 341, 347
  required
    362
lengthwise
    198, 306
less-Children
    431
lesson
    204, 316, 377, 405, 420, 430, 433
  extra
    392
  great
    393
  important
    315
  painful
    221
  safest
    377
letdown
    99
  initial
    90
lethargic
    25, 238, 360
Lethargy-excessive sleepiness
    79
lethargy, severe
    77
letter
    272, 275
leukemia
    42, 47
levels
    46, 80, 105, 113, 131, 138, 431
  armpit
    225
  chlorine
    372
  elevated

    80
  high
    80
  hormone
    131
  intelligence
    384
Levy, Stuart
    262
Liam
    391
lids
    213, 327
lid slams
    213
life
    1, 4, 9, 38, 47, 87, 93, 129, 261,
    267, 288, 290, 307, 330, 386
  baby's;babys
    7
  child's;childs
    247, 398, 413
  choking kids
    200
  first month of
    95, 140
  marine
    11
  person's;persons
    42
Lifebank
    47
life event
    154
  stressful
    131
life experiences
    383
lifetime
    296, 382
Life Vac
    199
lift

533

     117, 171, 176, 318, 431
light blanket
     323
light clothing
     354
light-colored eyes
     34
light fixture
     416
light layer
     362
lights
     25, 34, 138, 144, 152, 156, 163, 211, 214, 269, 277, 353, 355
  bili
     80
  black
     221
  bright
     171
  fluorescent
     79
  sparkling
     213
  special
     80
  special phototherapy
     80
light sensitivity
     180
light switches
     401
light tan
     219
light T-shirt
     74
lightweight
     57
light weight muslin, breathable
     139
likes
     74, 292, 301, 324, 342, 348
Lilly

     392
limbs
     173, 223, 335
limitations
     5, 374
limited availability
     17
limits
     126, 207, 283, 327, 341, 403, 412, 420, 425, 429
  establishing firm
     413
  reasonable
     404, 412
  setting
     413, 439
link
     293
  possible
     261
linked breathing issues
     372
lip balm
     22, 206, 368
lip quivers
     41
lips
     231, 256, 281, 306
  dry
     238
  infant's;infants
     96
  lower
     93
liquid baking extracts
     202
liquid charcoal
     204
liquid gold
     102
  precious
     99
liquids

97, 117
down
  238
  open
  109
liquids breast milk
  102
listeria
  11
listeria poisoning
  306
Listeriosis
  12
Little Genius Read article
  187
little girls
  388, 391, 395
  old
  395
little pellets, hard
  95
little piggy
  190
  this
  329
littlest feet
  66
little Thomas
  354
liver
  79, 81, 247, 313
  immature
  79
local anesthetic
  29
local drug
  70
local environmental protection
    agency
  11
local licensing agency
  347
location

227, 250, 342, 366
lochia
  114
lock
  207, 210, 213, 229, 377
  install toilet
  208
Logical consequences-Use
  427
Long lasting
  275
Loomans, Diane
  411
Loomas, Diane
  410
loss
  31, 96, 130, 247, 255, 287, 442
  large doses
  217
  rare cases
  306
lotions
  21, 69, 73, 247
  little
  276
  non-scented
  69
  scented baby
  69
Lotromin
  101, 242
Lott, Lynn
  525
Louisiana State
  287
love
  17, 264, 269, 286, 294, 296, 320,
    324, 333, 408, 412, 420, 423,
    446
love bites
  421
loved spending time
  394
Lovell, Patty

411
love Maggie
   124
love object
   160, 281
love relationships
   382
love rhythm
   285
love teaching
   447
love, unconditional
   296, 402
Love Very
   342
loving
   344
loving, compassionate
   391
loving nurturing mother
   383
low-grade fever
   248
low-keyed efforts
   274
Low staff turnover
   345
Low thyroid levels
   131
Lubriderm
   72
lump
   36
   bruising
      36
   sized
      99
lungs
   40, 201, 205, 371
   baby's;babys
      201

M

Macintosh
   302
mad
   289, 422
magazines
   323, 413
   illustrated
      310
Maggie
   125
Maggie's birth;Maggies birth
   124
magic
   68, 364
magical times
   9
magical way
   353
Magnesia
   119, 244
magnetic type
   207
makeshift instruments
   286
makeshift jungle gym
   416
Male fetuses
   384
Male Genitalia
   35
males
   27
   adult
      386
malignancies
   49
Malignant melanoma
   355
mama
   110, 182, 187, 190
   pregnant
      11
   tired new

4
mama gut
211
mammals
15, 275
mangos
301
manufacturers
54, 59, 217, 361
manufacturers guidelines
61
marbles
99, 199
Marc
526
Marc Weissbluth Healthy Sleep Habits Happy Child
164
market
52, 199, 252, 262, 368
marriage
351, 444
marshmallows
198
Maryland
12, 390
masculine
390, 398
mask
104, 128, 200, 258, 267
Mason, Mary
9
massage
73, 267, 334
  daily
336
  gentle
99
massage therapy
335
massaging
99, 114, 337
mastering

196, 410
Master ISR instructor
378
Mastitis
101
matching individuals
49
Maternal human placentophagy
15
mattress
55, 61, 82, 136, 139, 231
  firm flat
137
  new mesh style
56
  parent's;parents
136
  regular
56
  soft
136, 146
mattress air
56
maturing
68, 269, 273, 278
maturity
25
  emotional
374
  neurological
272
  physical
185
maximum group size
343
May call it their thinking spot
419
Mc Graw Hill
526
meals
82, 112, 122, 300, 303, 327, 397
  extra
122
  next

303
premade
112
prepared
112
mealtime
281, 303, 314, 413
mealtime LOL
177
meats
15, 302, 310
  jarred
  302
  lean
  240
meat sticks
198, 305
meat tenderizer
254, 364
meconium
68
meconium, black
94
meconium pass
95
meconium stools
94
Media
390
medical advantages, potential
27
medical help
220
medical monitoring
130
medical problems
219
  multiple
  5
medical value
48
medication
53, 84, 101, 104, 130, 204, 208,
    236, 242, 244, 267, 274, 354
  antifungal
  70
  fever-reducing
  78, 237
  spilled
  203
medicine dropper
367
medicines
50, 167, 201, 207
  daily
  204
Medicine's Prevention Research
    Center;Medicines Prevention
    Research Center
129
Mediterranean descent
39
Meg Meeker
411
Melanoma
353
Melanoma www.skincancer.org,
    developing
354
meltdown
393
  full-blown
  445
Meltzoff
194
members
46, 311, 351
  important
  414
memories
  best
  331
  long
  428
  sad
  386
memory

193, 329
infant's;infants
  193
 long term
  195
 long-term
  194
Meningitis
  87
Mennella's advice;Mennellas advice
  13
mental delays
  215
mental snapshot
  194
mental status
  256
 altered
  255
mercury
  11, 14, 106
Merlin
  158
Merlin Sleep Suit
  140, 158
mesh weave, small
  59
Metamucil
  119
Metformin/Insulin
  204
method
 cry it out
  153
 right
  133
methods measure
  31
Metzoff
  194
Mexican-style cheeses
  12
Mexico

  84
Miami Florida
  292
Michael Popkin PhD
  413
microorganisms
  371
microphone
  31
microwave
  12, 103, 112
microwave breast milk
  109
middle-of-the-night
  151
mildew
  218
milestones
  32, 169, 186
 developmental
  169, 196
 emotional
  276, 286, 292
milia
  39
milk
  53, 81, 84, 89, 96, 102, 297, 300,
   303, 307, 310
milk allergy
  307
milk collector cups haacaa
  65
milk flavoring
  312
milk intolerance
  106, 303
 cow's;cows
  106
Milk of Magnesia
  119, 244
milk production, increased
  16
milk protein

106
milk shoot
99
milk stools
94
milk supply
85, 90, 99, 103
milk supply fluctuates
92
milk tongue
101
milk volume
90
Miller, Frank
9
mimic
217, 315, 383
Mimicking
194
mimic seasickness
217
minerals
86, 308, 311
minerals titanium dioxide
357
mineral supplements
313
miniature scale
387
miniture football
392
Minnesota
390
minutes
90, 95, 103, 149, 152, 154, 204, 228, 238, 255, 274, 289, 335, 355, 359
miracle
9, 392
Miralax
119, 244
mirror
283, 324
  review

229
  safe
  422
  unbreakable crib
  318
mirror neurons
288
misbehavior
417, 435, 438
  aggressive
  444
miscarriages
12, 248
misconception, popular
310
misdeeds, minor
439
mistakes
3, 229, 349, 409, 423, 431, 433
  common
  418
mist, cool
63
Mistletoe
214
mix
94, 107, 109, 241, 299
mobile
161, 182, 194, 318, 385
mobile baby
421
mobile move
194
mobile, moving
385
mobility
336, 421
  newfound
  283
moderation
11, 311
moist
72, 199
moist heat

99
warm
  120
moisture
  72, 242
moisturizer
  72
molars
  264
  second
  263
mold
  218
moles
  254, 354
mom
  4, 13, 24, 35, 53, 105, 121, 147,
    200, 217, 282, 286, 291, 332,
    349, 378, 395, 411
  associates
  188
  better
  1
  immunity
  235
  maniacal
  360
  new
  129, 388
  parenting
  378
  pinch
  420
  pregnant
  13, 234
  realized
  429
  stay-at-home
  349
  strong
  5
  super
  132
  test

283
working
  349
mom and dad
  3, 144, 159, 188, 193, 280, 293,
    319, 329, 394, 403, 432
moments
  110, 118
  collected
  43
  loving cuddle
  329
  scariest
  200
moments count
  333
mommy
  187, 214, 286, 293, 418, 424, 425,
    430, 434
Mom's Diet;Moms Diet
  97
mom's milk;moms milk
  67
Monday
  394
Monell Chemical Senses Center
  13
money
  45, 53, 207, 351
Mongolian spot
  39
Monique
  2, 112
Monique Couillard Nelson BS
  1
monique@inelsons.com
  447
monique, sure
  241
monitor
  4, 40, 204, 240, 244, 255, 300,
    304, 349, 377, 392
  apnea/heart

4
television
  187
video baby
  64
monkeys
  383
  female
  383
  rhesus
  383
Montessori
  348
Montessori type setting
  348
months-Smiles
  187
moons
  246, 393
morning sickness
  14
Moro reflex
  26
Moro/startle reflex
  174
mos
  260, 287, 415
mosquitoes
  361
Most Drs
  95
motherhood
  3, 88, 110, 112, 349
mothers
  16, 81, 86, 88, 105, 113, 123, 290,
  293, 350, 383, 389, 424
  expectant
  248
  new
  119
  perfect
  19
  working

  351, 398
mother's attitude;mothers attitude
  350
mother's breast milk;mothers breast
  milk
  317
motion
  bicycle
  335
  raking
  180
  weak sucking
  98
motion sickness
  367
motor ability
  26
motor skills
  396
  fine
  185, 192, 314, 325
  large
  57, 176, 186, 384, 410
Motor vehicle crashes
  224
motto, great
  290
mouth
  93, 96, 100, 135, 160, 170, 173,
    199, 201, 210, 249, 256, 304,
    361, 420
mouth break
  93
mouth disease
  249
mouth muscles
  298
mouth secretions
  249
Mouth traumas
  256
mouth ulcers
  249
move furniture

212
movements
    41, 147, 170, 174, 237, 329, 384, 409
    arm-thrusting
        170
    baby's;babys
        271
    disorganized
        273
    jittery
        77
    little
        142
    newborn's;newborns
        170
    restless
        141
    rhythmic
        324
    slowed
        130
    smoother
        170
    strong reflex
        170
    uncontrolled body
        220
    uncoordinated
        175
    uncoordinated eye
        220
MRIs
    386
mucus
    114
Multi-racial people
    45
Munchkin brand miracle
    179
Munchkin miracle
    303
muscle control
    170
    large
        192, 318, 321, 324
muscles
    77, 97, 117, 167, 175, 180, 243, 320, 409
    abdominal
        117
    fine
        321
    large
        326
    small
        318, 322, 325
    strengthen neck
        138
    tight
        180
muscle tension
    336
Muscle twitching
    220
muscular dystrophy
    5
mushrooms
    203
    wild
        202
music
    21, 148, 286, 320, 324, 411
    played
        211
Musical greeting cards
    210
Musicology
    316
Muslim-majority countries
    29
Myelin
    336
myelin sheath
    336
Mylicon

40, 64

N

Nail clippers
    63
nail file
    63
nails
    72, 170, 199, 394
name
    5, 183, 187, 189, 214, 284, 294,
    324, 346, 376, 385, 388
name objects
    324
Nancy Marshall PhD
    349
nanny
    340, 348
  in-house
    339
  super
    435
Nanny/Sitter
    339
naps
    82, 121, 145, 152, 158, 211, 245
  cat
    153
  morning
    152
  solid
    163
  taking cat
    163
nap schedule
    152, 158, 163
nap time
    256, 279, 418
  next scheduled
    153
  normal
    256
nap wake

256
Nasal discharge
    230
nasal passages
    231
nasal stuffiness
    234
nasal swab
    234
National Academy of Early Child-
    hood Programs
    343
national accreditation
    345
national bone marrow registry
    44
National Day Care study
    343
National Fisheries Institute
    11
national guidelines
    133
National Highway
    225
National Highway Traffic Safety Ad-
    ministration
    223
National pesticide telecommunica-
    tions network
    363
national registry
    44
national TV
    425
Native American
    39
Natrapel
    363
natural alternatives
    362
natural analgesic
    99
natural instinct

320
natural lubricant
   100
natural ways
   267
nature
   293, 317, 382, 383, 389, 399, 405
   second
      421
   strong-willed
      393
nature's miracles;natures miracles
   293
naughty
   409, 422
nausea
   101, 217
N-diethyl-M-tolumide
   361
neck
   39, 52, 54, 69, 72, 219, 237, 318
neck, baby's;neck, babys
   61
neck stiff
   237
neck support
   138
neck torsion
   138
negotiating
   393, 417
negotiation
   351, 443
neighbors
   342, 376
Nelsen
   446, 525
Nelsen, Jane
   407
Nelson
   525
Nelson, Jane
   411, 414, 437
neonatal acne
   69
Neosporin
   255
Neosporin pain relief
   255
nerves
   36, 336
nervous system
   172, 269, 273, 278, 336
   central
      215
   immature
      40, 273
   overloaded
      273, 278
   overstimulated
      273
nervous system matures
   170
neural connections, new
   387
neural pathways
   332, 387
   early
      193
   new
      316
neural tube defects
   14
neurologist
   4
Newark
   295
newborn appearance
   33
newborn baby girls
   35
Newborn behavior
   40
newborn boys
   36, 67
newborn care
   41, 66
newborn girls

75
newborn hair
37
newborn head
165
Newborn Illness
66
newborn infants, healthy
49
newborn males
35
Newborn Necessities
52
newborns
3, 23, 31, 36, 43, 66, 73, 77, 81, 92, 142, 145, 170, 317
  average
  165
  dependent
  127
  studied
  385
newborns cartilage
34
newborn screening
29
newborn screening panel
29
newborn screening, universal
48
newborn's eyes;newborns eyes
34
newborn's head;newborns head
36
newborn size
63
newborns nurse
91
newborns sleep
140
newborns wake
140
New Jersey

193
New mattresses
56
newness wares
33
New Parents Survival Guide
111, 124
New pox
247
new RN
204
news
  good
  38, 76, 158, 239, 261, 273, 278, 307, 310
  old
  399
New Zealand
134
NICU
275
niece
53
nightmares
155, 161
nights
143, 154
nighttime
144
nighttime, exacerbate
159
nighttime fears
155
  mild
  156
nighttime separation
290
nighttime separation fears
160
nighttime separation, severe
160
nipples
53, 93, 100, 107, 298
  new

107
sore
100
nipple shields
100
No-Cry Sleep Solution
164
No-Cry- Sleep Solution
526
noise
    41, 77, 96, 148, 162, 171, 174, 189, 270, 292, 345
  background
    148
  barky
    233
  squealing
    178
noise hitting
    283
Noisy breathing
    231
nonexistent
    139
non-fussy times
    319
non-milk/non-soy
    105
non-REM sleep
    141
Non-REM sleep-Non-REM sleep
    142
non-skid soles/socks
    20
non-steroidal option
    72, 252
non-swim time
    375
nonverbal disapproval
    415
nonverbal ques
    422
normal awakenings
    145
normal color variations
    68
normal hunger cry
    293
normal pregnancy changes cause
    130
normal pulsing
    77
normal shape
    34
normal size
    88, 113
normal stressors
    336
normal time
    256
North Scottsdale Pediatric Associates
    77
North Scottsdale Pediatrics
    140, 448
nose
    34, 39, 76, 136, 191, 199, 220, 231, 235, 245, 250, 255, 287, 317
  child's;childs
    287
  runny
    234, 246
  saline
    231
  stuffy
    230
nose contact
    82
Nose Freda
    63
Nose Freida
    231
no-tip bracket
    208
nourishment
    111
Nubby

303
Nubby brand
  179
nudge, little
  124
nuggle time
  331
number
  cell phone
    214, 367
  final
    430
  growing
    48
  important phone
    223
  increasing
    261
  largest
    359
  pediatrician's;pediatricians
    342
  recommended daily
    311
  vehicle license plate
    224
numbness
  117, 220
  facial
    220
Num num
  65
nurse
  1, 4, 24, 80, 89, 92, 97, 111, 118, 124, 133, 146, 281
  full-time
    3
  new mothers
    90
  pediatric
    7, 84, 104
  pediatric triage
    3
  registered

    1
  triage/advice
    18
nursery
  56, 217, 289, 385
nursery Rhymes
  331
nursing
  3, 13, 80, 86, 89, 95, 114, 146, 152, 157, 246, 274, 298
nursing bra
  20
nursing career
  448
nursing degree
  3
nursing moms
  13, 97, 166
nursing mothers
  115, 171
nursing pads
  20
nursing pajamas
  20
nursing sessions
  150
nursing women
  98
nurture
  296, 382, 383, 389, 399
nurturing
  383, 397, 399
nurturing and compassion
  391
nurturing wives
  391
nutrients
  10, 105, 301, 313
nutrition
  90, 105, 297, 313
  best
    88
  extra

149
nutritional
    297
nutritional composition
    86
nutritional content
    309
nutrition babies
    297
nutritious
    89, 309
nuts
    118, 198, 305
nutshell, condensed
    3
Nystatin
    70, 101, 243

O

OAEs measure responses
    31
OAEs (Otoacoustic Emissions);OAEs (Otoacoustic Emissions)
    31
OB/GYN
    7, 130, 351
OB/Gyn, good
    131
object permanence
    282, 327
Object permanence and person permanence
    285
objects
    169, 173, 187, 198, 282, 285, 318, 322, 341
  bright
    318, 322
  colored
    277, 320
  colorful
    318, 321
  comfort/love

159
comfort objects/love
    160
dangling
    173
dropped
    181
familiar
    173, 280
favorite
    318
grab
    322
hidden
    181
hot
    257
moving
    168, 173, 318, 385
off-limits
    421
security
    160
sharp
    210
small
    168, 177, 322
stacking
    326
stationary
    385
visual
    321
obliterating
    262
Obstetricians
    10
Obstetrics
    9, 13
occasions
    2
occasions, multiple
    25, 70
occasions place

549

145
ocean water
371
odor
98, 115, 171, 203
  foul
  66, 116
Offering choices
425
office
18, 66, 125, 204, 237, 243, 250
  doctor's;doctors
  416
  pediatrician's;pediatricians
  67, 76, 235, 245, 250
office hours
18
office workers
349
Ohio State University School
167
oil diffuser
21
oils
69, 73, 218, 362
  baby-safe
  21
  coconut
  73, 363
  excessive
  69
  natural
  373
  soybean
  361, 362
  vegetable
  106
ointment
65, 69, 71, 74, 252
  antibiotic eye
  24
ok
110, 117, 143, 151, 392, 397, 406, 413, 419, 425, 431, 436
ok playing
333
old-fashioned way
91
Omega
12, 14
one-on-one interaction
343
onesies
22, 74
online monitoring
349
only one at a time
199
openers
211
  drain
  205
opinion
8, 17, 21, 41, 45, 229, 308, 346
  personal
  304
Opponents
439
oral hygiene, good
268
oral painkillers
116
oral steroids
233
oral suspension
101
Oral temp/pacifier temp
78
Oral Zyrtec
247
oranges
301
orchards
302
organic compounds
56
Organic fruits

309
organic material
258
organizations
47
organ, largest
361
Ornaments
213
orthodontic pacifier
55
orthotic pacifier
22
ory/newborn-screening/index.php
29
Osteoporosis
88
other-the-counter diaper rash creams
242
otitis media
87
Otoacoustic Emissions (OAEs);Oto-
   acoustic Emissions (OAEs
31
otolaryngology
235
ounces
111, 151, 239
  extra
90
outfits
111, 161
  princess
393
outgrow
5, 72, 82, 225, 307
outgrown
61, 309
outlet plugs
366
outstretched hands
177
oven

208, 427
hot
214
Overage soils
111
overbite, severe
55
over-bundle
147
overcast day
356
overfeeding
81
overheating
137
overload
273
 sensory
162
overprotect
283
overprotective
214
overreacting
211
Overstimulation
161
overwhelmed step
280
oxybenzone
357
oxygen
31, 128, 204, 351
oxygen mask
128, 351
oxygen mask analogy rings
128
oxygen, supplemental
4
oz
4, 12, 63, 81, 85, 91, 96, 108, 143,
   153, 165, 238, 297, 306
oz bottles

63
oz, couple of
90, 239
oz cup
12
oz glass
97
oz vinegar
310

P

PABA
358
pace
169, 185, 196, 348
pacifiers
22, 54, 90, 95, 101, 107, 137, 143, 146, 150, 154, 160, 364
pacifier shield
54
pacifiers use
55
pacifier thermometer
236
pack
21, 64
  cool
254
  gel
359
  gel ice
228
Paddles
443
pads
21, 114, 185
  bumper
61
  color bumper
194
  gauze
65, 74
  heating
114
  maxi
21, 111
  soft cotton
76
  thinnest
21
  waterproof
241
pails
328, 369
pain
96, 99, 101, 115, 118, 219, 232, 236, 254, 257, 274, 277, 364, 442, 444
  chest
217
  constant
238
  emotional
443
  increasing
116
  local
219
  muscle
223
  relieve
116
  severe
371
  severe abdominal
238, 240
painless sensor, small
31
pain medication
257
pain reliever
267, 360
  mild
114
pains, growing
336
paint

56, 209, 394
paint brush
  325
paint hazards
  215
paint, high-quality household enamel
  56
pajamas
  73, 161, 253
pale centers
  250
pale gold
  221
Palmer Reflex- Your
  26
palms
  26, 39, 180, 249
  stripping
    219
Pantley
  526
Pantley, Elizabeth
  164
paraben
  252, 358
paraffin wax
  258
Parental discipline
  446
Parent-child toddler
  374
parenthood
  5, 7, 110, 352
Parenting Article
  111
parenting classes
  1, 7, 192, 259, 380, 440, 447
  private
    2
parenting families
  267
parenting journey
  1, 3
parenting magazine
  124, 295
parenting principles
  425
  appropriate
    425
parents
  5, 27, 48, 155, 159, 187, 262, 294, 307, 337, 344, 373, 378, 388, 399, 412, 422, 430, 433, 439
  authoritative
    414
  best
    128
  child's;childs
    401
  deaf
    192
  expectant
    50
  new
    2, 3, 6, 17, 73, 83, 109, 128, 292
  perfect
    229
  scare
    211
  sex
    389
  spontaneous
    442
  ways
    277
  well-educated
    310
  well-meaning
    388
  working
    339
parent's ability;parents ability
  337
parent's absence;parents absence
  348
parents-Co-parenting
  440
parents discipline

414
parents fear
   83
parent's frustration;parents frustration
   442
parents magazine
   352
Parent's magazine;Parents magazine
   134
parents return
   288
parents sleep
   148
parents smile
   276
parents teach
   294
parents use
   133
Parent-Wise Solutions Inc
   526
park
   122, 410, 432
Parsol
   357
particulates
   215
parties
   164, 210, 213, 369
  slumber
    394
partner
   18, 22, 120, 123, 125, 339, 351
part-time basis
   350
parturition
   16
passage
   36, 69, 230
passenger-side airbag
   227
passing Maggie

125
passion
   3, 6
passive observers
   394
pass objects
   178
Passport Health- Website
   365
pasteurized milk
   12
pat
   70, 73, 241, 327, 365
pat-a-cake
   315, 326, 329
patches
   117, 252
  dry
    71
  white
    101
path, right
   151
patients
   5, 17, 43, 47, 49, 217, 292, 399, 449
  educating
    3
patient tones, pleasant
   345
patios
   122, 222, 393
Patricia Bauer PhD
   390
patterns
   81, 125, 141, 153, 157, 168, 264, 276, 319, 387
  baby's;babys
    276
  contrasting
    168, 318
  distinct sleep
    141
  immature sleeping

141
irregular
40
irregular breathing
40
nice
92, 142
regular
114
regular breathing
142
sleeping
172
pause
40, 422
PBS
390
peaches
300
peaches pears
243
peak age
55, 139
peanut butter powder
305
peanut, little
143, 289
peanuts
305, 307
pears
113, 300
  loved
300
peas
243, 265, 301, 308
  frozen
233
  green
301
  small
99
  uncooked
305
Pedialyte
235, 238, 249, 267
keeping down
239
plain
239
Pedialyte popsicle
256
pediatrician
17, 25, 36, 38, 66, 74, 94, 104, 146, 154, 159, 251, 258, 266, 312
pediatrician nothing
161
pediatric mentor
448
pediatric ophthalmologists
76
Pediatrics
2, 7, 48, 235, 292, 448
pediatrics call
274
pediatric triage protocol
77
peek
156, 159, 181, 283, 316, 323, 326
peek-a-boo
138, 315, 323, 329
peel
198, 258
  orange
317
peeling skin
69, 70
peers
295, 348, 390, 396
pelvic bone
37
penis
27, 36
pens
420
pediatric epinephrine
251
people respect

278
people's feelings;peoples feelings
  392
people sleep
  146
people stop
  382
people teaching parenting classes year
  2
percentages
  44
perception
  423
  depth
  168
perfumes
  69, 361
perineal soreness
  119
perineum
  115
period
  baby's sleep;babys sleep
  141
  brief
  83, 152, 168
  extended
  123
  long
  132, 276
  longer
  172, 183
  menstrual
  88, 131
  probationary
  341
  prolonged
  116, 120
  short
  130, 169, 172, 252
period-of-time
  9
Permanent color

34
permethrin
  361, 363
Perseus Books
  525
Persistence
  282
person
  17, 215, 219, 229, 287, 289, 376, 387, 399, 408, 414, 420, 444
  beautiful
  395
  morning
  158
  new
  278, 291
  right
  190
  small little
  293
personality
  2, 281, 296, 383, 390, 399
personal time
  349
person feeding
  54
person feeling
  401
person interview
  339
person permanence
  279, 283
perspective
  194, 433
  baby's;babys
  404
  husband's;husbands
  394
pesticides
  201, 310
  chemical
  309
pet dander

556

127
Peter Juscyzk PhD
187
petroleum-based products
205
pets
126, 209, 261, 341, 422
  household
  254
PET scans
386
PH
372
pharmacist
2, 104
phase
274, 312
PhD, Jill
525
PhD, Michael
525
Philadelphia
13, 404
philodendron
202
Phoenix Childrens Hospital
227
Phoenix Perinatal Associates
10
phone
22, 122, 210, 214, 332, 339, 372, 436
  cell
  229, 349
  smart
  349
photo album, safe
347
photos
22, 195
phototherapy
80
phrase
183, 190, 388, 422
physical abilities
409
physical appearance
396
physical blockers
358
physical health set
383
physical punishment
441
  safe
  443
physical setting
344
physical sunblock
357
physicians
8, 49, 76, 79, 82, 134, 205, 232, 244, 250, 252, 266, 449
  board-certified
  449
  brilliant
  2
  fabulous
  2
Physician's Assistant;Physicians Assistant
2
physiologic regulations
157
piano bench
209
PICC
3
Picking items
325
picky eater
312
picture books
323
pictures
57, 161, 195, 304, 318, 323, 330,

      344, 347, 352, 387, 409
  colorful
    331
  label
    295
  large
    328
Piedmont dermatologist
  357
Piglet toothbrush
  426
pill
  204
  grandmother's insulin;grand-
    mothers insulin
    204
pillows
  21, 61, 137, 145, 221, 396
pillows quilts
  137
pimples
  250
  little
    69
pincer
  180, 221
pinches
  420, 424, 438
Pink eye
  244
Pink eye and ear infections
  244
pink feather boa
  393
pin prick
  222
pins
  199, 214
pipes
  215
pipes call
  216
pitch

      331, 368
pitting, minor
  265
Pittsburg
  157
Pittsburgh
  155
PKU test
  30
placement fee
  50
placenta
  10, 12, 15, 35, 42, 49
placenta capsules
  16
placenta, desiccated
  16
placenta encapsulation
  15
Placental Encapsulation/Placento-
    phagy
  15
placentophagy
  16
place strings
  214
plan
  2, 20, 25, 84, 102, 112, 117, 142,
    149, 239, 316, 339, 347, 380
  escape
    215
  nap schedule
    153
plane
  128, 323, 365
Plantar
  26
plants
  202, 269, 317, 360, 406
  dangerous
    202
  holiday
    214
  medicinal

205
plasma
   42, 47
plastic
   21, 56, 199
plastic baggie
   368
plastic bags
   102, 199, 210
plastic containers
   327
plastic cookie cutters
   327
platelets
   4, 42
  low
    4
plate, small
   303
playground
   390, 406
playground equipment
   396
playing
   174, 177, 295, 303, 320, 327, 391, 393, 398, 402, 410, 416, 418
playing dress
   393
playing horsey
   83
playing peek
   291
playmate
   405, 434
playpens
   59, 415, 419, 438
  mesh
    59
playtime
   316, 333
  extra
    144
plenty

96, 237, 360, 397
pm
   147, 150, 276
pm bedtime
   158
pneumonia
   5, 87, 154, 215, 251
pocket, small
   136
poem
   410
  little
    191
Poinsettias
   214
Poison
   206
Poison control number- Poison help
   203
Poison helpline
   203
poisonings
   201, 205
pokes
   295, 420
policy, standard hospital
   24
policy statement
   48
polish
  wearing nail
    393
  wear nail
    392
pollen
   261, 307
ponds
   262, 369
pooh toothbrush
   426
pool
   265, 370, 375
  public

371
stagnant
361
swimming
221, 369
wading
210
pool fence
377
pool pumps
222
pool thinking
373
pool time
372
popcorn
198, 305
Popkin
414, 525
Popkin, Michael
414, 446
popsicles
235, 249, 267
Popular magazines
399
population
44
  widow
222
  world's;worlds
29
pores
69
  blocked-off skin
39
pork chop
304
position
  baby's;babys
34
  carriage
62
  crossed-legged

38
down
59
head shifts
26
highest
56
lower
351
lowest
57, 209
lying
135
middle
56
national
3
normal
35, 38
open
213
reclining
62
recommended back-lying
135
side-lying
135
supine
135
upright
174
positive adult-child interaction,
    frequent
343
positive discipline approach
444
positive discipline books
414
positive interactions
332, 423
positive outcomes, predicted
343
positive reinforcement

435
Positive reinforcement for Desired
    Behavior-;Positive reinforce-
    ment for Desired Behavior
435
positive self-confidence
409
positive way
440
posterior fontanel
37
post-partum
16
postpartum
7, 113
postpartum blues
127
  women experience
127
Post Partum Depression
129
post-partum, more energy
16
post-partum period
113
Post Partum Period
111
postpone menstruation
88
post-term
10
potatoes
301
  mashed
240, 302
  sweet
240, 243, 300, 312
potato sprouts
202
powder
73, 365
  baby cornstarch
73, 365
  fine

16
  treated black
205
Powdered form
107
power
211, 229, 383, 421, 436
power strip
209
pox
246
  chicken
246
  open
246
practice
  century-old
15
  common
29
  pediatric
266
praise
403, 406, 423, 435
praise character
408
praise children's character;praise
    childrens character
408
praise compassion
408
praise, honest
407, 423
preboard
365
precious jewels
52
predictability
316, 430
predictor, good
350
preemie, little
61
preemies

561

    37, 154, 167, 200, 275, 335
Prefers mother
    286
pregnancy
    3, 7, 13, 88, 98, 104, 113, 125, 129, 141, 234, 358
  duration of
    9
  high-risk
    3
  last trimester of
    13
  normal
    13
  second
    4
  started teaching
    3
Pregnant women
    15
Prelone
    233
preparedness
    345
preschool
    295, 348, 441
preschool age group
    162
preschool/daycare
    343
preschoolers
    193, 390
preschool setting
    386
prescribe
    70, 119
prescribe creams
    116
prescription
    84, 101, 333, 365
prescription cream
    252
prescription diaper rash cream
    70
prescription medication
    242
prescription, valid
    85
pressure
    34, 40, 55, 76, 99, 135, 234, 257, 269, 316, 348, 366, 408
pressure bar gates
    58
pressure, putting
    77
Preventable injuries
    197
prevention
    16, 221
  cavity
    264
  child abuse
    83
prevention division
    129
price, small
    76
Prickly Heat
    72
Prima publishing
    525
Prima Publishing1993
    525
princess dresses, wearing
    395
Prioritize
    352
Private banks
    49
Private cord blood banks charge
    50
privileges
    2, 17, 342
probiotics
    241
  purchase infant

241
problem
    131, 141, 145, 227, 262, 280, 291, 302, 396, 431, 441
  circulatory
    119
  decreased breathing
    335
  dental
    55
  increased behavioral
    215
  large scorpion
    221
  long-term
    23, 244, 252
  male
    397
  math
    386
  neurological
    26
  public health
    261
problem solving
    318, 322, 325
process
    143, 152, 157, 283, 385, 438
  cognitive
    279, 283
  developmental
    280
  gradual
    35
procrastinating
    118
products
    58, 64, 67, 138, 202, 212, 247, 262, 302, 304, 358, 361, 368
  cleaning
    201
  cow's milk;cows milk
    305
  dairy

239
  egg
    309
  first aid
    360
  lawn
    202
  natural
    362
  new favorite
    252
  plant-derived
    362
  plasma
    4
  vinegar
    218
progesterone
    131
program
    345, 376
  amazing
    378
  aquatic
    377
  learn-to-swim
    375
  progression
    247
  safe
    378
progressive aching sensation
    223
Promises
    432
prone
    52, 134, 234, 371
prone position
    135
proof
    13, 218
Prop
    323
pros

1, 27, 355, 437
protection
    67, 88, 102, 354, 357, 362, 374
protective coating
    75
protective substances
    87
protein
    10, 14, 16, 106
  allergic food
    308
  broken down
    107
protein hydrosolate formulas
    107
Protien Hydrosoalates
    105
provider
    8, 17, 26, 256, 259, 313, 347, 419
  healthcare
    17
prunes
    243, 300, 312
Psychiatry
    129
psychological adjustment
    129
Psychologists Michael Lewis
    287
psychology
    187, 287, 377, 406
  pediatric
    387
pubic bone
    33, 113
puddles
    262, 370
puffy
    34, 244
pull
    93, 101, 175, 180, 185, 210, 214,
    221, 227, 251, 254, 258, 322
pull moisture

    144
pull pool
    370
pull toys
    326
  music push
    328
pulse oximeter
    31
pulse oximeter measures
    31
pump
    59, 80, 84, 98, 104, 292
pumping
    85, 89, 99, 103, 173
pumping equipment
    107
pumpkin, little
    429
punish
    426, 446
punishment
    438, 446
  punitive
    414, 419, 437
punitive disciplinary approaches-
    Dictators
    414
punitive time
    437
Purple Crying
    274
purse
    206, 229, 368
pursuits
    349
  artistic
    278
pus
    39
  drains
    250
push
    173, 176, 179, 182, 203, 213, 298,

321, 326, 328, 331
final
1
least
239
Push cars and toys
185
pushed gates
58
push feet
335
pushing
113, 243, 438
push mom
428
push toys
185
Putt
324
Putting objects in containers-;Putting objects in containers
325
Putting window locks
208
puzzles
386, 396, 436
  chunky
  328

Q

Q-tip
101
quadruple birthweight
166
Quakers
247
queso Blanco
12
queso franco
12
Question List
17, 340
questionnaire
7
questions
  basic
  130
  medical
  8
  nurses
  41
  pediatrician interview
  17
  warmup
  340
Questran
70, 242
quickest
421, 446
quickest way
407
quivers
41, 170

R

rabies
254
rabies shots
254
rainbow
301, 394
raisins
200, 312
Rapid eye movement
141
Rapid flu cultures
18
rash
38, 68, 232, 237, 241, 245, 251, 364
  chicken pox
  246
  colored
  237
  common

        39
    distinct
        248
    localized
        253
    main
        242
    netlike
        248
    peeling
        241
    purple
        77
    red
        68
    severe skin
        107
    small pinpoint
        253
    yeast diaper
        70, 242
rash appointment
    252
rash guards
    355
raspberries
    177
    start blowing
        281
ratio, small
    348
rattle
    199, 321
raw
    16, 241
raw eggs
    12, 306
rays
    357
    harmful
        356
    sun's;suns
        356
    ultraviolet

        354
    rays UVA
        356
    razors
        207
    reabsorption
        81
    reactions
        26, 67, 280, 288, 307, 308
        anaphylactic
            307, 365
        baby's;babys
            288
        chemical
            210
        defense
            422
        drug
            267
        emotional
            131
    readiness
        346
        baby's;babys
            291
    Reading nook
        419
    rear wheels
        62
    reason
        5, 16, 20, 75, 85, 89, 136, 144,
        238, 245, 273, 378, 385
        best
            191
        good
            136
        main
            57
        medical
            146
        next
            156
        possible

135
reasonable science-based precautions, taking
148
reason babies
76
reassurance
160, 162, 293, 417, 422
Re- Bink
160
receipt
217
receptive learner
404
recharges
153, 293
reclines
59, 225
Recognition
406
recommendations
24, 59, 105, 135
  new
    147, 251, 305
  new FDA
    232
Recommendations for Water conditions
372
reconnecting
288
recovery
113
recovery, better cell
46
recovery mission
378
recovery room
124
rectal stitches
119
rectal suppositories
119
rectal temperature lubricate

78
red blood
114
red blood, bright
114
red blood cells break
79
red bumps
71
  small
    250
red cheeks
248
  bright
    248
red circular mark
223
redirect
416, 422, 438
redirections
419, 433, 437
redness
29, 36, 66, 116, 219, 244, 253
red rouge
287
reds
168, 365
red spots
247, 249
  small
    247
Reeder M, David J.;Reeder M, David J
449
reflex
25, 292, 298, 375, 421
  emotional
    293
  grasping
    26
  high gag
    304
  startle
    26, 41, 67
  stepping

26
tongue-thrust
    298
reflex responses
    23
reflux
    52, 82, 149, 274
  severe
    53, 107, 136
refrigeration
    103
regain
    96, 117
register
    49, 216
registration card
    224
regret
    214, 442
Regular cooking oatmeal
    247
Regularity-How
    282
reinforcements
    352
reinforcing
    408, 413
rein, tight
    126
relationship
    122, 296, 315, 404, 440, 446
  cherishing
    398
  close
    288
  healthy
    348
  personal
    287
  social
    315
  spatial
    396
  supportive

    382
  trusting
    413
relatives
    122
relax
    21, 159, 180, 243, 278, 320, 323, 338, 349, 445
  help mom
    337
relaxation help
    161
Relaxing music
    21
release
    48, 56, 334
release toxins
    364
relief
    120, 315
relieve
    99, 115, 442
relieved symptoms
    127
reminder
    195, 430
  gentle
    193
remotes, small
    211
removable pieces
    161
REM pattern
    142
REM sleep
    141, 270
REM sleep and non-REM sleep
    141
repellants
    362
  insect
    363
repellents

362
bug
361
combination sunscreen/insect
362
excellent
363
great natural
363
residual
362
repetition
330, 420
Repetitive forceful vomiting
109
Report Unrestrained Children
223
Reproductive Health
129
Reputable Cord Blood Banks
46
research
15, 42, 47, 57, 330, 349, 353, 378, 385, 391, 398
research journals
399
research organization
350
research scientist
349
research, swimming
376
resentment
439, 443
reserves
177, 239, 443
residual fumes
56
residue, possible
102
resilient
3, 5
resistance

262
bacterial
262
resources
7, 41, 132, 147, 163, 411
great
8
respect
292, 352, 367, 408, 414, 420, 425
respect, mutual
440
respect people's feelings;respect peoples feelings
295
respirations, rapid
233
respiratory distress
230, 233
respiratory rate
231
Respiratory Syncytial Virus
233
response
32, 139, 281, 393, 404, 431
echo
31
healthy
288
left-brain
446
loving
294
predictable physical
270
right brain
446
tests parental
286
responsibilities
121, 296, 342, 351, 396, 399, 428
age-appropriate
407
mom's;moms

89
restaurant
    200, 393, 416
restlessness
    130, 145, 220
restraint
    274, 444
restrictions
    224
restroom
    20, 119
resume
    273
  menstrual cycles
    115
  menstrual periods
    115
resume menstruation
    115
retention figures range
    378
retina
    167, 385
retract
    75
retractions
    75, 231, 233
return
    36, 88, 111, 117, 126, 288
  hormone levels
    127
  reproductive organs
    113
return home
    425
Reverse osmosis filters
    266
reward
    436
  child's favorite;childs favorite
    435
  greatest
    436
  lifelong

164
overuse
    436
pleasant
    435
reward kids
    389
Reye's syndrome;Reyes syndrome
    247
RH
    25
RH antibodies
    25
Rhea Paul PHD
    315
Rh factor
    81
rhymes
    275, 285, 330
  sounds sing nursery
    324
Rhythmic songs and games
    285
rhythms
    125, 183, 282, 285, 330
ribbons
    161, 199, 213, 321
rice cereal constipates
    299
Richard Ferber- Solve Your Child's
    Sleep Problems;Richard Fer-
    ber- Solve Your Childs Sleep
    Problems
    164
Richard MD
    526
Richmond, Maryanne
    411
rich sources
    15
ride
    153, 214, 226, 396, 424, 429
rinse

570

70, 74, 101, 218, 241, 310
Rinse in cold water and air
　　　102
rinse kids
　　　373
rinse, ocean
　　　364
rinsing
　　　115, 310
risk
　　　11, 24, 27, 135, 137, 236, 266,
　　　　304, 312, 353, 370, 439, 441
　drowning
　　　374
　high
　　　47, 258
　highest
　　　229
　lower
　　　27
　main
　　　311
　possible
　　　361
　reasonable
　　　407
　reduced
　　　88
risk benefits
　　　361
risk factors
　　　359
　high
　　　216
Rit Sun Guard
　　　356
RN
　　　1
road
　　　431
　bumpy
　　　83
robe

　　　20
Robert Mckenzie author
　　　439
rock
　　　60, 112, 126, 144, 320, 326
rocket ships
　　　386
rocking
　　　144, 148, 152, 157, 163, 272, 277
　gentle
　　　146
　staff members
　　　344
rocking chair
　　　277, 320
Rogers, Fred
　　　315
role
　　　120, 294, 387, 390, 398, 405
　critical
　　　390
　helper's;helpers
　　　120
　important
　　　398
role models
　　　398, 402
　good
　　　355
　positive
　　　410
roll
　　　102, 138, 175, 199, 317, 321, 326,
　　　　444
　alligator death
　　　430
Ron Fischler M
　　　448
room
　　　20, 118, 122, 147, 152, 162, 167,
　　　　178, 194, 207, 209, 415, 419
　child's;childs
　　　156
　darkened

274, 278
empty
  56
glass
  85
guest
  207, 445
hospital emergency
  55, 60
room temperature
  103, 109
  elevated
    137
Roosevelt, Eleanor
  197
Rooting reflex
  26
Roquefort
  12
Roseola
  245
Rosyln
  525
roughest time
  267
routine fluoride supplements, recommending
  266
routine formula supplements
  95
routines
  123, 127, 146, 157, 159, 188, 274, 277, 342, 352, 404, 414, 430
  child's;childs
    367
  daily
    153, 331
  normal
    159
  repeated
    316
  setting
    430
routine vitamins
  313
RSV
  233
RSV infection
  234
RSV vaccine, new
  234
rub
  37, 154, 220, 278, 322
  gentle head
    154
  menthol
    201
  rubber
    209
  smooth
    319
Rubbermaid type container
  327
rubbing
  26, 336
Rubin, Gretchen
  6
rules
  144, 152, 199, 405, 408, 413, 420, 423, 427, 430, 434
  firm
    92, 142
  important
    428
  society's;societys
    414
Run Naked
  408
runner, fast
  396
runny
  230
  longer
    306
rush
  160, 233, 396, 432
rush home

41
Rutgers University
193

S

sadness
  127, 295, 350, 397
Safe Drinking
  216
Safesleep
  139
safesleeptech.com
  139
safest place
  227
safest way
  305
safety
  138, 197, 212, 223, 226, 288, 318, 344, 363, 377, 404, 415
  kid's;kids
    155
  traffic
    223
safety administration
  225
safety belts
  224
safety council
  212
safety devices
  58, 366, 373
Safety First
  207
safety hint
  306
safety label
  361
safety latches
  415
safety lecture
  262
safety measure, extra
  366
Safety Numbers
  211
safety precaution
  376
safety proof
  283
safety regulations
  55
safety risks
  185
safety skills
  346
safety standpoint
  182
safety step
  377
safety strap
  214
safety sweep
  366
safety tip
  306
safety training
  340
sailing, smooth
  1
saline
  231, 367
saliva
  256
saliva, baby's;saliva, babys
  100
saliva triggering
  210
salmon
  12, 14, 106
salmonella
  12, 305
  growing conditions harbor
    305
salt
  300
Saltwater pools

373
samples
   30, 48
sand
   356, 363, 434
  child throwing
   427
  dried
   364
sanitation, modern
   261
sanity
   272, 351
Sassy
   276
satisfied call
   95
scab
   247
  dry brown
   247
  yellow
   36, 250
scalp
   36, 39, 69, 71, 73
  baby's;babys
   73
scare
   112, 229
scarlet fever
   253
scarring, bad
   257
scary
   39, 41, 256, 429
scary situation
   204
scent
   21, 160, 281
  baby's;babys
   126
scented soaps
   361
schedule
   149, 153, 159, 250, 278, 340, 346, 352
  predictable
   279
vaccine
   18
Schmidt, Barton
   2, 440
Schmitt
   417, 525
Schmitt, Barton
   34, 39, 77, 80, 162, 166, 269, 272, 411, 415, 435, 437
school
   3, 162, 232, 295, 331, 343, 348, 390, 401, 403, 406, 442
  elementary
   395
  high
   193, 200, 394, 395
school age children
   441
Schuster1985
   526
Schwindt, Angela
   129
scientists
   54, 193, 383, 387
scissors
   213
  small
   368
sclera
   244
sclerosis, multiple
   261
scoop
   376
  letting new people
   283
score
   23, 32
  maximum

23
scorpions
  219
  species of
  219
scorpion's food source;scorpions food source
  222
scorpion stings
  222
scrapes
  40, 254, 364, 371
Scream
  408
screaming
  124, 428
  full-on
  271
screams bloody murder
  288
screen
  31, 187, 356
  fine
  221
  mesh
  58
screening panel
  30
  state's newborn;states newborn
  29
screenings
  30
screen newborns
  31
screentime
  332
Screen time
  332
screwdriver
  209
Scribbling
  325
scrotum

35
seafood
  11
  refrigerated smoked
  11
  shelf-safe smoked
  11
seal
  72, 93, 96, 221
seat
  22, 59, 62, 136, 223, 359, 366, 403, 418, 425, 429
  assigned
  365
  cart
  429
  facing
  225
seat belts
  59, 213, 226
  regular
  226
seat information
  223
seat locator
  223
seat rear
  63
seats fit
  224
seat tipping
  58
Seattle
  135
Sea World
  214
seconds
  40, 78, 83, 149, 214, 262, 439
secretions
  41, 230, 245
security
  269, 288, 373, 392, 402, 430, 443
Sedona Arizona

575

371
self
  emerging
    294
  usual
    281
self-assurance
  401
self-comfort
  146
self-comforting
  278
self-control
  419, 440, 444
self-control, time learning
  414
self-control trick
  446
self-discipline
  412
self-esteem
  395, 401, 407, 409, 441
  child's;childs
    401
  healthy
    348, 406
  healthy/positive
    432
  low
    414
  parent's;parents
    402
  person's;persons
    407
  positive
    268, 402, 423
Self Esteem
  401
self-feeding utensils
  65
Self-image
  287
self-indulgent

349
selfish
  349
  little
    128
selfless people
  449
self soothe
  140, 173, 280
self-soothe
  133, 150
semesters
  4, 193
Senekot
  119
senior year philanthropy project
  193
sensitivity
  296, 354
sensitization
  306
sensory books
  330
Sensory threshold
  282
separation
  155, 159, 162, 288, 290
separation anxiety
  155, 159, 178, 283, 287, 289, 316
  nighttime
    159, 323
separation fears
  155, 347
Serena Gordon Health Day News
  441
Serotonin
  334
set activities
  344
set limits
  412
set nap times
  158
set schedule

152
severity
    76, 231, 258
sexes
    386, 397
sex roles
    392
sex-role stereotyping
    398
shades
    168, 354, 385
  blackout
    158, 163
shaking
    83, 190
shampoo
    21, 73
  anti- dandruff
    73
Shannon, Keith
    352
Sharing toys
    435
Shearer
    50
Shearer, William T.;Shearer, William T
    49
sheets
    61, 71, 139, 210, 377
  fitted
    137
  tight-fitting crib
    56
shellfish
    305, 307
Shelov
    526
shelves
    213
shiny
    98, 422
shock

307, 445
small
    210
shoes
    26, 118, 185, 221, 229, 232, 361, 363, 403, 445
  flexible
    185
  great
    185
  high-heeled princess
    393
  house princess
    392
  pink plastic princess
    393
shopping
    429, 436
shopping basket
    62
shopping carts
    213
shopping trip
    436
short break
    437
short excerpt
    15
Short goodbyes make dryer eyes
    290
short sleeves
    74
short time
    79, 273, 289
shots
    24, 233, 255
  antibiotic
    289
shoulder belt
    227
shoulder blades
    200
shoulder level

225
shoulders
    37, 71, 137, 172, 225, 248, 318
  baby's;babys
    96
shower
    21, 57, 99, 115, 206
shrimp
    14, 200
  cooked
    12
shy
    222, 286, 388, 414, 416
shyness, quiet
    278
sick hours
    18
sickle cell anemia
    47
side effects
    43
  long-term
    204
sidewalk
    128, 325
  bumpy
    83
side windows
    367
SIDS
    54, 76, 134, 139
  incidence of
    74, 135, 139
  risk of
    54, 74, 134, 148, 159
SIDS and swaddling Arizona Parenting
    139
SIDS Prevention Recommendations
    136
SIDS studies
    54
Siegel, Jeffrey

134
sight
    144, 147, 155, 195, 279, 282, 286, 291, 327
  long-range
    169
  short-range
    169
signed Dylan
    378
signing
    184, 192
sign language
    191, 433
  basic
    285
signs
    78, 107, 109, 115, 116, 119, 128, 192, 222, 230, 233, 250, 253, 258
  basic
    183
  danger
    233
  first
    265, 316
  good
    234, 292
  healthy
    289
  positive
    287
  severe
    231
signs and symptoms of dehydration
    238, 240
signs and symptoms of infection
    40, 219, 223, 255, 258
Signs and symptoms of respiratory distress
    230
Signs of illness
    77
Sigrid Leo

269
silence
    189
    vow
        112
Simethicone
    82
Simethicone gas
    64
Simethicone infant
    82
Simon
    526
sing
    138, 189, 277, 319
sing songs
    190
sink
    70, 136, 242, 344
sister
    1, 4, 45, 390, 392
    older
        394
sister-in-law
    53
site
    74, 219, 223, 253, 293
    pricked
        30
    surgical
        28
    web
        46
sitter
    290, 333
sitting position
    57, 172, 180, 279, 318, 324
    cradled
        319
    cuddled
        277
Sitz baths
    70, 242
size restrictions
    59
sizes
    older
        54
    standard
        55
skills
    140, 158, 196, 376, 386
    basic water survival
        375
    cognitive
        282
    coping
        410
    developing personal and social
        277, 319, 323, 326
    important
        140
    important life
        346
    important visual
        321
    intellectual
        377
    learned
        89
    new
        158, 407
    new large motor
        169
    physical
        410
    sensory motor
        377
    start building swim readiness
        374
    verbal
        185, 191
skim
    90
skin
    36, 38, 67, 75, 79, 206, 219, 222, 231, 250, 252, 256, 357
    bumpy

579

252
common
358
crusty
73
delicate
75, 241
dry
72
extra
35
irritate
241
little
365
reddened
257
rinse
73
sensitive
67
thin
356
white
359
skin call
253
skin cancer
353, 357, 359
  new cases of
353, 359
skin contact
335
skin damage
356
skin disorders
337
skin graft
257
skin irritation
355
skin sensitivity
257
skin symptoms
306
skin tastes
420
skin use tweezers
254
skin www.cancer.skincancer.org
353
skull
37
  baby's;babys
76
Slats
55
sleep
54, 103, 112, 120, 133, 161, 211, 256, 265, 270, 273, 448
  broken
132
  light sleepers
149
  longer
336
  nighttime
153
  restless
270
  safe
161, 342
  weighed
140
sleep approach
133
sleep book, perfect
163
sleep campaign
134
sleep deprivation
112
sleep disturbances
157
sleep drowsy
144
sleeper, good

90, 148
Sleepers
   22
sleep experts
   158
sleep experts call
   147
sleep guidelines
   138
sleep habits, good
   133, 143
sleeping through the night
   141
sleep issues
   148
sleep lecture
   199
sleep method
   164
sleep noises
   41
Sleep Patterns
   141, 159
  active
     141
  quiet
     142
sleep plan
   148
sleep positions
   136
sleep problems
   131
sleep regression
   156
Sleep Safety
   161
sleep saliva production
   265
sleep schedule
   153
sleep space
   137
sleep train

154, 159
sleep-train
   154, 163
sleep training
   142, 155, 162
Sleepwear
   211
sleepy, acting
   256
sleepy call
   256
slippers
   20, 118
slots, upper
   225
Small activity gym
   64
small amounts breast milk
   238
small amount thaws
   102
Smalley, Gary
   401
Small flashlight
   368
small toys
   199
smear
   265, 305
  small
     198, 305
smells
   13, 54, 67, 126, 147, 171, 286, 317
  everyday
     317
  pleasant
     317
  sugary
     171
smile
   172, 189, 263, 272, 276, 284, 292, 294, 318, 323, 326, 423, 435
  best

177
healthy
268
social
174, 292
smiling
272, 319, 418
smoke
215
smoke detectors, multiple
215
Smoked Seafood
11
smoke, secondhand
215
snacks
312, 366, 416
snags
66
Sneak
347
sneeze
41, 77
snow
354, 356
snowflakes
196
snug
137, 226
snuggling
289, 329, 404
soak
101, 258, 310
  baby's bottom;babys bottom
70
soaking
115, 120
soap
67, 73, 115, 252
  antibacterial
253, 257, 310
  mild
69, 253
  mild baby

252
unscented
72, 252
use baby
72
soap and water
206, 219, 258, 262, 362, 364
soapy H2O, hot
102
Social interactions start
295
socialization
314
social people
348
social ques
294
social skills
277, 319, 323, 326
social time
327
Societies
388
society
382, 388, 390, 395
  gender stereotypical
391
sock, old
247
socks
22, 73
soft fluffy
21
Soft music
321
Soft Robis
185
soft spots
37, 76, 237
soft surface
135
soft washcloth
115, 241, 264
Sognovello, Lisa

12
soles
    39, 249
  nonskid
    185
solid foods
    13, 67, 71, 98, 105, 156, 298
  started
    156
  withholding
    238
solids
    71, 108, 156, 238, 243, 297, 313
  giving
    299
  started
    156, 177, 243, 322
  withholding
    238
solids rule
    314
Solona
    139
Something Happy
    162
son
    5, 27, 36, 53, 74, 154, 200, 206,
    209, 325, 378, 389, 392, 397
son Dylan
    4, 388
songs
    157, 183, 320, 329, 377
  baby action
    329
  sang
    376
son playing dress
    393
son turn
    371
soothe
    150, 154, 162, 203, 276, 320, 323,
    326, 360, 402
Soothie

22
soothing
    100, 150, 274
soothing effect
    320
soothing music
    320
soothing tones
    319
  happy
    277
soothing words
    152
Sophie Bulk MD chair
    216
Sophomore
    5
sores
    70, 250
  open
    70
  yellow
    241
sounds
    21, 25, 31, 75, 138, 145, 170, 187,
    277, 281, 286, 291, 328
  crunchy
    319
  gentle
    321
  happy
    318
  putting
    281
sounds monitor
    163
sound stimulation
    330
sources
  excellent
    49
  good
    240
  great

14
main
297, 314
South Africa
29
South America
29, 335
Southern Connecticut State University
315
South Korea
29
soy
105, 305, 308
Soy formulas
106, 240
Soymilk formulas
106
soy protein
106
spacing
264, 268
spank
440
spanking
414, 437, 441
parents use
441
specialist
5, 32, 308
pediatric eye
354
Special Thank
448
Special time together-It
433
species
11, 15, 219
diff
221
spectrum
356
speech

55, 180, 185, 190, 268, 332
long
434
near-normal
32
slurred
220
SPF
356
SPF ratings
358
SPF sun protection
356
Spice
400
spills
350, 426
spit
41, 52, 71, 81, 109
baby's;babys
100
painful
82
spit bubbles
178
spitting
53, 81
spit-up
41, 82
normal
81
spit up/reflux
81
spoil
145, 277, 319
sponge
74
spoon
298, 303, 327
spoons, measuring
327
sporting events
332
sports

396, 410
sports bar
    393
sports, organized
    396, 409
spots
    59, 67, 71, 95, 119, 242, 247, 250,
        342, 360, 367, 445
  flat
    76, 138
  isolated
    364
  pink
    250
  safest
    224
  satellite
    70
  small
    250
  warm
    119
spotting
    74, 168
spouse
    120, 126, 179, 409, 422, 433, 440
sprays
    116, 363
  bug
    363
  repellent
    363
sprinkles
    73, 241, 364
squash
    240, 301
  yellow
    243
squeak
    77, 328
squeal
    280
squeeze

364, 426
Squirrels
    254
stability
    59
Stacking toys
    328
staff
    41, 343
staff/child ratio
    343
staff, good
    345
staff-infant ratios, low
    343
staff members
    346
staff ratio
    343
staff turnover
    345
stage
  normal
    392
  temporary
    446
staining, brown
    266
Stair gates
    58
stairs
    58, 438
Stall
    402
Stamm
    383, 525
Stamm, Jill
    288, 329, 332, 382, 387
Stamm's book;Stamms book
    383
standards
    55
  double

585

397
optimum
   343
standing
   120, 177, 179, 325, 405
standing position
   38, 57, 181, 324
standpoint
   249
  developmental
   192
start
   33, 84, 123, 142, 151, 155, 173, 178, 183, 267, 277, 294, 299, 338, 365, 400, 421
start eating
   67
start feeding
   91
startles
   77, 270, 278
start lessons
   374
start school
   414
start solids
   156, 279, 298, 313
start sprouting
   265
state laws
   17
statement
   22, 48, 395
state-of-the-art facility
   46
states
   1, 12, 29, 48, 224, 266, 270, 274, 369, 379, 408, 437, 439
  active
   271
  clear boundaries
   439
  local

224, 345
normal pre-pregnancy
   131
pre-pregnant
   113
wide-awake
   272
state screens
   31
stations
   59, 64, 77, 178, 279, 317, 323
statistics
   33, 45, 86, 124, 129, 350, 395
st-ban-oxybenzone-in-sunscreen-now
   358
St Christopher's Hospital;St Christophers Hospital
   404
STD
   27
steam
   198, 273
stem cells
   42
  mature bone marrow
   43
  precious
   51
Stem cell transplantations
   48
  hematopoietic
   49
step commands
   190
Stephany Watson
   106
stereotypes, traditional
   391
stereotypical
   390
steri-stips
   117
steri-strips

117, 259
stern
　417, 422
steroidal creams
　252
Steven
　526
Steven Shilov Chairman
　292
stick
　58, 195, 267, 302, 320, 352, 367
stickers, little
　32
sticking
　194, 393
stiff
　171, 180
stiffening, brief
　41
stillbirths
　248
stimulate language development
　188, 315
stimulate milk production
　88, 337
stimulation
　271, 278, 333, 387
　cognitive language
　　343
　extra
　　273
　natural sensory
　　336
　oral
　　299, 313
stimuli
　25, 273, 282
　negative
　　270
　new
　　291
　positive
　　270
sting

219, 254, 362, 372
stinger
　254, 364
sting site
　220
Stings- Wasps
　364
sting, yellow jacket
　254
Stock
　63
stomach
　79, 82, 118, 135, 140, 148, 158, 170, 203, 227, 231, 303, 318, 321
　3-chambered
　　15
　baby's;babys
　　82
stomach hurt
　118
stomach position
　134
Stone, Elizabeth
　42
stooling
　68, 134, 240
stools
　41, 68, 79, 94, 107, 235, 240, 243, 249
　baby's;babys
　　299
　black colored
　　68
　black tarry
　　68
　black thick sticky
　　94
　blood in
　　107, 238
　normal breastfed
　　244
　watery

240
 yellow
  240
stools call
 68
stools change
 94
Stools for BF babies
 94
stool softeners
 119
Stooping
 326
stop
 41, 45, 149, 273, 314, 317, 409, 416, 420, 422, 428
stop behavior
 422
stop breathing
 371
stop, helping child
 438
stop playing
 174, 410
Stop Reference Guide
 525
stops snowing
 128
storage
 45, 48
storage areas
 222
storage, baby's;storage, babys
 313
storage space
 48
stores
 310
 inadequate
  24
 maternal
  10
storms

 1, 429
story
 2, 6, 84, 118, 331, 370, 378, 393, 394, 421, 424, 445, 449
 little
  112
 long
  289
 personal
  2
 sharing
  8
 short
  331
straighten
 26, 38
straining
 41, 95
strains
 41, 119, 241
stranger anxiety
 291
strangers
 44, 122, 188, 283, 286, 290
 important
  283
strangle
 56, 60
Strangulation
 213
strangulation hazard
 56, 59
strapping
 85, 227
straps
 60, 209, 214, 225
 position harness
  225
 tether
  225
 waist
  60
straw

136
strawberries
　　　301
streaks
　　　95, 253
　red
　　　102
stress
　　　26, 86, 103, 110, 211, 314, 335
stress autonomy
　　　290
stress, extra
　　　85
stress hormones
　　　334
stretch
　　　152, 157, 173, 195
　long
　　　143
stretching
　　　98, 115
strides, new
　　　50
stridor
　　　232
strings
　　　161, 194, 321
　long
　　　54
string vowel
　　　190
strips
　　　304
　milk test
　　　98
stroke
　　　323, 338, 418, 422
stroller
　　　62, 82, 214, 366, 393, 418, 425
stroller canopy
　　　354
stroller ride
　　　83, 153
strolls

　　　122, 126
strong base
　　　61
strong caregiver qualifications
　　　343
Strong Fathers Strong Daughters
　　　411
strong foundation
　　　423
strong gender type
　　　392
strong healthy foundation
　　　296
strong insecticide
　　　222
Strong Mothers
　　　411
strong sense
　　　277
Strong Sons
　　　411
Stuart Fishoff PhD
　　　406
study mothers
　　　389
stuff
　　　229
　small
　　　6, 103
stung
　　　219, 378
sturdy bottom
　　　61
sturdy cardboard pages
　　　331
style
　　　270, 414
　nova
　　　11
subconscious stereotyping
　　　388
subjective feeling
　　　16
subjects

3, 7, 243, 377
substance
  81, 203
 harmful
  205
 ingested
  205
 poisonous
  203
 special
  81
substances, harmless
  261
substandard
  350
substitute
  55, 308
suck
  22, 26, 41, 54, 77, 91, 95, 234, 366
sucking
  54, 92, 96, 145, 171, 231, 234, 270, 298
sucking, active
  97
sucking call
  41
sucking movements
  41
suck reflex
  4, 84
sucrose
  106, 311
  refined sugars
  311
suction
  96, 200
suction cups release
  58
suffocate
  55, 59
suffocation
  146, 197
suffocation hazard

210
sugar
  86, 265, 300, 310, 400
sugar cane
  311
sugar milk
  311
sugar, refined
  311
summer
  72, 221, 249, 353, 356, 363
 warm
  365
summersaults
  396
Summertime lecture
  353
sun
  163, 228, 353, 358
sunburn
  258, 353, 356, 358
sunburns doubles
  354
Sunburn Soothers
  359
sun exposure
  353
sunglasses
  354
 expensive
  355
 wear UVA/UVB
  354
sunken
  77, 238
sunlight
 direct
  79, 122, 228, 354
 indirect
  80
sun protection
  355
sunscreen

355, 362
  chemical
    357
  fresh
    358
  non-barrier
    355
  organic
    357
sunscreen sample size
  368
sunscreens use
  355, 358
sunscreen types
  357
sun sensitivity
  354
suns, little
  353
suntan year
  353
superfoods
  14
superhero's help people;superheros help people
  395
Superman
  176
supervision
  308, 375, 407
  constant parental
    376
supervisors
  350
supplement
  95, 105, 298, 313
support
  120, 173, 177, 182, 296, 326, 351, 390, 394, 409, 448
  arch
    185
  lid
    209
  online
    132
support breastfeeding
  86
support groups
  132
support lid
  213
surfaces
  firm
    173
  flat
    26, 176
  smooth
    58
surgery
  28, 35, 424
surgical procedure
  28
surprises
  120, 142, 308
surroundings
  175, 194, 283, 291
  private
    120
survival
  374, 376
survival rate
  43
Survival Swimming
  369
suspect thrush call
  101
Suspension
  259
sutures
  255, 256
swaddle
  73, 137, 147
swaddling
  137
swaddling Arizona Parenting
  139
swallow

97, 198, 204, 233, 305, 366, 371
swallowing
    97, 199, 254, 298, 365
swallowing/anaphylaxis
    250
swat
    221, 443, 445
sweat glands
    72
Swedish women
    12
sweet friend
    118
sweets
    310
sweet solutions
    311
swelling
    36, 76, 99, 115, 119, 219, 247, 254, 306, 360, 364
  initial
    223
  joint
    77, 237
  natural
    259
swells
    1, 98
swim
    373, 378
swim attire
    356
swim lessons
    369, 374
  traditional parent child
    376
swimming
    373, 376
swimming lessons
    374
Swimming lessons and ISR
    374
swimming movements
    375
swimming programs
    376
swim overconfident
    373
swim party
    373
swimsuit rings
    373
swing
    59, 82, 136, 145, 152, 279, 317, 321
swinging
    416
swipe
    173, 321
switch blockers
    209
swollen
    35, 199, 221, 244
swollen breast tissue
    36
swollen labia
    35
swollen, red
    101
swollen tongue sensation
    220
syllables
    182, 186
symptoms
    101, 127, 130, 219, 222, 230, 233, 237, 247, 250, 254, 258, 306, 364, 525
  cold
    238, 253
  cold-like
    230
  initial
    223
  mask
    236
  severe

220, 238
Symptoms of carbon monoxide poisoning
217
symptoms of infection
116, 253
symptoms of respiratory distress
231, 233
Symptoms of RSV
234
synchronize
272
Syndrome, Reyes
247
syringe
25
  bulb
63, 231
syrup
204
system
  alarm
342
  circulatory
334
  healthy immune
261

T

table
3, 60, 214, 416
  changing
64, 82, 201
  coffee
179
table foods
302
  recommending offering
304
tablespoons
70, 242, 299, 303
tablets

259
tachycardia
4
tags
356, 396
  blue
388
  vaginal
35
tail
230, 427
talkers, advanced
184
Tall Mary Lou Mellon
411
tampons
21, 114
tans
356, 359
tantrums
192, 417, 419, 426, 433, 437, 444
Tanya M.D
525
tape
187, 258
tap water
310
  cool running
310
tarry
68, 94
  black
95
tasks
296, 348, 352, 407
  important
348, 352
  management
343
  undesired
435
tassels, free
212
taste

593

  13, 107, 171, 201, 301
 new
  298, 313
tasting
 317
Taylor
  4, 45, 51, 118, 193, 217, 389, 429,
  438, 444
Taylor mixing
 86
tbsp
 41, 238, 300
tea
 13, 15, 100, 360
 caffeinated
  12
 mother's milk;mothers milk
  84
teachers
 193, 211, 295, 343, 402, 444, 448
teachers reimbursement
 346
teachers, third-grade
 5
teacher/student ratio
 346
teach girls
 395
teach independence
 402
teaching
  3, 6, 138, 191, 261, 407, 420, 433,
  448
teaching Dylan sign language
 193
teaching parenting classes
 3
teaching responsibility
 442
teaching sign language
 183, 191
teach shy kids
 405
team
  385, 394, 410
 medical
  23
teammate
 410
tearfulness
 127
techniques
 cooling-off
  73
 good hand-washing
  104
 problem-solving
  403
 proceeding
  415
 stall
  150
 teach self-soothing
  402
tech TM, cool
 359
teenagers
 198, 247
teeth
  55, 179, 263, 298, 303, 312, 426
 adult
  268
 brushing
  157, 430
 first
  179, 235
 front bottom
  179
 lower front
  264
 next
  264
 permanent
  264
 primary
  264
 rinses

265
teether
  267, 331
 dual
  267
teething
  159, 175, 179, 235, 266, 298
teething biscuits
  235, 302
teething gels
  267
teething rings
  235, 267
Teething rings and toys
  267
teeth popping, new
  235
temp
  74, 360, 419
 axillary
  78, 236
 internal
  228
 oral
  236
 rectal
  78, 236
temperament
  2, 282, 295, 382, 399
 baby's;babys
  164, 278
 child's;childs
  415
 developing
  281
 emerging
  270
 unique
  163, 269, 399
temperature
  78, 108, 137, 147, 231, 235
 baby's;babys
  78
 best
  108
 low-grade
  234
 rectal
  63, 78, 237, 244
 right
  88
temperatures, extreme
  248
temporary time
  59, 419
temptation
  312, 416
temp time
  415
tendencies
  399
 behavioral
  383
 natural
  405
 school phobia
  404
testicles
  35
test limits
  413
tests
  18, 23, 26, 30, 38, 95, 98, 109, 215, 310, 312
 crash
  227
 first
  23
Tetanus
  255
tetracyclines
  354
Textured BPA-free silicone teething toys
  236
textured surfaces
  58
textures

595

298, 303, 313, 319, 321, 330, 385
  pleasant
    312
thanks you
  123
the1980s research studies
  134
thermometer
  63, 78, 211, 236, 368
  digital
    63, 78
Thermoscan
  63
thighs/hips, upper
  226
Think Baby
  358
thinking chair
  434, 444
thinking spot
  415
  makeshift
    445
thinner whiter milk
  98
Thomas, Marlo
  411
Thompson, Melissa
  449
thorns
  258
  cactus
    258
  long
    258
threats, repeated
  430
thrill seeker
  286, 399
throat
  41, 199, 210, 235, 245, 249, 267
  sore
    253
  strep
    252
Thrombocytopenia
  4
Thrombosis/Blood clots
  119
thrush
  101
thumb
  54, 73, 97, 301
thumb tacks
  199
thyroid
  131
tiara
  393
ticks
  361
  deer
    363
tie
  54, 64, 247, 321
tie backs
  212
tie strings
  161
Tighter weave cloths
  355
time
  44, 90, 112, 115, 123, 126, 138, 165, 193, 235, 261, 274, 278, 289, 346, 375, 419, 433, 445
time children
  332
time ins
  423
time latching
  99
timeline
  264, 314
time log
  153
time outdoors
  353
time-outs

439, 444
Time outs
   419, 437, 445
time period
   255
time playing
   397
times birthweight
   166
times infants
   92
time waving
   173
time zones
   367
tingling
   220
tip backward
   62
tip brackets
   209
tip furniture brackets
   209
tips
   58, 78, 93, 100, 110, 209, 213, 221
  great
   212
  little
   54
  metal
   236
tiredness
   127, 131
tissue
   259
  fatty
   40
  pink
   35
titanium dioxide
   358
toast

239
toddler classes
   3
toddlerhood
   294, 303, 316, 420, 422
toddler meltdowns
   445
toddlers
   190, 213, 316, 331, 369, 372, 378, 403, 406, 416, 419, 427, 429, 437
  active
   206
  daring
   399
  young
   426
toddler's head;toddlers head
   165
toddler sign language
   191
toddlers plenty
   425
toddler survival
   376
toes
   26, 57, 119, 190, 212, 249
toilet bowl cleaners
   205
Toiletries
   21
toilets
   208, 344, 370
Tomato
   202
tommee tippee
   54
tone
   189, 319, 417, 421
  disapproving
   418
  disrespectful
   423
  muscle

23, 336
tongue
    93, 194, 210, 249, 256, 298, 306, 320
  white
    101
Tonic neck reflex
    26
tools
    110, 181, 262, 316, 341, 405, 433
  effective
    431
  good
    419
  special
    24
  use neonatal assessment
    25
tooth
    257, 264
  decayed
    265
  permanent
    265
  sweet
    311
tooth decay
    266, 311
toothpaste
    206, 265, 266
  regular
    265
  use kid
    265
top
    36, 56, 58, 63, 67, 73, 76, 93, 102, 225, 229, 352, 357
top choking hazards
    198
topical anesthetics
    116, 120
Topical lotions
    201
topics
    7, 50, 229, 380
  multiple
    7
toss
    145, 326, 427
Tot- Lok
    207
touch
    37, 77, 116, 119, 122, 219, 278, 293, 338, 384, 420
touch books
    330
touch, gentle
    276
Touchpoints
    525
touch relaxation
    338
touch supervision
    372
touch therapy
    335
touch use
    78
towels
    70, 102, 241
  beach
    228, 359
  clean
    102
  wet
    221
toxins
    56, 205, 254, 306
  ingested
    203
toxoplasmosis
    12
toy- Bounce
    323
toy box
    191, 213
toys
    160, 173, 182, 281, 284, 295, 318,

332, 344, 370, 391, 396, 416, 426, 432
age-appropriate
 318
enticing
 318
expensive
 333
favorite
 321, 325
floating
 325
imported wooden
 209
musical
 318
noisy
 323
patterned
 321
safe
 322
small soft
 321
squeeze
 328
textured
 318
windup
 285
toy telephone
 329
track
 91, 168
 digestive
 358
training
 early
 261
 potty
 346
 supervised water
 377
 water survival skills

374
training programs
 345
trains
 293, 323, 354, 389
traits
 383, 399, 404
 female
 391
 male
 391
transition
 159, 270, 282, 430
 gradual
 278
 nice
 58, 140
Transitional stools
 94
transition object
 281
translucent
 221
transplantation
 48
transplants
 43, 47
 first successful
 43
 stem cell
 43, 45, 49
transporting
 85
trapped air/gas
 335
trapped underwater, becoming
 58
trash
 118, 395
trash cans
 208
trash compactor
 208
Travel/Vacations

599

365
tray
    59, 214, 324
treadmills, sure
    213
treatment
    30, 43, 55, 70, 80, 101, 220, 231,
        238, 242, 247, 265, 365
  aggressive
    102
  antifungal
    243
  best
    205
  effective
    129
  emergency
    247
  medical
    219
Treatment for diaper rash
    241
treatment heat rash
    72
tree nuts
    305, 307
trees
    213, 221, 323, 354, 386, 399, 424
  palm
    219
trembling
    41
trick, new
    177
Triclocarban
    262
Triclogan
    262
Triclogan blocks
    262
triple birthweight
    166
trucks

328, 395
trump card
    438, 440
trust
    8, 85, 92, 118, 142, 277, 288, 346,
        349, 404, 435, 443, 446
  building
    404
  developing
    404
  sense of
    403, 404
trusted advisors
    133
trusted pediatrician
    445
trusted provider/s
    1
tsp
    259
tub
    58, 67, 122, 242, 247, 251, 262,
        371
  clean
    120
  hot
    370, 372
  nonskid
    58
  small
    242
tubes
    65, 235
  60-gram
    242
  eustachian
    234
  neural
    14
tug
    371, 420
  stitches
    111
tugging

96, 411
tummies, sensitive
   145
tummy
   136, 147, 152, 158, 173, 240, 318
tummy bug
   241
tummy position
   135
tummy time
   64, 77, 138, 317
   encouraging
      321
   productive
      138
tummy, traditional
   135
tuna
   11, 106
   canned chunk light
      11
   fresh
      11
tune
   125, 421, 431
turbulence
   366
turn panhandles
   208
turn predisposes
   235
Tuteur, Amy
   84
TV
   342, 390
TV societies
   390
tweezers
   364, 368
Twitter
   297
two-step command
   191
Tylenol
   249
type pacifier
   22
Tyrant
   352

U

uh oh
   190
ulcerative colitis
   87
ulcers
   249
   small painful
      249
ultrasound tech
   392
ultraviolet
   356
Umansky, Warren
   296
Umbilical cord infections
   66
Unbreakable mirrors
   320, 328
uncircumcised partners
   28
Uncooked meats
   12
undernutrition
   92, 142
Unexpected
   275
unexplained fever
   245
unit
   217
   intensive care
      335
   new
      217
United Kingdom

29, 106
United States
    29, 129, 134, 198, 290, 378
University
    9, 46, 87, 157, 295
Unpasteurized juice
    306
unplug
    208, 210
unverifiable sources
    133
upper body strength
    138
upright
    172
  sitting
    322
upside
    85, 200
urinary incontinence
    117
Urinary tract
    117
urinate
    29, 118
urine
    18, 28, 35, 67, 75, 77, 313, 377
urine, expensive
    313
urine stream
    67
  strong
    67
US Bureau
    350
US Center
    129
use
    45, 50, 61, 67, 73, 104, 114, 137,
        160, 181, 187, 208, 213, 221,
        241, 262, 321, 360, 416, 444
use Acetaminophen
    236
use alcohol
    442
use Aquaphor
    71
use baking soda
    247
use clothing
    355
use diffusers
    218
use feedings
    272
use Hydrocortisone cream
    72
use ice packs
    120
use images
    386
use insect repellent
    360
use material reinforcers
    436
use milk shells
    99
use pads
    114
use repellent
    361
use soap
    72
use speech
    189
use straps
    209
use sunscreen
    355
use toys
    286
use tweezers
    258
use walkers
    57
use weather stripping
    221
use words

395
uterine lining
114
utero
13, 34
uterus
11, 38, 88, 100, 113
UTI
27
UVA
357
UVA rays
356
UVA/UVB
356
UVA/UVB sticker
355
UVB
356
UVB rays
356
UVB rays cause burns
357
UV rays
357
  sun's;suns
356

V

vacation
341, 351, 368
  sunny
356
vaccines
24, 246, 341
vacuum
53, 432
vagina
115
  baby's;babys
35
vaginal birth

114, 120
Valerie
125
Valerie Frankel Entitled
111
Vanicream
64, 71, 74, 252, 358
vanilla
171, 317
variation
34, 383
  great
185
  normal
170
Varicella
246
varicella vaccine
246
variety rhyming words
330
Vaseline
74, 78, 236
Vaseline-like coating
75
Vasoline
65
vegetables
13, 302, 309
vegetarian, strict
313
Veg/garden
202
veggies
300
  green
243, 300
  leafy
119
  yellow
243, 300
vehicle
63, 224, 339
  moving

224
vein-popping
124
Velcro bibs
64
Venmo
341
venom
254, 364
vent
217, 409
  internal
  53
ventilate
206, 218
ventilation holes
54
Verbal correction
417
verbal disapproval, mild
415
verbal messaging
417
verbal ques
190
verbal terms
386
Viacord.com
43
vial, small
30
videos
187, 332
vinegar
171, 218, 310, 317
  distilled
  310
violence
397, 442
viral conjunctivitis
244
Viral diarrhea
240
Virginia Medical School

235
virus
230, 232, 246, 248
  airborne
  246
  cold
  232
vision
163, 167, 169, 323, 367
  baby's;babys
  34, 169
  blurred
  255
  developing
  319
  full-color
  169
visitors
20, 113, 121, 159
visual acuity
177
visual development milestone, new
168
Visual disturbances
220
visual preferences
385
visual processing area
385
visual spatial abilities
386
Vit
105, 313
vitamins
14, 24, 86, 105, 116, 201, 297, 301, 308, 311
  extra
  105
  fat-soluble
  312
  little
  24
  prenatal

604

97
soluble
313
vitamin supplement
313
vivid scary dream
162
vocabulary
184, 191
  new
  330
vocal cords
233
vocalizations
292
voice
77, 167, 174, 178, 186, 211, 291, 329, 352, 417, 423
  familiar
  170, 293
  father's;fathers
  186
  happy light
  319
  hoarse
  232
  mother's;mothers
  186
  synthesized gender-neutral
  187
  woman's;womans
  186
volume
  increased blood
  11
  increased fluid
  11
  sheer
  329
vomited day
3
vomiting
87, 107, 205, 217, 235, 238, 255, 306
vomiting, last
239
Vomiting of petroleum-based products
205
vomits
136, 156, 205, 238, 256, 366
  blood-tinged
  109
  green
  238
vowel sounds
172, 187
vowel sounds ooh aah
187

W

wake
92, 140, 147, 149, 151, 155, 158, 256
wakefulness
276
wakening, next
151
wakes up
119
wakeup call
351
wake-up time
158
walker
57, 185
walkers, new
185
wall hangings
161
walls
58, 208, 213, 219, 344, 399, 427, 437, 444
Walmart
429
wander

167
warmer
    74, 108
Warm moist
    305
war, modern
    261
warm steeped tea bags
    100
warmth
    65, 253, 290, 353
warm water
    67, 70, 74, 115, 241, 247, 258, 275, 323, 364
warm water rinses
    69
Warner, Jeff
    51
warning
    11, 270, 283, 430, 434, 445
Warning Signs
    171, 174, 184, 273
Warren Umanky PhD
    269
wash
    64, 69, 73, 102, 115, 118, 206, 219, 253, 262, 310, 362
  antiseptic
    367
  human bite-;human bite
    253
washable fabric
    59
washcloths, cool
    73
wash dishes
    120
wash hands
    102
Washington
    226
wasp's nest;wasps nest
    378
waste

45, 79, 102
little
    68, 244
medical
    42, 51
solid
    95
watch
    169, 173, 250, 253, 258, 276, 282, 285, 318, 348, 364, 370, 410
watch for signs and symptoms
    250, 254
Watch for symptoms of allergic reactions
    364
water
    13, 58, 66, 70, 107, 206, 219, 253, 266, 297, 313, 325, 354, 361, 369
  boiling
    108
  bowl of
    99
  contaminate drinking
    216
  dumping
    325
  extra
    368
  fluorinated
    266, 297
  hot
    103, 216
  inhaled
    371
  lukewarm
    206
  nursery
    266, 297
  offering
    298
  parent-child
    375
  plain

218
public
266
squeezing
325
water conditions
372
water heaters
208, 216
water hose
257
water intoxication
370
watermelon
304
Waterproof
355
Waterproof pad/pads
64
Water Safety
371
water safety habits, good
374
water temp
372
water wings
373
  wearing
  373
watery
68, 240, 244
watery cottage cheese
94
waves
183, 285
way children
348
  primary
  315
way home
445
way males
387
weaning

304
  traditional
  304
wear
100, 104, 214, 356, 360, 373, 393
  wear clothes
  360
  wear shoes
  221
Weasel
329
weather
122
  humid
  72
webs
222, 249
  strong white
  222
website
192, 212, 223
  great
  212
wedge
136, 231
weekend hours
18
weekends
124, 211
weepy, open
241
weighing
108
  bruiser
  4
weight
10, 92, 95, 142, 146, 149, 165, 177, 224, 227, 322, 335
  baby's;babys
  95
  child's;childs
  342
  ideal

607

10
  pre-pregnancy
    88
weight gain
    16, 96, 131, 166, 335
  increased
    335
  normal
    92, 142, 166
weight restrictions
    63
Weissbluth
    526
Wellesley college
    349
wet burps
    81, 109
wet compress, cool
    220
wet diapers
    93, 237
wet T-shirt
    355
wet washcloth
    74
wheat
    300, 305
  creamed
    312
wheezing
    87, 232
  audible
    231
whites
    268
  egg
    305
whole milk
    91
WHO (World Health Organization);WHO (World Health Organization
    88
wife
    2, 289
wife Abbey
    2
wife, old
    232
wiggle
    60, 276, 286, 293
wind
    161, 285
window cords
    59, 211
  looped
    211
window lock
    56
windows
    56, 79, 206, 212, 217, 221, 367
window shades
    212
window shields
    359
Winnie
    426
winning state championships
    5
winter
    72, 139, 233, 378
  late
    248
wiping
    76, 261
wire
    316
  electrical
    209, 336
wisdom
    2, 399
  infinite
    445
withstand jolts
    61
woman
    84, 385
woman beginning

10
womb
   14, 34, 38, 98, 387
   tight
      33
women
   10, 88, 100, 104, 120, 125, 129, 187, 349, 355, 386, 391, 397
   pre-menopausal
      88
   successful
      398
women experience
   117
Womensheatlth.gov article
   130
women work
   349
Wonder Woman
   351
wood burning fireplace
   217
wood-burning furnaces
   216
woodpiles
   219, 222
word danger
   421
word decoration
   422
word discipline
   412
word love
   395
words
   180, 182, 187, 258, 281, 327, 330, 397, 401, 405, 415, 417, 421, 432, 435
   code
      342
   extra
      184
   imitate
      190
   link
      187
   new
      421
words chubby bunny
   199
work
   2, 3, 85, 89, 120, 123, 128, 152, 158, 258, 283, 339, 349, 360, 415
   extra
      352
   hard
      408, 447
work accounts
   350
work home
   349
work material
   259
work terms, flexible
   350
work time
   349
world
   169, 175, 178, 193, 201, 319, 321, 323, 330, 416, 420
world, comfortable
   291
world fit
   407
World Health Organization (WHO);World Health Organization (WHO
   88
world revolves
   406
wrists
   69, 71, 214
www.babycenter.com
   195
www.celebrationstemcellcenter.com

46
www.cordblood.com
46
www.cpsc.gov
212
www.cryo-cell.com
46
www.cryo-intl.com
47
www.epa.gov
363
www.handspeak.com
193
www.healthychildren.org
8, 50, 363, 448
www.infantswim.com
378
www.lifebankusa.com
47
www.nhtsa.gov
223
www.pbs.org
276
www.postpartum.net
132
www.postpartumprogress.com
132
www.ppdtojoy.com
132
www.safekids.org
212
www.savethecordfoundation.org
48
www.sign2me.com
193
www.viacord.com Cambridge
46
www.windowcoverings.org
212

Y

Yale child Study Center
315
Yale University School
129
Yarnell PhD Clinical, Thomas D.;Yarnell PhD Clinical, Thomas D
411
Yarnell PhD, Thomas D.;Yarnell PhD, Thomas D
407
year 500children ages
226
year career
448
year molars
264
year's list;years list
310
year subscription
331
yeast
70, 101, 241
Yeast infections
101
yell
431
yell help
214
yelling
423, 431
yellow jackets
364
yellow pigment
79
Yep
416
yolks
305
    egg
312
you can have a turn next
391
young adults
353, 447
    independent

5
young children breathe
   216
younger
   110, 157, 237, 277, 320, 332, 424,
      431, 434
Your Child's Health and Advice;Your
   Childs Health and Advice
   306

Z

Zeanah, Charles
   287
Zelle, monthly
   341
zinc oxide
   357
Ziplock
   241
Zoli
   267
Zoli Bunny
   267
Zyrtec
   250, 255, 259, 365
  children's;childrens
   299
  recommending
   259
Zyrtec for allergic reactions
   251

BIBLIOGRAPHY

Nelsen, Jane ED.D.,Erwin, Cheryl M.A., Duffy, Rosyln. Positive Discipline: The First Three Years. Prima publishing. 1998

Nelson, Jane, Lynn Lott, H. Stephen Glenn. Positive Discipline A to Z: 1001 Solutions to everyday patenting Problems. Prima Publishing1993.

Schmitt, Barton D. M.d. F.A.A.P. Your Child's Health. The Parents One Stop Reference Guide to Symptoms, Emergencies, Common Illnesses, Behavior Problems, Healthy Development. Second revised edition Bantam books 2005.

Schmitt, Barton D. M.d. F.A.A.P. Your Child's Health. The Parents One Stop Reference Guide to Symptoms, Emergencies, Common Illnesses, Behavior Problems, Healthy Development. Bantam books 1987.

Popkin, Michael PhD., Active Parenting Today. Active Parenting Publishers Inc 1993.

Brazelton, T. Berry M.D. Touchpoints: The Essential Reference: Your Child's Emotional and Behavioral Development. Perseus Books. 1992.

Stamm, Jill PhD. Bright From the Start. Gotham Books. 2007

Altman, Tanya M.D. FAAP, Hill, David L. MD FAAP. The complete and Authoritative Guide : Caring for your baby and young child: American Academy of Pediatrics. Bantam Books. 2019

Cohen, George J MD FAAP. American Academy of Pediatrics Guide to Your Child's Sleep: Birth through Adolescence.

Pantley, Elizabeth. The No-Cry- Sleep Solution: Gentle ways to help your baby sleep through the night. Mc Graw Hill 2002.

Weissbluth, Marc. M.D. Healthy Sleep Habits Happy Child. Ballantine Books 1987.

Ezzo, Gary M.A., Buckman Robert M.D. On Becoming Baby Wise. Parent-Wise Solutions Inc.2001

Shelov, Steven P. M.D. M.S. FAAP. Your Baby's first year. The American Academy of Pediatrics. Bantam Books1998.

Ferber, Richard MD. Solve Your Child's Sleep Problems. Simon and Schuster1985.

Karp, Harvey M.D. The Happiest Baby on the Block. Bantam Books 2002.

Made in the USA
Monee, IL
03 March 2025

13173278R00341